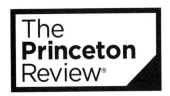

The Princeton Review®

D1194253

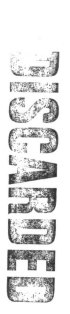

DISCARDED

Cracking the OAT®

2nd Edition

The Staff of The Princeton Review

Penguin
Random
House

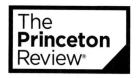

The Princeton Review
110 East 42nd St, 7th Floor
New York, NY 10017

Published in the United States by Penguin Random
House LLC, New York, and in Canada by Random House
of Canada, a division of Penguin Random House Ltd.,
Toronto.

Terms of Service: The Princeton Review Online Com-
panion Tools ("Student Tools") for retail books are
available for only the two most recent editions of that
book. Student Tools may be activated only twice per
eligible book purchased for two consecutive 12-month
periods, for a total of 24 months of access. Activation
of Student Tools more than twice per book is in direct
violation of these Terms of Service and may result in
discontinuation of access to Student Tools Services.

ISBN: 978-0-525-56756-1
ISSN: 2164-0327

Editor: Selena Coppock
Production Coordinator: Craig Patches
Production Editor: Liz Dacey

Printed in the United States of America on partially
recycled paper.

10 9 8 7 6 5 4 3 2 1

Editorial
Rob Franek, Editor-in-Chief
Mary Beth Garrick, Executive Director of Production
Craig Patches, Production Design Manager
Selena Coppock, Managing Editor
Meave Shelton, Senior Editor
Colleen Day, Editor
Sarah Litt, Editor
Aaron Riccio, Editor
Orion McBean, Associate Editor

Penguin Random House Publishing Team
Tom Russell, VP, Publisher
Alison Stoltzfus, Publishing Director
Amanda Yee, Associate Managing Editor
Ellen Reed, Production Manager
Suzanne Lee, Designer

CONTRIBUTORS

The Princeton Review would like to thank: Jes Adams, Neil Adams , Dave MacKenzie, Archana Murali, Juhi Shah, Dorothy Vandermolen, Joanna Yang, and Ryman Yeung.

CONTENTS

Get More (Free) Content

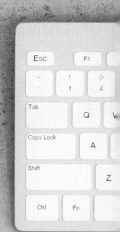

1 Go to **PrincetonReview.com/cracking**

2 Enter the following ISBN for your book: 9780525567561

3 Answer a few simple questions to set up an exclusive Princeton Review account. (If you already have one, you can just log in.)

4 Click the "Student Tools" button, also found under "My Account" from the top toolbar. You're all set to access your bonus content!

Need to report a potential **content** issue?

Contact **EditorialSupport@review.com**.
Include:

- full title of the book
- ISBN number
- page number

Need to report a **technical** issue?

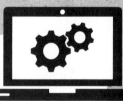

Contact **TPRStudentTech@review.com**
and provide:

- your full name
- email address used to register the book
- full book title and ISBN
- computer OS (Mac/PC) and browser (Firefox, Safari, etc.)

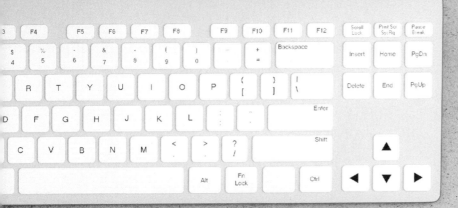

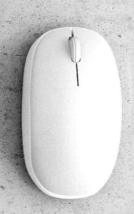

Once you've registered, you can...

- Take two full-length, scorable, OAT practice exams

- Get valuable advice about the college application process, including tips for writing a great essay and where to apply for financial aid

- Use our searchable rankings of *The Best 384 Colleges* to find out more information about your dream school

- Check to see if there have been any corrections or updates to this edition

- Get our take on any recent or pending updates to the OAT

Look For These Icons Throughout The Book

 ONLINE PRACTICE TESTS

 PROVEN TECHNIQUES

 APPLIED STRATEGIES

 STUDY BREAK

 OTHER REFERENCES

Chapter 1
Introduction

SO YOU WANT TO BE AN OPTOMETRIST

If you're reading this book, there's a pretty strong chance that you are giving serious thought to becoming an optometrist. Maybe your parents are optometrists and you always knew that you would grow up to be an optometrist. Maybe you were pre-health in college and flirted with the idea of becoming a doctor or a nurse before you decided that becoming an optometrist would suit you better. However you've come to this point, you've taken the required pre-optometry classes, and now all that remains before you can apply is to take the Optometry Admission Test (OAT).

Just the OAT.

The OAT is a long, complex, detailed exam of much of the basic biology, chemistry, and physics that you learned in your pre-optometry courses, together with math that you may not have seen since high school, and reading comprehension that only vaguely resembles any kind of reading that you've done before. And it's this monstrosity that is standing between you and optometry school.

Understandably, you may feel somewhat daunted. The path to a good OAT score is not necessarily as straightforward as the path to a good GPA or to a good letter of recommendation. While much of the OAT is about recalling facts that you learned at some point in school, much of it is not, and the test is as much about how you apply what you know as it is about what you know.

However, we would like to help. This book provides the details of the OAT that you need to know, eliminating the mystery about what is tested and how it appears. This means that we will discuss the core of the test structure and test-specific strategies. We will also review in detail the physics that you need to know and provide a high-level overview of the other subjects.

If you want a complete review of the subjects other than physics, you should buy Cracking the DAT as well. The Dental Admission Test (DAT) is extremely similar to the OAT, and, in fact, the biology, organic chemistry, general chemistry, quantitative reasoning, and reading comprehension cover the same content with the same question types. This book will describe what you do and do not need to know from Cracking the DAT and what differences there are between the DAT and OAT, and it will provide the hard-to-find but necessary coverage of OAT Physics. With this book as a supplement to Cracking the DAT, you will have everything you need to do well on the OAT.

We lay it out for you here, because you want to be an optometrist. And we want to help.

WHAT IS THE OAT... REALLY?

Many students approach studying for the OAT like studying for a final exam in college. This can mean cramming lots and lots of science and math facts into your head in the few days leading up to the exam and hoping just to regurgitate what you've memorized on test day. This might have worked in college (although even then it probably wasn't the best way to go about taking a test), but it generally leads to disappointing results on the OAT.

The OAT is not a purely content-based, fact-recall test. If optometry school admission committees wanted that, they could just look at your transcript. What they want to see is both how much you know and how well you think under the intense pressure of a timed admission exam. The combination of the two is what they will try to determine from your OAT score.

The nature of the test impacts how you must study for it. Making lots of flashcards to memorize o-chem reactions (or whatever) will help you get part of the way on this exam, but it will only get you part of the way. After all, there are no facts to memorize for reading comprehension, and even on the sciences and math, you must be able to apply your knowledge to (potentially) new situations. So what else do you have to do to study for this exam, other than memorize lots of facts?

You must also practice applying the knowledge that you have to OAT-style questions. Taking the OAT is a skill in itself, and this skill, like any other, requires practice. This is much like learning to play a musical instrument or speak a foreign language; you learn to play the piano by practicing playing for an hour or two every day, not by reading about playing the piano all day before a big recital. This book contains a great many practice questions inside, and more are available online. Other questions are available from the makers of the test, the American Dental Association (ADA) directly. (The test is sponsored by the Association of Schools and Colleges of Optometry, ASCO, but it is actually made by ADA, which is part of why it looks so much like the DAT.) Practice as much as you can, because it is through practice that you will get better and your score will improve.

HOW TO USE THIS BOOK

Hopefully, you've picked this book up at the beginning of your OAT preparation, and you have at least two or three months to study before you take the test. If you're planning to take the test in a very short time, such as a week from now, it is unlikely that you will be able to read the whole text and do all of the practice that comes with it. Thus, how you use this book will depend on where you are in relation to your test date.

Further, how you use this book will depend on whether you also have Cracking the DAT. This book is not intended to be complete on its own. We list topics and facts for the subjects that the OAT shares with the DAT, but we do not explain them in detail. The only subject that we explain in detail is physics, which the DAT does not share with the OAT and you therefore couldn't find in Cracking the DAT.

Long-Term Prep with Cracking the OAT and Cracking the DAT

If the test is still at least a month from now, try to read the two books cover to cover, skipping only the Perceptual Ability portion of Cracking the DAT (since the OAT does not have a Perceptual Ability Test). Begin with the introduction, and progress through the sections on the different subjects in a staggered fashion (that is, read a little bit of Bio, then a bit of O-Chem, then a bit of G-Chem, and so on, until you come back to Bio). Work the chapter-end practice questions as you go, since these are important to solidify the information that you're reviewing, and read the solutions both for questions you get right and questions you get wrong, so that you can make sure you understand the proper reasoning for the questions.

Access the online practice material as soon as you can, because the most important thing you can do is take the tests that come with this book and determine your strengths and weaknesses. If you're scoring a 380 in a subject, you probably don't need to practice it much if at all, but if you're scoring a 230, it needs some serious shoring up before you take the test, and you don't know which subjects are which until you take a practice test. Thus, you should not leave the tests until the end of your practice. Take one in the middle to gauge your status, and one near the end for another assessment.

Shortly before the test, you should read the introduction again, because you'll want to remind yourself of test-day procedures, and frankly, you should read the optometry admissions information because you want to get excited for the test! You will do better if you think of this as your first step on the road to a great career in the field of optometry than if you think of this as a horrible, time-consuming, draining, boring, standardized test (which it probably is, but it's better not to think of it that way!).

More Great Books

The Princeton Review publishes Cracking the DAT which is chock full of information that's useful to you, even as a book buyer who is taking the OAT. We also have assorted flashcards and coloring books for reviewing anatomy—check them all out at PenguinRandomHouse.com.

Short-Term Prep with Cracking the OAT and Cracking the DAT

If the test is very soon (e.g., a week from now), then read the introduction (you could skip the admissions information if you want, although, as noted above, it might be best not to), and take one of the online practice tests. Use this to identify your areas of weakness, which could be as general as "I'm not good enough at O-Chem" or as specific as "I forget how to use sine and cosine in math," and read up on those areas. Make sure that you work some of the practice questions in those subjects.

If you don't feel comfortable with these topics even after some practice, you might consider postponing your test date to give yourself a little more time to do more detailed review and additional practice. However, don't postpone indefinitely, because then you'll never be able to go to optometry school. Choose a specific test date to move to, and prepare for that date. If you learn everything that is in this book and study the practice questions carefully, you will not be surprised by anything on the test, and you should be able to do your best. Good luck!

Prep with only Cracking the OAT

If you do not wish to purchase Cracking the DAT as well, you can use this book as an overview of most of the subjects and a detailed guide to physics. Read through the introduction and the physics portion, working through the problems. While you go, read over the lists in the other subjects, and make sure you know those topics. If you feel uncomfortable with any of them, consult some source—maybe your old class notes, maybe an online resource—to re-familiarize yourself with those topics. If there are a lot of them, though, and you feel you need a complete review, you really should purchase Cracking the DAT as well and use this book alongside that one.

OAT NUTS AND BOLTS

Sections (Sub-Tests)

There are four timed groups of questions on the OAT. These groups of questions are called "tests" by ADA, but we will usually call them "sections." Before these sections is a tutorial, in the middle is a break, and after is a survey, so the overall structure of the test is as follows.

Section	Number of Questions	Time
Tutorial		15 minutes
Survey of Natural Sciences Biology General Chemistry Organic Chemistry	100 total 40 30 30	90 minutes total
Reading Comprehension Test	50	60 minutes
Break		15 minutes
Physics Test	40	50 minutes
Quantitative Reasoning Test	40	45 minutes
Survey		15 minutes

The sections are always in this order. The test is a computer-based test (CBT), though it is fixed-form (not adaptive). You can move around within a section at your discretion, and the questions in any given test form are set before the test begins, just as on a pencil-and-paper exam.

Note that there are a few differences between the OAT and the DAT. Most obviously, the DAT has a Perceptual Ability Test that the OAT does not, and the OAT has a Physics Test that the DAT does not. Thus, you do not have to worry about Perceptual Ability when you are studying for the OAT, and you do have to worry about Physics. This is the reason that the Physics Test is covered in detail in this book.

The other difference is the order of the sections. On the DAT, the second section is Perceptual Ability and the third is Reading Comprehension. On the OAT, the second section is the Reading Comprehension Test and the third is Physics. On both the DAT and the OAT, the Survey of the Natural Sciences (SNS) is the first section, and the Quantitative Reasoning Test (QRT) is the last section.

Scoring

You receive eight scores after taking the OAT, six for different subjects and two multi-subject scores. OAT scores range from 200 to 400 and go in increments of 10. You will receive a numerical score for each individual section:

- Biology
- General Chemistry
- Organic Chemistry
- Physics Test
- Reading Comprehension Test (RCT)
- Quantitative Reasoning Test (QRT)

Next, you receive a total science score for the four science subjects (biology, both chemistries, and physics). This score is an average of your four science scores, rounded to the nearest 10. Finally, the scores for all six individual subjects are averaged and rounded to the nearest 10, and this score is called the Academic Average.

Typically, optometry schools care most about the Academic Average. Even if the Academic Average is high, though, they will also look for any outlier scores. For example, if your four science scores are each 350, but your RCT score is 240 and your QRT score is 400, your Academic Average will be 340. However, schools may worry about your RCT score, which is 100 points lower than your Academic Average. If the difference is minor, schools will generally overlook it. For example, if your Academic Average is 340 and your QRT score is 330, it is unlikely that any school will give that small difference a second thought.

You might ask, "What's a good score?" This question is not as easy to answer as you might imagine. It varies somewhat from school to school. However, a score around the mid-300's is competitive for most schools, and for any more detail, you should consult the specific schools to which you would like to apply. Be sure to look at your percentile, as well as your numerical score, in order to get a sense as to where you stand with respect to other test takers.

As a general rule, bell curves tend to slant down dramatically away from the center. That is, a very large percentage of people score close to 300, and moving your score from a 320 to a 330 or from a 330 to a 340 will put your score past a lot of other test takers. There is an enormous premium, therefore, on eking out every last point that you can, and we will discuss how to do this.

Non-Scored Questions

ADA says: "Each test includes equating and pretest questions. The purpose of the equating questions is to form a link among collections of items, so that examinee's standard scores can be placed on the same measurement scale. Because of these equating questions, examinee's scores have the same meaning regardless of the test they were administered. Unscored pretest questions are included on the test in order to gather information. This information is used in the test construction process to insure that these questions are appropriate before they are included among the scored items."

(from the OAT Examinee Guide)

What does this mean for you? Well, certain questions will not count towards your score. There is no way to know how many or which ones. However, it does mean that you should not spend too much time on any one question, because it may not even count. As a rule of thumb, you should never spend more than three times as long on any one question as you average on the other questions. For example, if you average about 1 minute per QRT question, you should never spend more than 3 minutes on any one QRT question, unless you've already finished every other question in the section.

Registration and The Test Experience

The OAT is created by ADA, and you can register at www.ada.org/oat.aspx. It is offered by appointment at Prometric computer testing centers, which also offer many other tests, including the GRE. In fact, other test takers in the room with you will be taking many other tests, unrelated to the one you are taking. Appointments are available for a variety of different dates and times, usually including mornings, afternoons, and evenings. Some weekend dates may be available. Convenient locations and dates often fill up well in advance, so you should sign up early (ideally at least a month or two before you are planning to take the test, just in case).

The testing center contains two parts, a waiting room and a secured computer area. In the waiting room, you are greeted by an administrator who checks your identification and signs you in. You must have two forms of identification, the primary a government issued ID with a signature and photograph (such as a driver's license), and the secondary anything with a signature (such as a credit card). Expired identification cannot be used. Test takers are checked in as they arrive, so you may have to wait a short time before being checked in.

You will be given a small locker in which to store whatever items you brought with you (such as a small snack). Literally anything that you brought with you, other than your clothing and your IDs, must go into your locker, including books, calculators, cell phones, bags of any kind, writing implements, or food. (ADA specifically notes that, among other things, "[g]ood luck charms, statues, religious or superstitious talismans" cannot be brought into the computer room.) ADA is very explicit about the items that can and can't be brought and when they can be accessed, so make sure to read their guidelines before you go.

The security verifications during check-in can be somewhat involved and intimidating, but they are nothing to worry about (unless you are trying to cheat somehow—which you shouldn't, because you'll get caught!). Prometric testing centers are equipped with video and audio recording devices that can see and hear every part of the center, and you will be asked to sign in and out every time you enter and exit the computer room. You may also be asked to turn out your pockets, and other basic security procedures may be followed. Don't worry; they're standard.

During check-in, you will be provided with noteboards and two dry-erase markers. You may or may not be given an eraser. These noteboards are typically two sheets of laminated, letter-sized graph paper. The two dry-erase markers are fine-tipped, usually pencil-sized but sometimes larger. The eraser works, but the noteboards often don't erase very cleanly on the first swipe without pressing fairly hard, so don't plan to erase a great deal during the middle of a section. You can, however, get a fresh set of noteboards during the break in the middle of the test, so feel free to fill up the sheets during the SNS and RCT.

Once you are checked in, you will be allowed to enter the computer room. You will be taken to a seat and asked to verify that your name is on the computer screen. At the computer will be a screen, a keyboard, a mouse, and noise-canceling headphones (which are bulky but very effective). The mouse is a two-button mouse. Once you sit down and click forward, the tutorial will begin.

During the test, other test takers will be checking in and taking breaks sporadically. Test takers are checked in one-by-one, so even if someone else has exactly the same appointment time as you, he or she will start the test before or after you, and most other test takers do not have the same appointment time (and are not even taking the same test). Thus, don't worry about anyone else at the center. They are completely irrelevant to your test.

After the test, your scores pop up on the screen instantly, so steel yourself mentally when you finish the QRT. You are also given a printout of your scores. This printout is technically unofficial, since ADA must review them before they become official, though this step is usually just a formality.

TEST STRATEGIES

There are a few overall test strategies that you should be familiar with at the outset.

CBT Tools

You will have several resources at your disposal on test day, in addition to the noteboards mentioned above. It is important to make good use of these resources. Keep your noteboards neat and organized. Here are some additional suggestions on how and when to use your noteboards:

- summarize a question stem or take key notes, if you need help understanding what a question is asking
- write down equation manipulations or calculations in G-Chem, Physics or QRT
- write down molecules, reactions and/or mechanisms in O-Chem
- generate your passage maps in RCT

A Mark button is available for each question and allows you to flag a question as one you would like to review later, if time permits. When clicked, the "Mark" button turns red and says "Marked."

A Review button is found near the bottom of the screen, and when clicked, brings up a new screen showing all questions and their status (either "answered" or "unanswered," and "marked" or not). You can then choose one of three options: "review all," "review unanswered," or "review marked." You can only review questions in the section of the OAT you are currently taking.

If you click a question on the Review screen, you will be taken directly to that question. Because of this, the Review screen is a good way to quickly navigate through a section. For the most part, you will use the Mark and Review buttons for the "Two-Pass Technique" described below. No matter what, as time runs short in a section, use the Review button to make sure that you have selected an answer for every question before time runs out. You should never, ever, ever leave a question blank on the OAT, as the "Guessing" discussion below will explain.

Clicking the Exhibit button on the SNS will open a periodic table. The periodic table is large and covers most of the screen. However, this window can be resized so you can see the questions and a portion of the periodic table at the same time. The table text will not decrease, but scroll bars will appear on the window so you can center the section of the table of interest in the window. On the QRT, this button says "Calculator" instead, and it pops up the on-screen calculator. This calculator will be discussed in detail later, when we discuss the QRT. Note that you do not have access to a calculator during the SNS or Physics Tests!

You can highlight words in question stems and can also highlight RCT passages. To do this, click and drag over text, or double click to select a single word. Once you have some text selected, an icon shows up below the text and after clicking the icon, the word(s) you have selected are highlighted yellow. These markings will be retained for the entire section, even if you navigate around. You can remove highlighting by clicking it again. If you are struggling to understand what a question is asking, you should highlight some key words in the question stem. Many students answer questions more accurately if they highlight words in the question stem such as least, most, not, except, true, or false. Highlighting RCT passages will be discussed in Chapter 17. You can also electronically strikeout answer options when you are using Process of Elimination (POE).

To do this, right click on a word in an answer option, and that answer option will change to having a line through it, like this:

A. ~~An example of striking out~~

If you right click the answer option again, the strikeout will be removed, and if you left click, the strikeout will be removed and the option will be selected as the correct answer. Finally, strikeouts are retained as you navigate around a section of the OAT.

Process of Elimination

Since the OAT is a multiple-choice test, knowing that one answer is right is helpful, but knowing that all of the other answers are wrong is equally helpful. You might not be sure what the primary purpose of the first paragraph of a reading passage is, but you might be able to tell what it's not, and whatever is left over after you eliminate what it cannot possibly be must be the right answer. The same is true throughout the other sections of the OAT.

As you are doing Process of Elimination (POE), strike out answers you are sure are definitely wrong. Leave answers that you are not sure about or that you don't understand. Hopefully, on your first pass through the answers, you will eliminate between 2 and 4 options. If you only have one answer left, read it quickly to make sure it makes sense, then select it and move on. Beware that you will see questions on test day where you are sure four answers are wrong but you're not sure why the option that is left is correct. If the other answers are definitely wrong, the last answer must be right, so don't waste time worrying about it and move on.

If you have more than one answer left, slow down a little and focus. Try to find a something that is true and answers the question. If you're working on the RCT, the correct answer should also be supported by the passage. You can also compare the remaining answer choices to each other, to help you spot differences between them. Once you've decided on the best answer, select it and move on.

Guessing

There are no penalties for wrong answers, so you should never leave blanks; a blank question is treated the same as a wrong answer, but a question with a guessed answer could be right. On some questions, you can eliminate answers and guess among the remaining choices. For the rest, choose your favorite guessing letter. We call this the Letter of the Day. Select your Letter of the Day for any question you can't or don't have time to answer. No letter is more often right than any other letter, but there is a statistical advantage to guessing consistently. Thus, if your Letter of the Day is A, guess A for every question you skip or can't answer in every section of the test. Finally, keep in mind that most questions on the OAT will have five options (A through E), but some may have only three or four.

SCORING AND PACING

Introduction

Many students approach the OAT the way that they would approach tests in school: they attempt to answer every question to the best of their abilities, which in the OAT usually amounts to rushing at top speed through most sections. They expect that they will get almost all of the questions right, and that this is what they need to do to get a good score. Then they are shocked by what their actual score is.

The reason for this is that the OAT is not scored like tests in school. If you are accustomed to getting at least an A– (or possibly a B+) in your classes, you probably spend time on all test questions and aim to get at least 90% of them correct. A score around a 350 is competitive for most optometry schools, and, depending on the section, and, you typically need between 75% and 85% correct to get a 350. In addition, there are likely to be some questions that, no matter how much time you spend on them, you just don't know how to answer. Overall, you must come to the realization that you have to approach this test differently than other tests you've taken in your life.

Consider the following scoring grid, which converts numbers of questions answered correctly into scaled, standard scores. (This grid changes slightly from test to test, by the way, but it is often much like this one.)

Raw Score (i.e., how many questions you answered correctly)						
STD SCORE	Biology [/40]	General Chem [/30]	Organic Chem [/30]	RCT [/50]	Physics [/40]	QRT [/40]
400	40	30	30	49–50	39–40	39–40
390	39	29	29	48	38	38
380	38	28	28	47	37	36–37
370	37	27	27	46	36	35
360	36	26	26	45	34–35	34
350	35	25	25	43–44	33	33
340	34	24	23–24	40–42	32	32
330	32–33	23	22	37–39	31	30–31
320	30–31	22	21	33–36	29–30	28–29
310	28–29	20–21	19–20	30–32	26–28	25–27
300	25–27	18–19	16–18	27–29	23–25	22–24
290	22–24	15–17	14–15	25–26	22	21
280	19–21	12–14	12–13	22–24	19–21	19–20
270	17–18	11	11	18–21	18	18
260	15–16	10	9–10	15–17	16–17	16–17
250	14	8–9	8	13–14	14–15	14–15
240	13	7	7	11–12	13	12–13
230	12	6	6	9–10	12	11
220	11	5	5	7–8	10–11	10
210	8–10	3–4	3–4	5–6	8–9	8–9
200	0–7	0–2	0–2	1–4	0–7	0–7

Skip-Some Strategy

Now, let's do some calculations with the above numbers, specifically with the QRT section for the sake of discussion. To get a competitive score of 360 on the QRT, you need about 34 questions correct. You could answer all 40 questions in the time allotted (45 minutes), at an average speed of a little over a minute per question, and hope to get 85% (34 questions) correct. This is certainly a possibility, and it is what many test takers try to do.

However, it is not the only way to get this score. Consider slowing down and skipping some questions instead. If you completed only 35 of the 40 questions, you would have more time per question (an extra 10–12 seconds on average). You can get 1 or 2 of the 35 wrong because if you guess on the 5 hardest questions, you would probably get 1 or 2 of those questions right. Remember, if you guess consistently, you have a 1 in 5 chance of getting the question correct.

Now, a difference of 10–12 seconds per question may not sound like very much. However, bear in mind that if you guess on 5 questions, you get to skip questions that you don't know how to do. You will have more time to answer the questions you do know how to do, instead of rushing through everything. If you're answering fewer questions, your accuracy rate has to increase, but this is likely going to happen anyhow if you're skipping the hardest questions and focusing on your strengths.

Overall then, pacing yourself to finish all the questions in every section may not be the best strategy for you. Instead, make pacing goals for each OAT section of each practice test (or section) you complete. A pacing goal is a total number of questions to attempt in a given section, perhaps combined with goals for times at which to finish each group of questions (e.g., finish the first 15 questions in 8 minutes, then the next 15 in 10 minutes, and so on). For example, if you just scored a 300 on Biology (meaning you got 25 to 27 questions right out of 40), it's fairly unlikely that you will immediately jump to getting all 40 questions right. On your next practice test, you should try to gain a few scaled points,

Proven Techniques

perhaps 20, which means that your total pacing goal should be to answer about 30 questions and guess on the rest. This is an achievable goal, and it will improve your score. Once you score a 320, you can pace yourself to answer more questions, and more, and more, until you get to your desired final score.

Similar advice applies to each of the other sections as well. On the RCT, answering all the questions on two passages completely and finishing about half of a third passage with a similar accuracy will result in 40 questions correct and a score of 340. To get a 350 on the SNS sections, you can miss about 5 biology questions and 5 questions from each Chemistry section. Instead of rushing through everything, mark questions that you can't answer or questions that will take a long time to answer. If you have time for these at the end of the section, great. If not, answer them using your Letter of the Day. Keep in mind that Biology, General Chemistry, and Organic Chemistry are scored individually as well as together, and that you must complete all three in 90 minutes total. Many students find the Chemistry questions more difficult than the Biology questions, so you will probably need more time per question for the 60 Chemistry questions than the 40 Biology questions.

Two-Pass System

In the SNS, Physics, and QRT, you should move through the section in two passes. On the first pass, categorize questions as Now, Later, or Never. Now questions are those that you know how to answer quickly and accurately. Later questions are those that you can probably figure out how to answer, but they will take more time. Never questions are those that you probably don't know how to answer at all, at least not within a few minutes (and you should not spend more than a few minutes on any one question on the test).

While you are categorizing questions on the first pass, complete the Now questions as soon as you see them, and mark the Later questions in some way (either on your noteboard or with the Mark button) so that you can come back to them. Guess on the Never questions, because you don't want to spend any more time thinking about them. On your practice exams, make some indication on your simulated noteboard that you guessed on a question, so that you will know on review why you chose your answer, although this is not necessary on the real OAT.

Then, on the second pass, come back for the Later questions. At this point, you can have a good idea how much time you have left for each remaining question. For example, if you categorize 25 QRT questions as Now and 10 as Later (with 5 Never questions), and if you finish the Now questions in 25 minutes (which is fast), then you know that you have 20 minutes left for the remaining 10 Later questions and should spend about 2 minutes on each question. On the other hand, if you just tried to complete the Later questions as you came to them, you would not know whether 2 minutes was too long to spend on a single question.

Conclusion

In essence, much of this advice boils down to four simple words: accuracy first, speed second. Getting questions wrong quickly is not much better than getting questions wrong slowly; first, get them right, and then you can worry about getting them right quickly. Students who rush through easier questions, to questions that are hard (or impossible) for them, often make preventable mistakes on the easy questions. First you must focus on answering the questions that you know how to answer, and then you can work on answering the rest of the questions.

Of course, if you do get to the point where you are consistently scoring a 350 or higher on a section and are shooting for an extremely high score, you need to answer all of the questions and get pretty much all of them right. (To give some frame of reference, on many sections you need better than 90% correct on all the questions in order to score a 360 or above.) In that case, you don't need to worry about guessing letters, but you will still probably want to take the section in two passes and follow much of the rest of the advice above. Even if you answer all of the questions, there is an advantage to having the last few questions you work be the hardest questions, so that you know exactly how much time you can allot to working them. This might, in extreme cases, mean that your first pass consists of about 35 questions, and the second pass consists of about 5 questions; just make sure that your question sequence makes sense.

OPTOMETRY OVERVIEW

Pre-Optometry Curriculum

Before you take the OAT, you have to take certain classes in college. These are the pre-optometry prerequisites. These may vary somewhat from school to school, but in general, you are required to take at least a year of English, general chemistry, organic chemistry, physics, and biology. Schools may also require classes in calculus, biO-Chemistry, or other fields, such as psychology or statistics.

Most schools require you to have completed a bachelor's degree in some subject from an accredited college or university, though most do not recommend any particular major over any other, as long as you complete your prerequisite coursework. You will also find it useful in the long term to take classes that develop your interpersonal communication and business skills, as well as your core science knowledge. Thus, in addition to advanced courses in biology, chemistry, and physics, you may find it useful to take courses that require extensive reading and writing, as well as courses in statistics, accounting, or economics. Such courses are not required for admission to optometry school, but they are useful to optometrists.

As you are choosing your undergraduate courses, bear in mind that rigorous courses are viewed very positively in admissions. While GPA is important, schools also consider the context in which you earned your GPA. The strength of your overall course history is a very significant factor, perhaps as significant as your personal statement or recommendations. If you took GPA-boosting easy classes, while another student took challenging and rigorous classes, then the other student may get the benefit of the doubt even on a slightly lower GPA.

Also, sometimes students pursue graduate degrees before applying to optometry school. Such degrees are helpful, even though your undergraduate GPA will be the primary GPA considered, not your graduate GPA. Having a Master's or Ph. D. is definitely a modest advantage in admissions, in part because it shows additional academic ability.

Optometry Admissions Information

Applications for optometry school are usually processed through the Optometry's Centralized Application Service (OptomCAS), which is sort of like a Common App for optometry schools. All components of a primary application go through this service. This application usually becomes available in July each year, and you must fill it out in the year before you intend to matriculate. Admissions is rolling at most optometry schools, so applying in the summer, especially early in the summer, is advantageous.

The components of an optometry school application include several numbers (termed "hard factors") and a variety of information ("soft factors" or "softs"). The main hard factors are your undergraduate GPA, potentially with emphasis on your science or major GPA, and your OAT scores, potentially with emphasis on your Academic Average score. The soft factors include a personal statement, letters of recommendation (often three), and a resume.

Optometry admission is typically holistic, meaning that no single factor is conclusive either way. For example, even if you have a great GPA, if your OAT is low and your personal statement is written poorly, you will likely be denied admission at most schools. Likewise, if you have an excellent overall application but one portion is a little worse than the others, that weak aspect may not hold you back. However, some optometry schools do have minimum numbers for GPA or OAT scores, so be sure to check the specific schools' admission standards to make sure that you are eligible for admission.

Despite holistic admissions, the hard factors are usually the first consideration in evaluating an applicant. If your GPA and OAT scores are above average for what the school usually accepts, you have a very good chance, but if they are both below average for the school, your chances are low. Once admission committees have examined your numbers, they will also scrutinize the rest of your application. Many also request more information through a secondary application.

If you are in serious consideration after many applications are sifted and many candidates are eliminated, you will likely be asked to interview at the school. The interview usually involves going to the school, meeting with current students and faculty, and being asked extensive personal questions about your career goals and many other topics, sometimes including specific aspects of your application. (If there are any specific weaknesses or if there is anything unusual in your application, be prepared to address it.) Being granted an interview at all is a very good sign, though it does not guarantee admission.

The interview season lasts through late fall and winter after you have submitted your application. Regular decisions (acceptance, rejection, or waitlist) are usually completed by March or April of the year in which you intend to matriculate, although some may not be given until later.

Overview of Optometry School

There are about 20 different optometry schools in the United States, and their educational methods are diverse, but some generalizations can be made. Optometry school programs are typically four years long, ending with a grant of the O.D. (Oculus Doctor) degree. The programs usually cover a mixture of classroom and clinical courses. Students learn about optics, visual perception, diseases of the eye, and many other topics relating to optometry. After you graduate, you can look forward to taking the national exam administered by the National Board of Examiners in Optometry.

After graduating from general optometry school, some students decide to pursue specialties. These typically involve one-year or two-year residencies. Additionally, some students pursue joint degrees. Some optometry schools offer Master of Science degrees alongside their O.D. degrees, which may be pursued concurrently or consecutively.

After Graduation

Many optometrists work in private practice. This can be in the offices of optometrists, physicians (including ophthalmologists), or health and personal care stores (including optical goods stores). Some work in other contexts, including hospitals. Some teach and do research at universities. Roughly one-quarter of optometrists are self-employed.

In general, optometrists are extremely well compensated. The Bureau of Labor Statistics says that the median annual wages of salaries for optometrists in 2017 was approximately $110,000. In 2015, the average annual income for self-employed optometrists was closer to $150,000. In addition, job opportunities are excellent, because the employment of optometrists is expected to grow much faster than the average for all occupations.[1]

---

[1] This information is from the BLS's *Occupational Outlook Handbook*, 2018 Edition.

Physics

Chapter 2
Units and Vectors

TOPICS IN OAT PHYSICS

Physics on the OAT is the one topic that differentiates it from the DAT, which is why it's set out in such detail in this book. ADA describes the content of the OAT as follows[1]:

- Units and Vectors
- Linear Kinematics
- Statics   } (40%)
- Dynamics
- Rotational Motion
- Energy and Momentum   (10%)
- Simple Harmonic Motion
- Waves   } (10%)
- Fluid Statics   (5%)
- Thermal Energy and Thermodynamics   (7.5%)
- Electrostatics
- D.C. Circuits   } (15%)
- Optics   (12.5%)

You should pay at least some attention to the weight of the topic as you study. If fluid statics seems fairly complicated for you, note that it only makes up roughly 5% of the physics section, or about two questions. You can get a fairly high score on OAT Physics without studying that particular topic. On the other hand, the chapters "Units and Vectors" and "Linear Kinematics" are weighted fairly heavily on the OAT. If you're not solid on concepts within these areas, you're likely to miss a lot of points. Note also the relatively high weight of optics (not surprising on the OAT) as an individual topic. These three topics make up roughly one-third of the physics section.

2.1 SCALARS AND VECTORS

Some quantities are completely described simply by a number (possibly with units). Examples include constants (like –2, 9.8, 0, and π) and physical quantities such as mass, length, time, speed, energy, power, density, volume, pressure, temperature, charge, potential, resistance, capacitance, frequency, sound level, and refractive index. All of these quantities are known as **scalars**, which you can think of as just a fancy word for *numbers*.

On the other hand, there are other quantities which are completely specified only when they're described by a number *and a direction*. Examples include displacement, velocity, acceleration, force, momentum, and electric and magnetic fields. All of these quantities are known as **vectors**. A vector is a quantity that involves *both* a number (its magnitude, which is a scalar) *and* a direction.

Here's an example: If I say the wind is blowing at 5 m/s, I'm giving the wind's *speed*, which is a *scalar*.

---

[1]   Source: *OAT User Guide*

However, if I say the wind is blowing at 5 m/s to the east, I'm giving the wind's *velocity*, which is a *vector*. (By the way, the distinction between speed and velocity is easy to remember: speed is a scalar, while velocity is a vector.)

Since a vector is determined by a number and a direction, we represent a vector by an arrow. The length of the arrow we draw represents the number, and the direction of the arrow represents the direction of the vector. For example, the wind velocity *5 m/s to the east* might be drawn as an arrow like this:

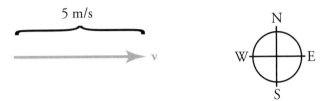

The symbol **v** is the name of this vector. In books, vector names are written as boldface letters; in handwritten work, we'd put a small arrow over the letter—like this: $\vec{v}$ or $\vec{v}$—to signify that the quantity is a vector.

The number (or scalar) associated with a vector is its **magnitude**; it's the length of the arrow. For instance, for the vector **v** = 5 m/s to the east, the magnitude would be the scalar 5 m/s. Here's another example: if we push on something with a force of 10 N to the left,

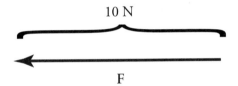

then the magnitude of the vector **F** = *10 N to the left* would be 10 N. Magnitudes are never negative.

There are two common ways to denote the magnitude of a vector. The first is to change the bold letter for the vector to an italic letter. Using this notation, the magnitude of the vector **v** would be written as *v*. As another example, the magnitude of the vector **F** would be written as *F*. The second way to denote the magnitude of a vector is to put absolute-value signs around the letter name of the vector. In this notation, the magnitude of the vector **v** would be written as $|\mathbf{v}|$ (or, in handwritten work, as $|\vec{v}|$) and the magnitude of the vector **F** would be $|\mathbf{F}|$.

2.2 OPERATIONS WITH VECTORS

For the OAT, the three most important operations we perform with vectors are (1) addition of vectors, (2) subtraction of vectors, and (3) multiplication of a vector by a scalar.

Vector Addition

To add one vector to another vector, we use the **tip-to-tail method**. The **tail** of a vector is the starting point of the arrow, and the **tip** of a vector is the ending point (the sharp point of the arrow head):

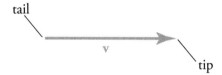

To add two vectors, we first put the tip of one of the vectors at the tail of the other one (tip-to-tail). Then we connect the exposed tail to the exposed tip; that vector is the sum of the vectors. The following figure shows this process for adding the vectors **A** and **B** to get their sum, **A** + **B**:

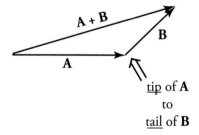

We could have put the tip of **B** at the tail of **A**, and the answer would have been the same:

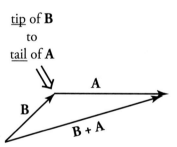

We can see from these two figures that the vector **A** + **B** has the same length *and* the same direction as the vector **B** + **A**. Therefore, the vectors are the same: **A** + **B** = **B** + **A**. We say that vectors obey the *commutative law for addition*; this means we can add them in either order, and the result is the same. (Actually, vectors *automatically* obey the Commutative Law for addition, by definition; that is, if **A** and **B** are vectors, then **A** + **B** will always be the same as **B** + **A**. There actually are quantities that are specified by a number and a direction but which do not obey the law **A** + **B** = **B** + **A**. Because of this failure, these quantities are not called vectors. However, you won't have to worry about such peculiar quantities for the OAT.)

Vector Subtraction

To subtract one vector from another vector, we use the familiar *scalar* equation $a - b = a + (-b)$ as motivation. That is, for any two vectors **A** and **B**, we say that **A** − **B** is equal to **A** + (−**B**). So, we first have to answer the question: Given a vector **B**, how do we form the vector −**B**? By definition, the vector −**B** has the same magnitude as **B** but the opposite direction:

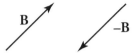

Therefore, to form the vector difference **A** − **B**, we just add −**B** to **A**:

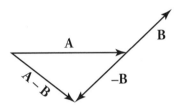

The following figure shows how to form the vector difference **B** − **A**, which is **B** + (−**A**):

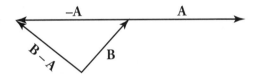

Notice that **B** − **A** is *not* the same as **A** − **B**, because their directions are not the same. That is, in general, **B** − **A** ≠ **A** − **B**; vector *subtraction* is generally *not* commutative. In fact, **B** − **A** will always be the *opposite* of **A** − **B** (same magnitude, opposite direction): **B** − **A** = −(**A** − **B**).

Another procedure you can use to subtract the vectors **A** and **B** is to put the tail of **A** at the tail of **B**, then connect the tips. (Vector *addition* uses the *tip*-to-tail method; vector *subtraction* (by this alternate procedure) uses the *tail*-to-tail method.) If you draw the resulting vector from the tip of **B** to the tip of **A**, you've constructed the vector **A** − **B**. On the other hand, if you draw the resulting vector from the tip of **A** to the tip of **B**, you've drawn the vector **B** − **A**.

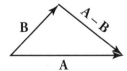 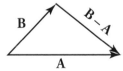

Notice that the figure on the left also illustrates the tip-to-tail vector addition **B** + (**A** − **B**) = **A**, while the figure on the right illustrates the tip-to-tail vector addition **A** + (**B** − **A**) = **B**.

Scalar Multiplication

To multiply a vector by a scalar, we consider three cases: that is, whether the scalar is positive, negative, or zero.

If k is a positive scalar, then $k\mathbf{A}$, the product of k and some vector $\mathbf{A}$, is a vector whose magnitude is k times the magnitude of $\mathbf{A}$ and whose direction is the same as that of $\mathbf{A}$. In short, multiplying a vector by a positive scalar k just changes the magnitude by a factor of k (but leaves the direction of the vector unchanged). If k is less than 1, the scalar multiple $k\mathbf{A}$ is shorter than $\mathbf{A}$; if k is greater than 1, then $k\mathbf{A}$ is longer than $\mathbf{A}$.

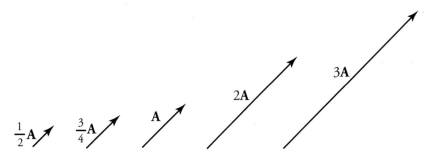

If k is a negative scalar, then $k\mathbf{A}$, the product of k and some vector $\mathbf{A}$, is a vector whose magnitude is the *absolute value* of k times the magnitude of $\mathbf{A}$ and whose direction is *opposite* the direction of $\mathbf{A}$. In short, multiplying a vector by a negative scalar k changes the magnitude by a factor of $|k|$ and reverses the direction of the vector.

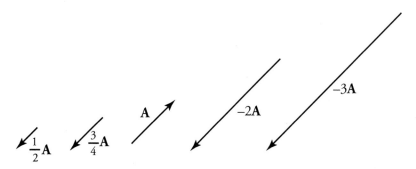

If k is zero, then the product $k\mathbf{A}$ gives $\mathbf{0}$, the **zero vector**. This unique vector has magnitude 0 and has no direction. Rather than being pictured as an arrow, the zero vector is simply pictured as a dot.

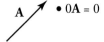

Example 2-1: Consider the vectors $\mathbf{A}$, $\mathbf{B}$, and $\mathbf{C}$ shown below:

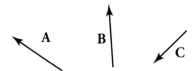

Construct each of the following vectors:

a) $\mathbf{A} + \mathbf{B}$

b) $\mathbf{A} - 2\mathbf{C}$

c) $\dfrac{1}{2}\mathbf{A} - \mathbf{B} + 3\mathbf{C}$

Solution:

a)   Using the tip-to-tail method for vector addition gives

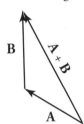

b)   Since $\mathbf{A} - 2\mathbf{C} = \mathbf{A} + (-2\mathbf{C})$, we first multiply $\mathbf{C}$ by -2, then add the result to $\mathbf{A}$:

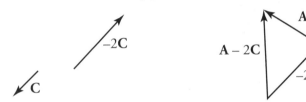

c)   We multiply $\mathbf{A}$ by 1/2, then $\mathbf{B}$ by -1, then $\mathbf{C}$ by 3, and add the three results:

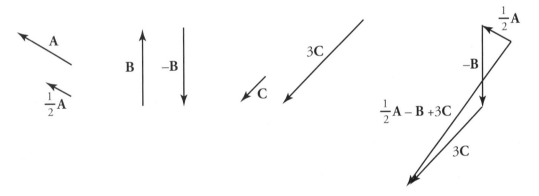

Example 2-2: Consider the vectors $\mathbf{A}$, $\mathbf{B}$, and $\mathbf{C}$ shown below:

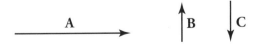

Construct each of the following vectors:

a) $-\mathbf{A} + \mathbf{B}$

b) $\mathbf{B} + \mathbf{C}$

c) $\mathbf{A} + 2\mathbf{B}$

2.2

Solution:

a) Multiplying **A** by –1 then using the tip-to-tail method to add the result to **B**, we get

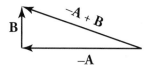

b) Since **C** has the same length as **B** but the opposite direction, **C** is equal to –**B**. So, adding **B** + **C** gives us **B** + (–**B**), which is **0**, the zero vector. You can also see that the sum of **B** and **C** will be **0** using the tip-to-tail method for vector addition: if we put the tip of **B** at the tail of **C**, then the tail of **B** *coincides* with the tip of **C**, so the vector sum is **0**.

c) Multiplying **B** by 2 then using the tip-to-tail method to add the result to **A**, we get

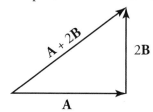

Example 2-3: Add these four vectors:

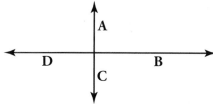

Solution: The vectors **A** and **C** have equal magnitudes but opposite directions, so **A** + **C** is **0**; that is, **A** and **C** cancel each other out. Now, since **D** points in the direction opposite to **B**, if we place the tail of **D** at the tip of **B**, then connect the tail of **B** to the tip of **D**, we get **B** + **D**, which is a vector in the same direction as **B**, but much shorter. This vector is **B** + **D**, which is also the sum **A** + **B** + **C** + **D** (since **A** + **C** = **0**):

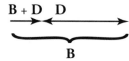

2.3 VECTOR PROJECTIONS AND COMPONENTS

In the preceding section, we performed the basic vector operations geometrically. In this section, we'll see how we can perform these operations with algebra and trig.

Let's imagine a vector **A** in a standard *x-y* coordinate system, with the tail of **A** at the origin. We construct perpendicular segments from the tip of **A** to the *x*-axis and to the *y*-axis. The resulting **vector projections** of **A** are denoted by $\mathbf{A}_x$ and $\mathbf{A}_y$; the vector $\mathbf{A}_x$ is the horizontal projection of **A**, and $\mathbf{A}_y$ is the vertical projection. Notice that $\mathbf{A} = \mathbf{A}_x + \mathbf{A}_y$. Therefore, *any vector* **A** *in the x-y plane can be written as the sum of a horizontal vector and a vertical vector (namely, its horizontal and vertical projections).*

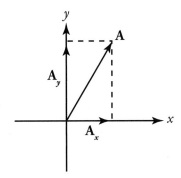

We now want to find a way to write $\mathbf{A}_x$ and $\mathbf{A}_y$ algebraically. Since any vector is specified by giving its magnitude and its direction, we need an algebraic way of describing the directions of these vectors. We do this by constructing two special vectors, one of which points in the horizontal direction, the other in the vertical direction. These two vectors are called **i** and **j**, and each has length 1:

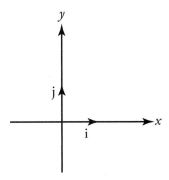

Any horizontal vector is some multiple of **i** ($\mathbf{A}_x = A_x\mathbf{i}$), and any vertical vector is some multiple of **j** ($\mathbf{A}_y = A_y\mathbf{j}$). Therefore, *any vector* A *in the x-y plane can be written as the sum of a multiple of* **i** *plus a multiple of* **j**:

$$\mathbf{A} = A_x\mathbf{i} + A_y\mathbf{j}$$

These multiples, A_x and A_y, are called the **components** of **A**. Notice that projections are vectors, while components are scalars.

For example, the horizontal vector of magnitude 3 that points to the right is 3**i**, and the horizontal vector of magnitude 3 that points to the left is 3(–**i**) or –3**i**. The vertical vector of magnitude 4 that points upward is 4**j**, and the vertical vector of magnitude 4 that points downward is 4(–**j**) or –4**j**. For the vector **A** = –3**i** + 4**j**, we would say that its horizontal projection is –3**i** and its horizontal component is –3; similarly, its vertical projection is 4**j** and its vertical component is 4.

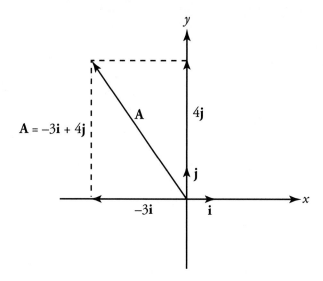

The great advantage of writing vectors algebraically is that it gives us the ability to perform vector operations quickly and precisely without having to draw the vectors (and using such procedures as the tip-to-tail method).

Magnitude

The magnitude of a vector can be found from its horizontal and vertical components using the Pythagorean Theorem:

$$A = \sqrt{(A_x)^2 + (A_y)^2}$$

For example, the magnitude of the vector **A** = –3**i** + 4**j** is $A = \sqrt{(-3)^2 + 4^2} = 5$.

Direction

The direction of a vector can be described by giving the angle, θ, which the vector makes with positive x-axis. Since the components of a vector **A** are given by the formulas

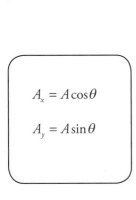

$$A_x = A\cos\theta$$

$$A_y = A\sin\theta$$

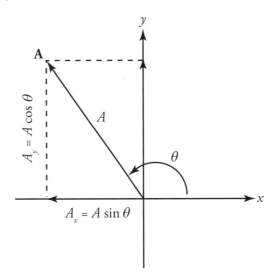

we see that

$$\frac{A_y}{A_x} = \frac{A\sin\theta}{A\cos\theta} = \tan\theta \rightarrow \boxed{\theta = \tan^{-1}\frac{A_y}{A_x}}$$

Vector Addition and Subtraction

The operations of addition and subtraction of vectors is made especially easy by the use of components. To add the vector $\mathbf{A} = A_x\mathbf{i} + A_y\mathbf{j}$ to the vector $\mathbf{B} = B_x\mathbf{i} + B_y\mathbf{j}$, we simply add the horizontal components and add the vertical components; and to subtract the vectors, we just subtract their components:

$$\mathbf{A} + \mathbf{B} = (A_x + B_x)\mathbf{i} + (A_y + B_y)\mathbf{j}$$
$$\mathbf{A} - \mathbf{B} = (A_x - B_x)\mathbf{i} + (A_y - B_y)\mathbf{j}$$

Scalar Multiplication

To multiply a vector by a scalar, just multiply each component by the scalar:

$$k\mathbf{A} = (kA_x)\mathbf{i} + (kA_y)\mathbf{j}$$

2.3

Example 2-4: Let **A** = –22**i** + 16**j**, **B** = 30**j**, and **C** = –10**i** – 10**j**.
Find each of the following vectors:

a)   **A** + **B**

b)   **A** – 2**C**

c) $\frac{1}{2}$**A** – **B** + 3**C**

Solution:

a)   **A** + **B** = (–22 + 0)**i** + (16 + 30)**j** = –22**i** + 46**j**

b)   Since 2**C** = 2(–10**i** – 10**j**) = –20**i** – 20**j**, we get:

   A – 2**C** = [–22 – (–20)]**i** + [16 – (–20)]**j** = –2**i** + 36**j**

c)   Since $\frac{1}{2}$**A** $= \frac{1}{2}$(–22)**i** $+ \frac{1}{2}$(16)**j** $= -11$**i** $+ 8$**j** and 3**C** = 3(–10**i** – 10**j**) = –30**i** – 30**j**, we find that

   $\frac{1}{2}$**A** – **B** + 3**C** $= (-11 - 0 - 30)$**i** $+ (8 - 30 - 30)$**j** $= -41$**i** $- 52$**j**

Compare this example (and its results) with Example 3-1.

Example 2-5: What's the magnitude and direction of the vector **A** = 3**i** – 3**j**?

Solution: If we draw the vector starting at the origin, then

the vector points down into Quadrant IV. Its magnitude is

$A = \sqrt{3^2 + (-3)^2} = 3\sqrt{2}$, and its direction is given by

$$\theta = \tan^{-1}\frac{A_y}{A_x} = \tan^{-1}(\frac{-3}{3}) = \tan^{-1}(-1) = 315° \text{ or } -45°$$

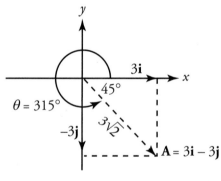

Example 2-6: Let **A** be the vector of magnitude 6 that makes
an angle of 150° with the positive *x*-axis. Sketch this vector, determine its components, and write **A** in
terms of **i** and **j**.

Solution: The figure at the right is a sketch of this vector.
Its components are

$$A_x = A\cos\theta = 6\cos 150° = 6(-\frac{\sqrt{3}}{2}) = -3\sqrt{3}$$

$$A_y = A\sin\theta = 6\sin 150° = 6(\frac{1}{2}) = 3$$

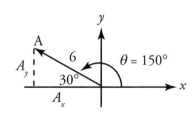

Therefore, since for any vector **A** we have $\mathbf{A} = A_x\mathbf{i} + A_y\mathbf{j}$, we can write

$$\mathbf{A} = -3\sqrt{3}\mathbf{i} + 3\mathbf{j}$$

Example 2-7: Any vector whose magnitude is 1 is called a **unit vector**. (For example, both **i** and **j** are examples of unit vectors.) Let **C** be the unit vector that makes an angle of 225° with the positive *x*-axis. Sketch this vector, determine its components, and write **C** in terms of **i** and **j**.

Solution: The figure at the right is a sketch of this vector. Its components are

$$C_x = C\cos\theta = 1\ \cos\ 225° = -\frac{\sqrt{2}}{2}$$

$$C_y = C\sin\theta = 1\ \sin\ 225° = -\frac{\sqrt{2}}{2}$$

Therefore, since for any vector **C** we have $\mathbf{C} = C_x\mathbf{i} + C_y\mathbf{j}$, we can write

$$\mathbf{C} = -\frac{\sqrt{2}}{2}\mathbf{i} - \frac{\sqrt{2}}{2}\mathbf{j}$$

Example 2-8: The figure below shows a vector **W** of magnitude 100 and its projections, $\mathbf{W}_1$ and $\mathbf{W}_2$, onto two mutually perpendicular directions, such that $\mathbf{W} = \mathbf{W}_1 + \mathbf{W}_2$. Find the magnitudes of $\mathbf{W}_1$ and $\mathbf{W}_2$.

Solution: By definition of the sine and cosine, we have

$$W_1 = W\cos\theta = 100\cos 60° = 100(\frac{1}{2}) = 50$$

$$W_2 = W\sin\theta = 100\sin 60° = 100(\frac{\sqrt{3}}{2}) = 50\sqrt{3}$$

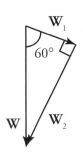

2.4 UNITS AND DIMENSIONS

Before we begin our study of physics, we'll briefly go over metric units. Scientists —and the OAT—use the Système International d'Unités (the International System of Units), abbreviated **SI**, to express the measurements of physical quantities. The **base units** of the SI that we'll be interested in (at least for most of our study of OAT Physics) are listed below:

SI base unit	abbreviation	measures	dimension
meter	m	length	L
kilogram	kg	mass	M
second	s	time	T

This system of units is also referred to as the **mks system** (m for meters, k for kilograms, and s for seconds). Each **dimension** is simply an abbreviation for the quantity that is being measured; it does not depend on the particular unit that's used. For example, we could measure a distance in miles, meters, or furlongs— to name a few—but in all cases, we're measuring a *length*. We say that distance has the dimensions of length, L. As another example, we could measure an object's speed in miles per hour, meters per second, or furlongs per fortnight; but regardless of what units we use, we're always dividing a length by a time. Therefore, speed has dimensions of length per time (L/T).

Any physical quantity can be written in terms of the SI base units. Here are some examples:

quantity	symbol	units	dimensions
speed	v	m/s	L/T
density	ρ	kg/m^3	M/L^3
work	W	kg·m^2/s^2	ML^2/T^2

Multiples of the base units that are powers of ten are often abbreviated and precede the symbol for the unit. For example, "n" is the symbol for nano-, which means 10^{-9} (one billionth). Thus, one billionth of a second, 1 nanosecond, would be written as 1 ns. The letter "M" is the symbol for mega-, which means 10^6 (one million), so a distance of one million meters, 1 megameter, would be abbreviated as 1 Mm.

Some of the most common power-of-ten prefixes are given in the following list:

prefix	symbol	multiple
pico	p	10^{-12}
nano-	n	10^{-9}
micro-	μ	10^{-6}
milli-	m	10^{-3}
centi-	c	10^{-2}
kilo-	k	10^{3}
mega-	M	10^{6}
giga-	G	10^{9}

You should memorize this list.

On the OAT, you won't need to convert between the American system of units (which uses things like inches, feet, yards, and pounds) and the metric system, so don't bother memorizing conversions like 2.54 cm = 1 inch or 39.37 inches = 1 meter, etc. You will need to be able to convert within the metric system using the powers-of-ten prefixes.

Example 3-1: Express a density of 5500 kg/m^3 in g/cm^3.

Solution: All we want to do with this physical measurement is to change the units in which it's expressed. For that, we need conversion factors. A **conversion factor** is simply a fraction whose value is 1, that multiplies a measurement in one set of units to give the equivalent measurement in a different set of units. In this case, we'd write

$$\rho = 5.5 \times 10^3 \, \frac{\text{kg}}{\text{m}^3} \times \left(\frac{10^3 \, \text{g}}{1 \, \text{kg}} \right) \times \left(\frac{1 \, \text{m}}{10^2 \, \text{cm}} \right)^3 = 5.5 \, \frac{\text{g}}{\text{cm}^3}$$

Notice that each of these conversion factors is written so that the unit we want to change (that is, the unit we want to eliminate) cancels out. The fraction

$$\frac{1 \, \text{kg}}{10^3 \, \text{g}}$$

is also a conversion factor for mass, but writing it like this would not have been helpful in this particular problem because then the "kg" would not have canceled.

Example 3-2: If a ball is dropped from a great height, then the force of air resistance it feels at any point during its descent is given by the equation $F = KD^2v^2$, where D is the diameter of the ball and v is its speed. If the units of F are kg·m/s^2, what are the units of K?

Solution: If the equation $F = KD^2v^2$ is to be valid, then the units of the left-hand side must be the same as the units of the right-hand side. To specify the unit of a quantity, we put brackets around it; for example, $[F]$ denotes the units of F; that is, $[F] = $ kg·m/s^2. So we need to make sure that $[F] = [KD^2v^2]$, which means

$$[F] = [K][D]^2[v]^2$$
$$\frac{\text{kg} \cdot \text{m}}{\text{s}^2} = [K] \cdot \text{m}^2 \cdot \left(\frac{\text{m}}{\text{s}} \right)^2$$
$$= [K] \cdot \frac{\text{m}^4}{\text{s}^2}$$
$$\text{kg} \cdot \text{m} = [K] \cdot \text{m}^4$$
$$\therefore [K] = \frac{\text{kg}}{\text{m}^3}$$

Chapter 3
Linear Kinematics

3.1 KINEMATICS

Kinematics is the description of motion in terms of an object's position, velocity, and acceleration. The OAT will expect not only that you can answer mathematical questions about these quantities but also that you know the definitions of these quantities.

Displacement

The **displacement** of an object is its change in position. For example, let's say we were measuring an object moving along a straight line by laying a meter stick along the object's line of motion. If the object starts at, say, the *10 cm* mark on the meter stick and moves to the *70 cm* mark, then its position changed by 70 cm – 10 cm = 60 cm, so we'd say its displacement is 60 cm.

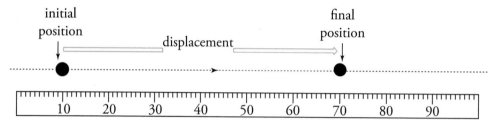

We find the displacement by subtracting the object's initial position from its final position:

$$\text{displacement} = \Delta(\text{position}) = \text{position}_{\text{final}} - \text{position}_{\text{initial}}$$

Now, what if the object moved from the *70 cm* mark on the meter stick to the *10 cm* mark? Then its displacement would be 10 cm – 70 cm = –60 cm.

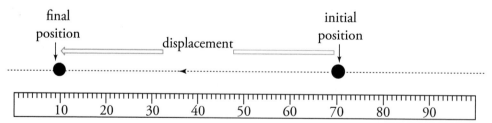

In both cases, the object moved a distance of 60 cm, but in the first case it moved to the right, and in the second case, it moved to the left. Displacement is a vector, so it takes direction into account. If we call *to the right* the positive direction (so *to the left* automatically becomes the negative direction), then in the first case, we'd say the displacement is +60 cm, and in the second case, it's –60 cm.

The motion of the object can be more complicated. For example, what if the object started at the *10 cm* mark, moved to the *50 cm* mark, back to the *40 cm* mark, and then over to the *70 cm* mark?

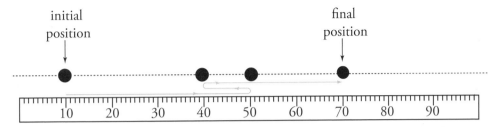

This example brings up a crucial point about displacement. The *total* distance that the object travels is (40 cm) + (10 cm) + (30 cm) = 80 cm, but the object's displacement is still

$$\text{displacement} = \Delta(\text{position}) = \text{position}_{\text{final}} - \text{position}_{\text{initial}}$$

$$= (70 \text{ cm}) - (10 \text{ cm})$$

$$= +60 \text{ cm}$$

Displacement gives us the *net* distance traveled by the object, which may very well be less than the total distance. So, the displacement is a vector that always points from the object's initial position to its final position, *regardless of the path the object took*, and whose magnitude is the *net* distance traveled by the object. There are multiple different symbols that are used to represent the displacement vector, but the most common one is the single letter **d**. Sometimes, we use $\Delta\mathbf{x}$ if we know the displacement is horizontal, or $\Delta\mathbf{y}$ if we know the displacement is vertical. Be aware that the OAT also uses the word *displacement* to mean just the magnitude of the displacement vector (that is, just the net distance traveled by the object without regard for direction); the question will make it clear which meaning is intended.

Displacement

$$\mathbf{d} = \text{position}_{\text{final}} - \text{position}_{\text{initial}} = \text{net distance plus direction}$$

For example, if a sprinter runs 400 meters around a circular track and returns to her starting point, she has covered a *total* distance of 400 meters, but her *displacement* is zero. If a sprinter runs 300 meters north, then 400 meters east, he's covered a total distance of 700 m, but his displacement is only 500 meters.

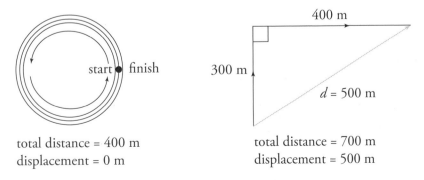

total distance = 400 m
displacement = 0 m

total distance = 700 m
displacement = 500 m

Example 3-3: The object shown below begins at the *90 cm* mark on the meter stick, moves to the *20 cm* mark, then to the *70 cm* mark.

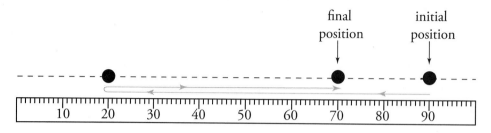

a) What's the total distance traveled by this object?
b) What's the object's displacement?

Solution:

a) In traveling from the *90 cm* mark to the *20 cm* mark, the object moved a distance of 70 cm. Then, in traveling from the *20 cm* mark to the *70 cm* mark, the object moved a distance of 50 cm. Therefore, the total distance traveled by the object is (70 cm) + (50 cm) = 120 cm.

b) Displacement: **d** = position$_{final}$ − position$_{initial}$ = (70 cm) − (90 cm) = −20 cm. Notice that the displacement here is negative, which indicates that the object's change in position was in the negative direction (it ended up to the *left* of where it started).

Velocity

Displacement tells us how much an object's position changes. **Velocity** tells us how *fast* an object's position changes. If you're in a car traveling at 60 miles per hour along a long, straight highway, then this means your position changes by 60 miles every hour. To calculate velocity, simply divide how much the position has changed by how much time it took for it to change; in other words, divide displacement by time.

Average Velocity

$$\text{average velocity} = \frac{\text{displacement}}{\text{time}}$$

$$\bar{\mathbf{v}} = \frac{\Delta \mathbf{x}}{\Delta t} = \frac{\mathbf{d}}{\Delta t}$$

This is actually the definition of **average velocity**, and we place a bar above the **v** to signify that it's an *average*. So, **v** is velocity and $\bar{\mathbf{v}}$ is average velocity. (If the velocity happens to be constant, then there's no distinction between *velocity* and *average velocity*, and we don't need the bar.) Notice right away that velocity is a vector; after all, we're dividing a vector (the displacement, **d**) by a number, so we're left with a vector. In fact, because Δt is always positive, $\bar{\mathbf{v}}$ always points in the same direction as **d**.

The magnitude of the velocity vector is called the **speed**. Speed is a scalar; it has no direction and can never be negative. (Notice that the speedometer in your car is well-named; it only tells you how fast the car is moving, not the direction of motion. It's not a "velocity-o-meter.") Velocity is a vector that specifies both speed and direction.

> **Velocity**
>
> $$\mathbf{v} = \text{speed \& direction}$$

In the figure below, each vector represents the car's velocity. Both cars have the same speed (let's say 20 m/s), so the magnitudes of their velocity vectors are the same. Nevertheless, they have different velocities, because the directions are different. (By the way, if the car on the right looks bigger than the car on the left, it's an optical illusion. Grab a ruler and check it for yourself. They're the same size!)

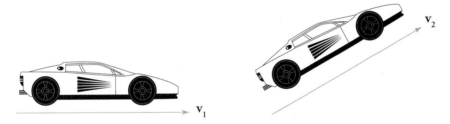

These two cars have the same speed but different velocities. Is it possible for two cars to have the same velocity but different speeds? No. Velocity is speed plus direction, so if the velocities are the same, then the speeds (and the directions) are the same.

Example 3-4: The object shown below begins (time $t = 0$) at the *90 cm* mark on the meter stick. At time $t = 3$ sec, it has moved to the *20 cm* mark, and at time $t = 5$ sec, it's at the *70 cm* mark.

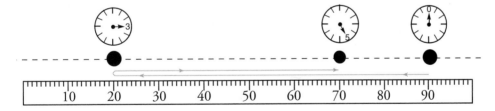

a) What was the average velocity of this object?
b) What was the object's average speed?

Solution:

a) We figured out in Example 3-3(b) that the object's displacement was –20 cm. Therefore,

$$\mathbf{v} = \frac{\mathbf{d}}{\Delta t} = \frac{-20 \text{ cm}}{5 \text{ s}} = -4 \text{ cm/s or } -0.04 \text{ m/s}$$

The minus sign indicates the direction of $\overline{\mathbf{v}}$ the object's displacement was to the left, so its average velocity is also to the left.

b) *Average speed* is not the magnitude of the average velocity. (Confusing, but true.) By definition, **average speed** is the *total* distance traveled divided by the time. We figured out in Example 3-3(a) that the total distance traveled by this object was 120 cm, so the object's average speed is (120 cm)/(5 s) = 24 cm/s = 0.24 m/s.

Example 3-5: A sprinter runs 400 meters around a circular track and returns to her starting point, covering a total distance of 400 meters in 50 seconds. What was her average speed? What was her average velocity?

Solution: The sprinter's average speed was (400 m)/(50 s) = 8 m/s. However, because her displacement is 0, her average velocity was zero.

Example 3-6: A sprinter runs 300 meters north, then 400 meters east, which takes 100 seconds.

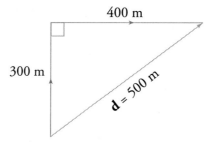

What was his average speed? What was the magnitude of his average velocity?

Solution: The sprinter's average speed was (700 m)/(100 s) = 7 m/s. However, because his displacement is 500 m, his average velocity has a magnitude of (500 m)/(100 s) = 5 m/s.

Example 3-7: An object moves from Point A to Point B in 4 seconds.

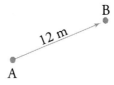

What was the object's velocity?

A. 3 m/s
B. 8 m/s
C. 6 m/s
D. 48 m/s

Solution: Notice that the question is asking for velocity (which is a vector) but all the choices are scalars. Strictly speaking, the answer should include the correct direction as well as the magnitude. However, the OAT (as well as textbook authors and teachers) will often use the word *velocity* when they mean *speed*; usually, it won't cause confusion. From the choices given, we know it's the magnitude of the velocity that is the desired quantity, and this is

$$v = \frac{d}{\Delta t} = \frac{12\ m}{4\ s} = 3\ m/s$$

Choice (A) is the answer we'd choose.

Acceleration

Velocity tells us how fast an object's position changes. **Acceleration** tells us how fast an object's *velocity* changes.

Average Acceleration

$$\text{average acceleration} = \frac{\text{change in velocity}}{\text{time}}$$

$$\bar{\mathbf{a}} = \frac{\Delta \mathbf{v}}{\Delta t}$$

Acceleration is a little trickier than velocity. Even though both involve how fast something changes, acceleration is how fast velocity changes, and an object's velocity changes if the speed *or* the direction changes. So, for example, an object can be accelerating even if its speed is constant. This is a very important point and a potential OAT trap.

In everyday language, we use the word *acceleration* to describe what happens when we step on the gas pedal and go faster. Well, that's certainly an example of acceleration even from the "proper" physics perspective, but it isn't the only example of acceleration.

What happens when you step on the brake? You slow down. Is that acceleration? Yes, although we might also call it a *deceleration*, because our speed changes.

Now, imagine that you set the car on cruise control at, say, 60 miles per hour. Up ahead you see a curve in the road, so as you approach it, you slowly turn the wheel to stay on the road. Even though your speed remains constant, your direction of motion changes, which means your velocity vector changes. Thus, you experience an acceleration.

Let's try this one. Throw a baseball straight up into the air. It rises, gets to the top of its path, then falls back down. At the moment it's at the top of its path, its velocity is zero. What is the ball's acceleration at this point?

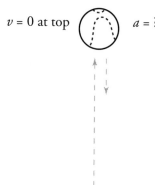

$v = 0$ at top $a = ?$

A common answer is, "If the velocity is 0, then the acceleration is 0 too." Let's see why this isn't the case here. What's happening to the baseball's velocity at the top of the path? Its direction is changing from up to *down*. The fact that the velocity is changing means there's an acceleration, so the acceleration can't be zero at the top of the path. Here's another way of looking at it: What if the acceleration *were* zero at the top? Zero acceleration means no change in velocity, so if $a = 0$ at a certain point, then whatever velocity there is at that point will stay constant. Does the velocity of the baseball remain zero? No, because the ball immediately starts to fall toward the ground.

Example 3-8: The velocity of an object moving along a straight line changes from $v_i = 4$ m/s at time $t_i = 0$ to $v_f = 10$ m/s at time $t_f = 2$ sec.

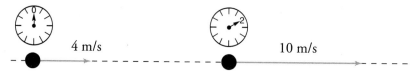

What was the object's average acceleration during this time interval?

Solution: By definition of average acceleration, we have

$$\bar{\mathbf{a}} = \frac{\Delta \mathbf{v}}{\Delta t} = \frac{\mathbf{v}_f - \mathbf{v}_i}{t_f - t_i} = \frac{10\,\text{m/s} - 4\,\text{m/s}}{(2\,\text{s}) - 0\,\text{s}} = 3\,\text{m/s}^2$$

Notice that $\bar{\mathbf{a}}$ is positive, which means that it points to the right, just like $\mathbf{v}_i$. If the acceleration points in the *same* direction as the initial velocity, then the object's speed is *increasing*.

Example 3-9: The velocity of an object moving along a straight line changes from v_i = 7 m/s at time t_i = 0 to v_f = 1 m/s at time t_f = 3 sec.

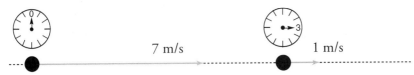

What was the object's average acceleration during this time interval?

Solution: By definition of average acceleration, we have

$$\overline{a} = \frac{\Delta v}{\Delta t} = \frac{v_f - v_i}{t_f - t_i} = \frac{1 \text{ m/s} - 7 \text{ m/s}}{(3 \text{ s}) - 0 \text{ s}} = -2 \text{ m/s}^2$$

Notice that $\overline{a}$ is negative, which means that it points to the left, in the direction opposite to v_i. If the acceleration points in the direction *opposite* to the initial velocity, then the object's speed is *decreasing*.

Example 3-10: The velocity of an object moving along a straight line changes from v_i = −2 m/s at time t_i = 0 to v_f = −5 m/s at time t_f = 2 sec.

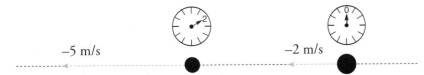

What was the object's average acceleration during this time interval?

Solution: By definition of average acceleration, we have

$$\overline{a} = \frac{\Delta v}{\Delta t} = \frac{v_f - v_i}{t_f - t_i} = \frac{-5 \text{ m/s} - (-2 \text{ m/s})}{(2 \text{ s}) - 0 \text{ s}} = -1.5 \text{ m/s}^2$$

Notice that $\overline{a}$ is negative, which means that it points to the left, just like v_i. If the acceleration points in the *same* direction as the initial velocity, then the object's speed is *increasing*.

Example 3-11: The velocity of an object changes from v_1 at time t_i = 0 to v_2 at time t_f = 2 sec.

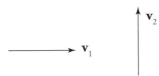

Which of the following best illustrates the object's average acceleration during this time interval?

A.

B.

C.

D.

Solution: By definition of average acceleration, we have

$$\bar{\mathbf{a}} = \frac{\Delta \mathbf{v}}{\Delta t} = \frac{\mathbf{v}_2 - \mathbf{v}_1}{t_f - t_i} = \frac{\mathbf{v}_2 - \mathbf{v}_1}{2\,\mathrm{s}}$$

The direction of $\bar{\mathbf{a}}$ is (always) the same as the direction of $\Delta \mathbf{v} = \mathbf{v}_2 - \mathbf{v}_1 = \mathbf{v}_2 + (-\mathbf{v}_1)$. The following diagram shows how we find $\mathbf{v}_2 + (-\mathbf{v}_1)$:

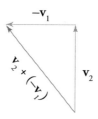

Therefore, choice (B) is the best answer.

The direction of **a** tells **v** how to change; the following diagrams summarize the possibilities:

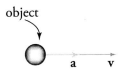

a in the same direction as **v** means object's speed is increasing.

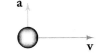

a perpendicular to **v** means object's speed is constant.

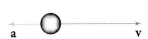

a in the opposite direction from **v** means object's speed is decreasing.

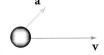

a at an angle between 0° and 90° to **v** means object's speed is increasing and direction of **v** is changing.

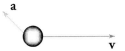

a at an angle between 90° and 180° to **v** means object's speed is decreasing and direction of **v** is changing.

Example 3-12: The velocity and acceleration of an object at a certain point are shown in the diagram below.

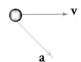

Describe the object's velocity a short time later.

Solution: We split the acceleration vector into components, one along the direction of **v** and one perpendicular to the direction of **v**:

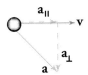

The component $\mathbf{a}_{\parallel}$ points along the line of the object's motion, so the *speed* of the object will change; in particular, the speed will *increase*, since $\mathbf{a}_{\parallel}$ points in the *same* direction as **v**. The component of **a** that's perpendicular to **v**, $\mathbf{a}_{\perp}$, will make the *direction* of **v** change; in particular, it will turn downward (since $\mathbf{a}_{\perp}$ points downward). Therefore, we'd expect the object to increase in speed as it turns downward.

3.2 UNIFORMLY ACCELERATED MOTION

In the last section, we defined the principal quantities of kinematics: displacement, velocity, and acceleration. In this section, we'll summarize the mathematical relationships between them in the special but important case of **uniformly accelerated motion**. This is motion in which the object's acceleration, **a**, is constant.

The definition of average velocity is $\bar{v} = \Delta x / \Delta t$. We can rewrite this equation without a fraction like this: $\Delta x = \bar{v} \Delta t$. To simplify the notation, let's agree to (1) use **d** for displacement, (2) use t, rather than Δt, for the time interval, and (3) abandon the bolding for vectors (although we'll still specify the direction of a vector by either a plus or a minus sign). With this change in notation, the equation reads simply $d = \bar{v}t$. In the case of uniformly accelerated motion (which means a is constant), the average velocity, $\bar{v}$ is just the average of the initial and final velocities: $\frac{1}{2}(v_i + v_f)$. Using t instead of Δt for the time interval means that we're setting the initial time, t_i, equal to 0 and that we're letting t stand for the final time, t_f (notice that $\Delta t = t_f - t_i = t - 0 = t$). The initial velocity is then the velocity at time 0, which we write as v_0 (pronounced "v zero" or "v naught") and the final velocity is v (dropping the subscript "f" on v_f just like we're dropping the subscript "f" on t_f). Therefore, the average velocity can be written as $\bar{v} = \frac{1}{2}(v_0 + v)$, and the equation for d becomes $d = \frac{1}{2}(v_0 + v)t$.

The definition of average acceleration is $\bar{a} = \Delta v / \Delta t$. We can rewrite this equation without a fraction like this: $\Delta v = \bar{a} \Delta t$. Now, since we are specifically looking at uniformly accelerated motion (motion in which the acceleration is constant), then there's no need for the bar on the **a**. After all, if **acceleration** is a constant, there's no distinction between **a** and $\bar{a}$. So, removing the bar and using the simplified notation described in the last paragraph, the equation becomes $\Delta v = at$, or $v = v_0 + at$.

The two equations $d = \frac{1}{2}(v_0 + v)t$ and $v = v_0 + at$ follow directly from the definitions of average velocity and acceleration. There are three other equations that relate these quantities, but they would require more algebra to derive them. Instead of boring you with the details, we'll just state them. Since there are five equations, we call them **The Big Five**:

The Big Five

1. $d = \frac{1}{2}(v_0 + v)t$ missing a

2. $v = v_0 + at$ missing d

3. $d = v_0 t + \frac{1}{2}at^2$ missing v

4. $d = vt - \frac{1}{2}at^2$ missing v_0

5. $v^2 = v_0^2 + 2ad$ missing t

Notice that these equations involve *five* quantities, d, v_0, v, a, and t, and there are *five* equations. Each equation has exactly one of those quantities missing, and this is how you decide which equation to use in a particular problem. A quantity is *missing* from the problem if it's *not given and not asked for*. For example, if a question does not give or ask for v, then use Big Five #3; if a question does not give or ask for t, then use Big Five #5. On the OAT, the Big Five equations that are used most frequently are #2, #3, and #5.

Example 3-13: An object has an initial velocity of 3 m/s and a constant acceleration of 2 m/s² in the same direction. What will the object's velocity be at $t = 6$ s?

Solution: We're given v_0, a, and t, and asked for v. Since the displacement, d, is neither given nor asked for, we use Big Five #2:

$$v = v_0 + at = 3 \text{ m/s} + (2 \text{ m/s}^2)(6 \text{ s}) = 15 \text{ m/s}$$

Example 3-14: A particle has an initial velocity of 10 m/s and a constant acceleration of 3 m/s² in the same direction. How far will the particle travel in 4 seconds?

Solution: We're given v_0, a, and t, and asked for d. Since the final velocity, v, is missing, we use Big Five #3:

$$d = v_0 t + \tfrac{1}{2}at^2 = (10 \text{ m/s})(4 \text{ s}) + \tfrac{1}{2}(3 \text{ m/s}^2)(4 \text{ s})^2 = 64 \text{ m}$$

Example 3-15: An object starts from rest and travels in a straight line with a constant acceleration of 4 m/s² in the same direction until its final velocity is 20 m/s. How far does it travel during this time?

Solution: We're given v_0, a, and v, and asked for d. Since the time, t, is neither given nor asked for, we use Big Five #5. Because the object starts from rest, we know that $v_0 = 0$, so we get

$$v^2 = v_0^2 + 2ad \;\rightarrow\; v^2 = 2ad \;\rightarrow\; d = \frac{v^2}{2a} = \frac{(20 \text{ m/s})^2}{2(4 \text{ m/s}^2)} = 50 \text{ m}$$

Example 3-16: A particle has an initial velocity of 6 m/s and moves with constant acceleration in the same direction for 5 seconds until its final velocity is 16 m/s. How far does it travel during this time?

Solution: We're given v_0, t, and v, and asked for d. Since the acceleration, a, is missing, we use Big Five #1:

$$d = \tfrac{1}{2}(v_0 + v)t = \tfrac{1}{2}(6 \text{ m/s} + 16 \text{ m/s})(5 \text{ s}) = 55 \text{ m}$$

Example 3-17: An object whose final velocity is 24 m/s traveled for 4 seconds at a constant acceleration of 2 m/s² in the same direction. How far did it travel?

Solution: We're given v, t, and a, and asked for d. Since the initial velocity, v_0, is neither given nor asked for, we use Big Five #4:

$$d = vt - \tfrac{1}{2}at^2 = (24 \text{ m/s})(4 \text{ s}) - \tfrac{1}{2}(2 \text{ m/s}^2)(4 \text{ s})^2 = 80 \text{ m}$$

3.3 KINEMATICS WITH GRAPHS

The OAT will expect you to not only handle kinematics problems algebraically (as we did in the last five examples) but also *graphically*. There are two types of graphs that we'll look at: the **position vs. time** graph and the **velocity vs. time** graph.

Consider the following graph, which gives an object's position, x, as a function of time, t:

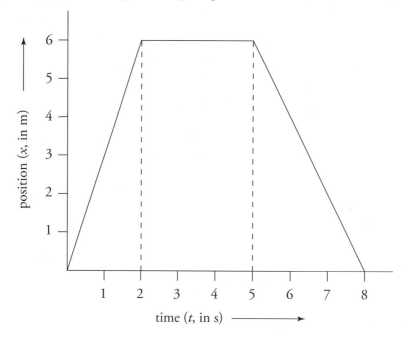

The object starts at $x = 0$, then moves to $x = 6$ m at $t = 2$ s. From $t = 2$ s to $t = 5$ s, it remains at position $x = 6$ m. Then, from $t = 5$ s to $t = 8$ s, the object moves from $x = 6$ m back to $x = 0$.

Let's figure out its velocity during these time intervals. From $t = 0$ to $t = 2$ s, its velocity is

$$v = \frac{\Delta x}{\Delta t} = \frac{x - x_0}{t_f - t_i} = \frac{(6\text{ m}) - (0\text{ m})}{2\text{ s}} = 3\text{ m/s}$$

Note that Δx is the vertical change in this graph and Δt is the horizontal change, from $t = 0$ to $t = 2$ s. Dividing a vertical change by the corresponding horizontal change gives the *slope* of a graph. So, we have this rule:

> The slope of a position vs. time graph gives the velocity.

From $t = 2$ s to $t = 5$ s, the object remained at position $x = 6$ m. Since the object didn't move, we expect its velocity during this time interval to be zero. But notice that the graph is flat here, and the slope of a flat line is 0.

Finally, from $t = 5$ s to $t = 8$ s, the velocity is

$$v = \frac{\Delta x}{\Delta t} = \frac{x - x_0}{t_f - t_i} = \frac{(0 \text{ m}) - (6 \text{ m})}{(8 \text{ s}) - (5 \text{ s})} = -2 \text{ m/s}$$

This is the slope of the graph from $t = 5$ s to $t = 8$ s.

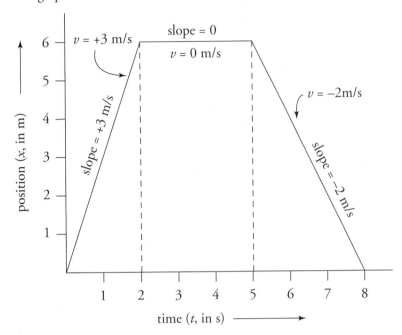

Now consider the following graph, which gives an object's velocity, v, as a function of time, t:

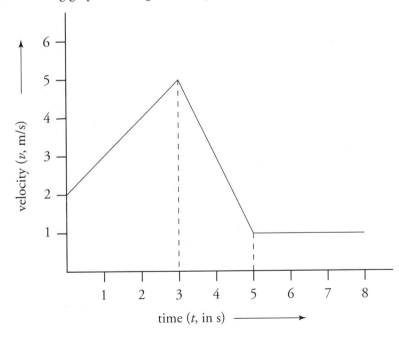

The object's velocity at $t = 0$ is $v = 2$ m/s, and steadily increases to $v = 5$ m/s at time $t = 3$ s. From $t = 3$ s to $t = 5$ s, the velocity decreases to $v = 1$ m/s. Then, from $t = 5$ s to $t = 8$ s, the object's velocity remains constant at $v = 1$ m/s.

Let's figure out the object's acceleration during these time intervals. From $t = 0$ to $t = 3$ s, its acceleration is

$$a = \frac{\Delta v}{\Delta t} = \frac{v - v_0}{t} = \frac{\left(5 \text{ m/s}\right) - \left(2 \text{ m/s}\right)}{3 \text{ s}} = 1 \text{ m/s}^2$$

Note that $\Delta \mathbf{v}$ is the vertical change in this graph and Δt is the horizontal change, from $t = 0$ to $t = 3$ s. Once again, dividing a vertical change by the corresponding horizontal change gives the slope of a graph. So, we have this rule:

The slope of a velocity vs. time graph gives the acceleration.

From $t = 3$ s to $t = 5$ s, the acceleration is

$$a = \frac{\Delta v}{\Delta t} = \frac{v - v_0}{t_f - t_i} = \frac{\left(1 \text{ m/s}\right) - \left(5 \text{ m/s}\right)}{\left(5 \text{ s}\right) - \left(3 \text{ s}\right)} = -2 \text{ m/s}^2$$

This is the slope of the graph from $t = 3$ s to $t = 5$ s.

Finally, from $t = 5$ s to $t = 8$ s, the object's velocity remained constant at $v = 1$ m/s. Since the object's velocity didn't change, we expect its acceleration during this time interval to be zero. The graph is flat here, and the slope of a flat line is 0.

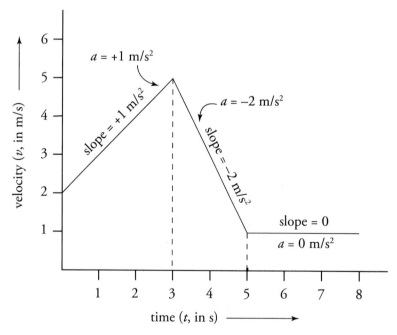

Besides asking about the object's acceleration, there's an additional type of question we could be asked given an object's velocity vs. time graph. For example, what was the object's *displacement* from $t = 5$ s to

$t = 7$ s? Since the object's velocity was a constant $v = 1$ m/s, we just use the basic equation *distance = rate × time* (which is really just Big Five #1 in the case where v is constant) to find that $d = (1$ m/s$)(2$ s$) = 2$ m. But if we look at the graph, we realize that what we've just found is the *area* under the graph from $t = 5$ s to $t = 7$ s. After all, the area under the graph is just a bunch of squares whose height is a velocity and whose base is a time. The area of a square is *base × height* (*bh*), so we're multiplying velocity × time, and that gives us displacement. The same rule applies even if the graph isn't flat:

> The area under a velocity vs. time graph gives the displacement.

What is the object's displacement from $t = 0$ to $t = 3$ s? It will be the area under the velocity vs. time graph from $t = 0$ to $t = 3$ s. The figure below shows that we can split this area into two pieces: a triangle whose area is $\frac{1}{2}bh = \frac{1}{2}(3\,\text{s})(3\,\text{m/s}) = \frac{9}{2}$ m, and a rectangle whose area is $bh = (3\,\text{s})(2\,\text{m/s}) = 6$ m. Therefore, the object's displacement from $t = 0$ to $t = 3$ s, which is the *total* area under the graph between $t = 0$ and $t = 3$ s, is $\left(\frac{9}{2}\,\text{m}\right) + \left(6\,\text{m}\right) = 10.5\,\text{m}$.

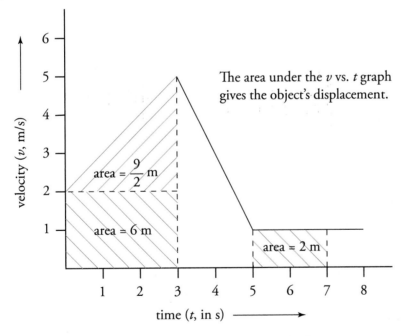

The area under the v vs. t graph gives the object's displacement.

We can check this result using Big Five #1:

$$d = \frac{1}{2}(v_0 + v)t = \frac{1}{2}(2\text{ m/s} + 5\text{ m/s})(3\text{ s}) = 10.5\,\text{m}$$

Example 3-18: For the object whose velocity vs. time graph is shown below, what is its displacement from $t = 2$ s to $t = 5$ s?

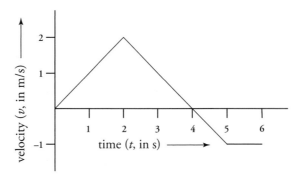

Solution: The area under the graph (or, more precisely, the area between the graph and the t-axis) gives the object's displacement. The area under the graph from $t = 2$ s to $t = 4$ s is $\frac{1}{2}bh = \frac{1}{2}(2\,\text{s})(2\text{ m/s}) = 2\,\text{m}$. After $t = 4$ s, the graph is *below* the t-axis, so any area here counts *negative*. From $t = 4$ s to $t = 5$ s, the area is $\frac{1}{2}bh = \frac{1}{2}(1\,\text{s})(-1\text{ m/s}) = -0.5\,\text{m}$. Therefore, the total area between the graph and the t axis, from $t = 2$ s to $t = 5$ s, is $(2\text{ m}) + (-0.5\text{ m}) = 1.5\text{ m}$.

3.4 FREE FALL

The Big Five are used only in situations where the acceleration is constant. The most important "real life" situation in which motion takes place under constant acceleration is **free fall**, which describes an object moving only under the influence of gravity (ignoring any effects due to the air, such as air resistance and buoyancy).

Near the surface of the earth, the magnitude of **g**, the **gravitational acceleration**, is approximately equal to 9.8 m/s². *For the OAT, we can use the simpler approximation of 10 m/s².* The term "free fall" might make you think that the Big Five apply only to objects that are actually falling, but if we throw a baseball up into the air (and ignore effects due to the air), then the ball is still experiencing the downward acceleration due to gravity, so it, too, would be considered in free fall. So, think of free fall not as a description of a downward velocity but as a description of a downward *acceleration*.

The way we decide which Big Five equation to use is to figure out which one of the five kinematics quantities (d, v_0, v, a, or t) is missing from the question, and then use the equation that does not involve this missing quantity. Often, in questions asking about objects in free fall, the acceleration will not be given because it's known implicitly. As soon as you realize the question involves an object moving under the influence of gravity, then you know that a is automatically known; on Earth, the magnitude of this a is about 10 m/s².

However, there is one thing you will have to decide on once you've selected which Big Five equation to use. Gravitational acceleration, like any acceleration, is a vector, so it has magnitude and direction. We know the magnitude is 10 m/s² and the direction is downward, but is it *down* the positive direction or the negative direction? The answer is: it's up to you. I suggest letting the direction of the object's displacement be the positive direction in every problem (this is almost always the simplest, most intuitive, decision). If the object's displacement is *down*, then call *down* the positive direction, and use $a = +g = +10$ m/s^2 in whichever Big Five equation you've selected. If the object's displacement is *up*, call *up* the positive direction (and thus *down* is automatically the negative direction) and use $a = -g = -10$ m/s^2.

It's important to remember that once you make your decision about which direction, up or down, is the positive direction, your decision applies to all other vectors in that problem: namely, v_0, v, and d. Therefore, if *down* is positive, for example, then in addition to the downward acceleration being positive, a downward initial velocity is positive, a downward final velocity is positive, and a downward displacement is positive. (This would mean that an upward initial velocity is negative, an upward final velocity is negative, and an upward displacement is negative.) Of course, if you follow the suggestion of always calling the direction of the displacement positive, then d will always be positive.

Example 3-19: An object is dropped from a height of 80 m. How long will it take to strike the ground?

Solution: We're given v_0, a, and d, and asked for t. Since the final velocity, v, is neither given nor asked for, we use Big Five #3. Because the object is falling, its displacement is downward, so let's call *down* the positive direction; this means that $a = +g = +10$ m/s^2. Since the term *dropped* means that the object's initial velocity is 0 m/s, we find that

$$d = v_0 t + \tfrac{1}{2} at^2 \rightarrow d = \tfrac{1}{2} at^2 \rightarrow t = \sqrt{\frac{2d}{a}} = \sqrt{\frac{2d}{+g}} = \sqrt{\frac{2(80\ \text{m})}{+10\ \text{m/s}^2}} = 4\ \text{s}$$

Example 3-20: An object is dropped from a height of 80 m. What is its velocity as it strikes the ground?

Solution: (Don't make the common mistake of thinking that the answer is 0 because once the object hits the ground, it stops. The question is really asking for the velocity of the object *as* it slams into the ground, and this won't be zero.) We're given v_0, a, and d, and asked for v. Since the time, t, is neither given nor asked for, we use Big Five #5. Because the object is falling, its displacement is downward, so let's call *down* the positive direction. This means that $a = +g = +10$ m/s^2. Since the term *dropped* means that the object's initial velocity is 0, we find that

$$v^2 = v_0^2 + 2ad \rightarrow v^2 = 2ad \rightarrow v = \sqrt{2ad} = \sqrt{2(+g)d} = \sqrt{2(+10\ \text{m/s}^2)(80\ \text{m})} = 40\ \text{m/s}$$

Example 3-21: A ball is thrown straight upward with an initial speed of 30 m/s. How high will it go?

Solution: We're given v_0, a, and v, and asked for d. (We know v because the question is asking how high the ball will go; at the top of the ball's path, its velocity at this point is 0.) Since the time, t, is missing, we use Big Five #5. Since we're interested only in the object's upward motion, let's call *up* the positive direction. This means that $v_0 = +30$ m/s and $a = -g = -10$ m/s^2. Because the velocity of the ball is 0 at its highest point, we find that

$$v^2 = v_0^2 + 2ad \rightarrow 0 = v_0^2 + 2ad \rightarrow d = -\frac{v_0^2}{2a} = -\frac{v_0^2}{2(-g)} = -\frac{(+30\ \text{m/s})^2}{2(-10\ \text{m/s}^2)} = 45\ \text{m}$$

Notice that the displacement d turned out to be positive; that's because we chose *up* to be our positive direction, and the ball moves *up* to its highest position.

Example 3-22: A ball of mass 10 kg and a ball of mass 1 kg are dropped simultaneously from a tower of height 45 m. If air resistance could be ignored, which ball will hit the ground first and how long does it take?

Solution: We're given v_0, a, and d, and asked for t. Since the final velocity, v, is missing, we use Big Five #3. Because each object is falling, its displacement is downward, so let's call *down* the positive direction. This means that $a = +g = +10$ m/s². Remembering that the term *dropped* means that $v_0 = 0$, Big Five #3 becomes $d = \frac{1}{2}at^2$, so

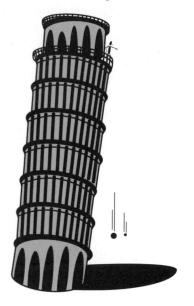

$$t = \sqrt{\frac{2d}{a}} = \sqrt{\frac{2d}{+g}} = \sqrt{\frac{2(45 \text{ m})}{+10 \text{ m/s}^2}} = 3 \text{ s}$$

Because none of the Big Five equations involves the *mass* of the object, this is how long it takes *each* ball to strike the ground. The free-fall acceleration of an object does not depend on its mass (or size or shape), so in the absence of effects due to the air, both objects will hit the ground *at the same time*.

3.5 PROJECTILE MOTION

The examples we've worked through so far have involved objects that move along a straight line, either horizontal or vertical. However, if we were to throw a baseball up at an angle to the ground, the path the ball would follow (its **trajectory**) would not be a straight line. If we neglect effects due to the air, the path will be a *parabola*. Although this technically doesn't fall under linear kinematics, it does involve constant acceleration (due to gravity). So, we feel it best to include it here to round out the discussion on uniformly accelerated motion.

In this case, the motion of an object, experiencing only the constant, downward acceleration due to gravity (free fall), is called **projectile motion**. This is also a case of uniformly accelerated motion.

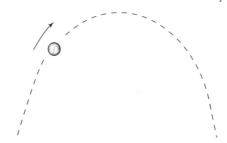

Because the projectile is experiencing both horizontal and vertical motion, we'll need to analyze both. But the trick is to analyze them *separately*. We'll use the Big Five to look at the horizontal motion, simply specializing the variables to horizontal motion; for example, we'll use x instead of d, we'll use v_{0x} and v_x instead of v_0 and v, and we'll use a_x instead of a. We'll use the Big Five to look at the vertical motion, too, and simply specialize the variables to vertical motion; we'll use y instead of d, v_{0y} and v_y instead of v_0 and v, and a_y instead of a. In this case, a_y will be equal to the gravitational acceleration.

In order to make an object follow a parabolic path, we'll need to launch the object at an angle to the horizontal. Therefore, the initial velocity vector $\mathbf{v}_0$ will have a nonzero horizontal component (v_{0x}) *and* a nonzero vertical component (v_{0y}). In terms of the **launch angle**, θ_0, which is the angle the initial velocity vector makes with the horizontal, we have $v_{0x} = v_0 \cos \theta_0$ and $v_{0y} = v_0 \sin \theta_0$.

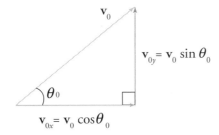

Let's first take care of the horizontal motion. This is the easier of the two for one important reason: once the projectile is launched, it no longer experiences a horizontal acceleration. That is, a_x will be zero throughout the projectile's flight. If the horizontal acceleration is zero throughout the projectile's flight, then *the horizontal velocity will be constant throughout the flight.* (This is a very important point and something the OAT loves to ask about.) If the horizontal velocity does not change, then whatever it was initially is all it'll ever be; that is, the horizontal velocity of the projectile at any point during its flight will be equal to the initial horizontal velocity, v_{0x}. Finally, if v_x is always equal to v_{0x}, then by using Big Five #1, we have $x = v_{0x}t$ (this is just *distance = rate × time* in the case where the rate is constant).

For the vertical motion, we realize that there *is* an acceleration; after all, the gravitational acceleration is vertical. In order to write down the equations for the vertical motion, we need to make a decision about which direction is positive. Let's call *up* the positive direction, so that *down* is the negative direction; this will mean that $a_y = -g$. Big Five #2 now tells us that the vertical component of the velocity, v_y, will be $v_{0y} + a_y t = v_{0y} + (-g)t$ at time t. Big Five #3 tells us that the vertical displacement of the projectile, y, will be $v_{0y}t + \dfrac{1}{2}a_y t^2 = v_{0y}t + \dfrac{1}{2}(-g)t^2$.

3.5

Projectile Motion

	Horizontal Motion	**Vertical Motion**
displacement:	$x = v_{0_x}t$	$y = v_{0_y}t + \frac{1}{2}(-g)t^2$
velocity:	$v_x = v_{0x}$ (constant!)	$v_y = v_{0_y} + (-g)t$
acceleration:	$a_x = 0$	$a_y = -g$
	$(v_{0x} = v_0 \cos\theta_0)$	$(v_{0_y} = v_0 \sin\theta_0)$

In addition to these formulas (which are really nothing new, since they're just a few of the Big Five equations), there are a couple of other facts worth knowing. The first involves the projectile's velocity at the top of its trajectory. Since the top of the parabola is the parabola's turning point, and an object's velocity is always tangent to its path (whatever the shape of the trajectory), the projectile's velocity will be horizontal at the top of the parabola. This means that the vertical velocity is zero. (*Be careful* not to say that the velocity is zero at the top. For a projectile moving in a parabolic path, it's only the *vertical* velocity that's zero at the top; the horizontal velocity is still there!)

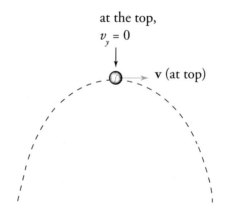

at the top,
$v_y = 0$

v (at top)

The second fact reflects the symmetry of the parabolic shape of the path. If we were to draw a vertical line up from the ground through the top point on the parabola, we'd notice that the left and right sides are just mirror images of each other. One of the consequences of this observation is that the time the projectile takes to reach the top will be the same as the time it takes to drop back down (to the same height from which it was launched). Therefore, *the projectile's total flight time will be twice the time required to reach the top*. So, for example, if the time it takes the projectile to reach the top of the parabola is 3 seconds, then the total flight time will be 6 seconds, because it'll take another 3 seconds to come back down.

Example 3-23: A cannonball is shot from ground level with an initial velocity of 100 m/s at an angle of 30° to the ground.

a) How high will the cannonball go?
b) What is the cannonball's velocity at the top of its path?
c) What will be the cannonball's total flight time?
d) How far will the cannonball travel horizontally?

Solution:

a) The maximum height reached by the projectile is the displacement y at the moment the cannonball is at the top of the parabola. What does it mean for the projectile to be at the top of the parabola? It means the vertical velocity is zero. So, we'll set the vertical velocity equal to zero:

$$v_y = v_{0y} + (-g)t \text{ with } v_y = 0 \rightarrow v_{0y} + (-g)t = 0 \rightarrow t = \frac{v_{0y}}{g} = \frac{v_0 \sin\theta_0}{g}$$

This is how long it'll take the projectile to reach the top. If we plug in $v_0 = 100$ m/s, $\theta_0 = 30°$, and $g = 10$ m/s², we find that

$$t = \frac{v_0 \sin\theta_0}{g} = \frac{(100 \text{ m/s}) \sin 30°}{10 \text{ m/s}^2} = 5 \text{ s}$$

So now the question is, "What is y when $t = 5$ s?" All we need to do is take the equation for the vertical displacement of the projectile and plug in $t = 5$ s:

$$y = v_{0y}t + \tfrac{1}{2}(-g)t^2$$
$$= (v_0 \sin\theta_0)t + \tfrac{1}{2}(-g)t^2$$

$$\therefore y \text{ (at } t = 5 \text{ s)} = (100 \text{ m/s} \cdot \sin 30°)(5 \text{ s}) + \tfrac{1}{2}(-10 \text{ m/s}^2)(5 \text{ s})^2 = 125 \text{ m}$$

b) At the top of its path, the cannonball's velocity is horizontal, and the horizontal velocity is the same throughout the flight, equal to the initial horizontal velocity:

$$v_x = v_{0x} = v_0 \cos\theta_0 = (100 \text{ m/s}) \cos 30° \approx (100 \text{ m/s})(0.85) = 85 \text{ m/s}$$

c) The projectile's total flight time is just equal to twice the time required for it to reach the top. Since we found in part (a) that it takes 5 seconds for the cannonball to reach the top, its total flight time will be 2 × (5 s) = 10 s.

d) The question is asking for the horizontal displacement at the time when the cannonball strikes the ground. We found in part (b) that the cannonball's horizontal velocity is a constant 85 m/s, and we found in part (c) that the cannonball's total flight time is 10 seconds. Therefore, the total horizontal displacement is

$$x = v_{0x}t = (85 \text{ m/s})(10 \text{ s}) = 850 \text{ m}$$

(The total horizontal displacement is called the **range** of the projectile.)

Example 3-24: A projectile is launched from a height of 5 m with an initial velocity of 80 m/s at an angle of 40° to the horizontal. If v_{x1} is the horizontal velocity of the projectile 1 second after launch, and v_{x2} is the horizontal velocity 2 seconds after launch, what is the value of $v_{x2} - v_{x1}$?

Solution: Sounds complicated, doesn't it? The OAT would love this question, because although it seems like solving it would be messy, the solution actually requires only applying one simple fact. You remember that once a projectile is launched, its horizontal velocity remains constant during the entire flight. Therefore, $v_{x2} = v_{x1}$, and the value of $v_{x2} - v_{x1}$ is zero.

Example 3-25: A rock is thrown horizontally, with an initial speed of 10 m/s, from the edge of a vertical cliff. It strikes the ground 5 s later.

    a)   How high is the cliff?
    b)   How far from the foot of the cliff does the rock land?

Solution:

    a)   The height of the cliff will be the vertical distance the rock falls. Because the rock is thrown horizontally, it has no initial vertical velocity: $v_{0y} = 0$. Therefore, the equation for the projectile's vertical displacement becomes $y = \frac{1}{2}(-g)t^2$. Considering the time it takes the rock to fall is $t = 5$ s, we have $y = \frac{1}{2}(-10 \text{ m/s}^2)(5\text{s})^2 = -125\text{m}$. This tells us that the rock falls 125 m in 5 s, so the height of the cliff is 125 m.

    b)   The horizontal displacement of the rock is given by the equation $x = v_{0x}t$. Since $v_{0x} = 10$ m/s and $t = 5$ s, we get $x = (10 \text{ m/s})(5\text{s}) = 50\text{m}$.

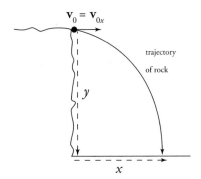

$\mathbf{v}_0 = \mathbf{v}_{0x}$

trajectory of rock

y

x

Example 3-26: A ball is kicked from ground level, travels as an ideal projectile in a parabolic path, and hits the ground 4 seconds after it was kicked. If its initial vertical speed was 20 m/s, how high did the ball go?

Solution: If the total flight time was 4 seconds, that means it took half that time, 2 seconds, to reach the top of the parabola (its highest point). Therefore, since we're given that $v_{0y} = 20$ m/s, the vertical displacement of the ball at $t = 2$ s was

$$\begin{aligned}
y &= v_{0y}t + \tfrac{1}{2}(-g)t^2 \\
&= (20 \text{ m/s})(2 \text{ s}) + \tfrac{1}{2}(-10 \text{ m/s}^2)(2 \text{ s})^2 \\
&= 20 \text{ m}
\end{aligned}$$

Summary of Formulas

displacement $\quad$ $\mathbf{d} = \Delta x = (\text{final position}) - (\text{initial position}) =$ *net* distance [plus direction]

average velocity: $\quad \bar{\mathbf{v}} = \dfrac{\Delta x}{\Delta t} = \dfrac{\mathbf{d}}{\Delta t}$

average acceleration: $\quad \bar{\mathbf{a}} = \dfrac{\Delta \mathbf{v}}{\Delta t}$

The **BIG FIVE** [for Uniformly Accelerated Motion: a = constant]:

1. $d = \dfrac{1}{2}(v_0 + v)t$

2. $v = v_0 + at$

3. $d = v_0 t + \dfrac{1}{2}at^2$

4. $d = vt - \dfrac{1}{2}at^2$

5. $v^2 = v_0^2 + 2ad$

Position [x] vs. time [t] graph: slope = velocity [v]

Velocity [v] vs. time [t] graph: slope = acceleration [a]
$\qquad\qquad\qquad\qquad$ area under graph = displacement [d]

Projectile Motion :

[Downward = Negative Direction]

	Horizontal Motion	**Vertical Motion**
displacement:	$x = v_{0x}t$	$y = v_{0y}t + \frac{1}{2}(-g)t^2$
velocity:	$v_{0x} = v_x$ [constant!]	$v_y = v_{0y} + (-g)t$
acceleration:	$a_x = 0$	$a_y = -g$
acceleration:	$(v_{0x} = v_0 \cos\theta_0)$	$(v_{0y} = v_0 \sin\theta_0)$

$v_y = 0$ at the top of the trajectory

$v_x \neq 0$ at the top of the trajectory

Chapter 4
Statics and Dynamics I

4.1 MASS, FORCE, AND NEWTON'S LAWS

In the preceding chapter, we studied kinematics, which is the description of motion in terms of an object's position, velocity, and acceleration. In this chapter, we'll begin our study of **dynamics**, which is the *explanation* of motion in terms of the forces that act on an object.

Simply put, a **force** is a push or pull exerted by one object on another. If you pull on a rope attached to a crate, you create a *tension* in the rope that pulls the crate. When a sky diver is falling through the air, the earth exerts a downward pull called the *gravitational force*, and the air exerts an upward force called *air resistance*. When you stand on the floor, the floor provides an upward, supporting force called the *normal force*. If you slide a book across a table, the table exerts a *frictional force* against the book, so the book slows down and eventually stops. Static cling provides a simple example of the *electrostatic force*. (In fact, all of the forces mentioned above, with the exception of gravity, are due ultimately to the electromagnetic force.)

> ### Newton's First Law
>
> An object's state of motion—its *velocity*—will not change unless a net force acts on the object.
>
> That is, if no net force acts on an object, then:
>
> > **if the object is at rest, it will remain at rest;**
> >
> > *and*
> >
> > **if the object is moving, then it will continue to move with constant velocity**
>
> (constant speed in a straight line).
>
> Or, more simply: **no net force = no acceleration**.

How forces affect motion is described by three physical laws, known as **Newton's laws**. They form the foundation of mechanics, and you should memorize them.

The First Law says that objects naturally resist changing their velocity. In other words, objects at rest don't just suddenly start moving all on their own. Some external source must exert a force to make them move. Also, an object that's already moving doesn't change its velocity. It doesn't go faster, or slower, or change direction all by itself; something must exert some force on it to make any of these changes happen. This property of objects, their natural resistance to change in their state of motion, is called **inertia**. In fact, the First Law is often referred to as the *Law of Inertia*.

It's important to note that the First Law applies when there is no *net* force on an object. This could mean there are no forces at all, though that couldn't happen in our universe; more commonly, it means the forces on an object balance out, in other words, the total of all the forces, in each dimension, is zero. We'll work examples of computing net force when we get to Newton's Second Law.

The **mass** of an object is the quantitative measure of its inertia; intuitively, mass measures how much matter is contained in an object. Mass is measured in *kilograms*, abbreviated kg. (Note: An object whose mass is 1 kg weighs a little more than 2 pounds on Earth, but be careful not to confuse mass with weight; they're different things.) Compared to an object whose mass is just 1 kg, an object whose mass is 100 kg has 100 times the inertia. Intuitively, we'd find it 100 times more difficult to cause the same change in its motion than we would with the 1 kg object. This point will be clearer after we state the second of Newton's laws.

Newton's Second Law

If F_{net} is the net—or total—force acting on an object of mass m, then the resulting acceleration of the object, a, satisfies this simple equation:

$$F_{net} = ma$$

Notice that the First Law is really just a special case of the Second Law: the case in which $F_{net} = 0$.

Forces are represented by vectors, because a force has a magnitude and a direction. If two different forces (let's call them F_1 and F_2) act on an object, then the total—or *net*—force on the object is the sum of these individual forces: $F_{net} = F_1 + F_2$. Since forces are vectors, they must be added as vectors; that is, their directions must be taken into account. The following figures show some examples of obtaining F_{net} from the individual forces that act on an object:

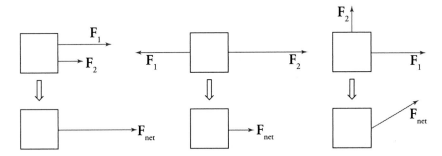

Note the following facts about the equation $F_{net} = ma$:

1. F_{net} is the sum of all the forces that act *on* the object; namely, the object whose mass, m, is on the other side of the equation. Any force exerted *by* the object is *not* included in F_{net}.

2. Because m is a *positive* number, the direction of a is always the same as the direction of F_{net}. Therefore, an object will accelerate in the direction of the net force it feels. This does not mean that an object will always *move* in the direction of F_{net}. Be sure that this distinction makes sense because it can be a source of confusion, and therefore a potential OAT trap. Newton's Second Law tells us about the direction of an object's *acceleration* but does not define the direction of an object's velocity.

3. What if $F_{net} = 0$? Then $a = 0$. What does $a = 0$ mean? It means that the object's velocity does not change, which is also what Newton's First Law says. But how about this question: Does $F_{net} = 0$ mean that $v = 0$? Not necessarily! $F_{net} = 0$ means that an object won't *accelerate*, not that it won't move. This is a key point and another potential OAT trap. If the object is already moving at, say, 100 m/s toward the north, then it will continue to move at 100 m/s toward the north as long as the net force on the object remains zero.

4. Because $\mathbf{F}_{net} = ma$ is a vector equation, it automatically means that the components of both sides must be the same. In other words, $\mathbf{F}_{net}$ could be written as the sum of a force in the horizontal direction, ($\mathbf{F}_{net,\,x}$) plus a force in the vertical direction ($\mathbf{F}_{net,\,y}$); these would be the horizontal and vertical components of $\mathbf{F}_{net}$. The equation $\mathbf{F}_{net} = ma$ would then tell us that $\mathbf{F}_{net,\,x} = ma_x$ and $\mathbf{F}_{net,\,y} = ma_y$. So, dividing the horizontal component of the net force by m gives us the horizontal component of the object's acceleration, and dividing the vertical component of the net force by m gives us the vertical component of the object's acceleration.

5. The unit of force is equal to the unit of mass times the unit of acceleration:

$$[F] = [m][a] = \mathrm{kg} \cdot \mathrm{m/s^2}$$

A force of 1 kg·m/s² is called 1 **newton** (abbreviated N). A force of 1 N is about equal to a quarter of a pound, or about the weight of a medium-sized apple (on Earth).

Newton's Third Law

If Object 1 exerts a force, $\mathbf{F}_{1\text{-on-}2}$, on Object 2, then Object 2 exerts a force, $\mathbf{F}_{2\text{-on-}1}$, on Object 1. These forces, $\mathbf{F}_{1\text{-on-}2}$ and $\mathbf{F}_{2\text{-on-}1}$, have the same magnitude but act in opposite directions, so

$$\mathbf{F}_{1\text{-on-}2} = -\mathbf{F}_{2\text{-on-}1}$$

and they act on different objects. These two forces are said to form an **action–reaction pair**.

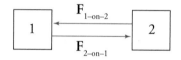

This is the law commonly stated as, "For every action, there is an equal but opposite reaction." Unfortunately, this popular version of Newton's Third Law can lead to confusion. Essentially, Newton's Third Law says that the *forces* in an action–reaction pair have the same magnitude and act in opposite directions (and on "opposite" objects). It does *not* say that the *effects* of these forces will be the same. For example, suppose that two skaters are next to and facing each other on a skating rink. Let's say that Skater 1 has a mass of 50 kg and Skater 2 has a mass of 100 kg. Now, what if Skater 1 pushes on Skater 2 with a force of 50 N? Then $\mathbf{F}_{1\text{-on-}2} = 50$ N and $\mathbf{F}_{2\text{-on-}1} = -50$ N, by Newton's Third Law.

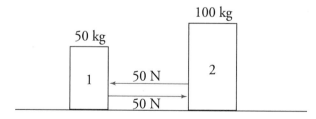

But will the *effects* of these equal-strength forces be the same? No, because the masses of the objects are different. The accelerations of the skaters will be

$$\mathbf{a}_1 = \frac{\mathbf{F}_{2\text{-on-}1}}{m_1} = \frac{-50 \text{ N}}{50 \text{ kg}} = -1 \text{ m/s}^2 \quad \text{and} \quad \mathbf{a}_2 = \frac{\mathbf{F}_{1\text{-on-}2}}{m_2} = \frac{+50 \text{ N}}{100 \text{ kg}} = +0.5 \text{ m/s}^2$$

So, Skater 2 will move away with an acceleration of 0.5 m/s², while Skater 1 moves away, in the opposite direction, with an acceleration of twice that magnitude, 1 m/s².

Therefore, while the forces are the same (in magnitude), the effects of these forces —that is, the resulting accelerations (and velocities)—are not the same, because the masses of the objects are different. Newton's Third Law says nothing about mass; it only tells us that the action and reaction forces will have the same magnitude. So, the point is not to interpret "equal but opposite reaction" as meaning "equal but opposite effect," because if the masses of the interacting objects are not the same, then the resulting accelerations (and velocities) of the objects will not be the same.

The key to distinguishing Newton's First Law from Newton's Third Law is to focus on the description of the forces. In Newton's First Law, all of the forces must be acting on a *single* object; thus, the net force on a single object is calculated by adding those vectors. However, in Newton's Third Law, each force must be acting on a *different* object in an action-reaction pair.

There are two aspects of Newton's Third Law that frequently give students trouble. First, just because two forces are equal and opposite does *not* mean they form an action-reaction pair; the forces also have to be from two objects acting on each other, not two objects acting on a third object. Second, the Third Law applies even when the objects are accelerating; even if one object is accelerating, the second object pushes or pulls just as hard on the first as the first pushes or pulls on the second.

Example 4-1: An object of mass 50 kg moves with a constant velocity of magnitude 1000 m/s. What is the net force on this object?

Solution: If the object moves with constant velocity, then the net force it feels must be zero, regardless of the object's mass or speed.

Example 4-2: The net force on an object of mass 10 kg is zero. What can you say about the speed of this object?

Solution: If the net force on an object is zero, all we can say is that it will not accelerate; its velocity may be zero, or it may not. Without more information, we cannot determine the object's speed; all we know is that whatever the speed is, it will remain constant.

Example 4-3: For 6 seconds, you push a 120 kg crate along a frictionless horizontal surface with a constant force of 60 N parallel to the surface. If the crate was initially at rest, what will its velocity be at the end of this 6-second time interval?

Solution: Using Newton's Second Law, we find that the acceleration of the crate is $a = F/m = (60 \text{ N})/(120 \text{ kg}) = 0.5 \text{ m/s}^2$. Using Big Five #2, we now find that $v = v_0 + at = 0 + (0.5 \text{ m/s}^2)(6 \text{ s}) = 3 \text{ m/s}$.

Example 4-4: For 6 seconds, you pull a 120 kg crate along a frictionless horizontal surface with a constant force of 60 N directed at an angle of 60° to the surface. If the crate was initially at rest, what will its horizontal velocity be at the end of this 6-second time interval?

Solution: To find the horizontal velocity, we need the horizontal acceleration.

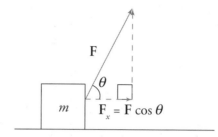

$$F_x = F \cos \theta$$

Using Newton's Second Law, we find that the horizontal acceleration of the crate is $a_x = F_x/m = (F \cos \theta)/m = (60 \text{ N} \cos 60°)/(120 \text{ kg}) = (30 \text{ N})/(120 \text{ kg}) = 0.25 \text{ m/s}^2$. Using Big Five #2, we now find that $v_x = v_{0x} + a_x t = 0 + (0.25 \text{ m/s}^2)(6 \text{ s}) = 1.5 \text{ m/s}$.

Example 4-5: Two crates are moving along a frictionless horizontal surface. The first crate, of mass $M = 100$ kg, is being pushed by a force of 300 N. The first crate is in contact with a second crate, of mass $m = 50$ kg.

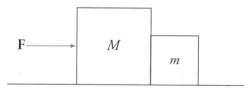

a)   What's the acceleration of the crates?
b)   What's the force exerted by the larger crate on the smaller one?
c)   What's the force exerted by the smaller crate on the larger one?

Solution:

a)   The force **F** is pushing on a combined mass of 100 kg + 50 kg = 150 kg, so by Newton's Second Law, the acceleration of both crates will be $a = (300 \text{ N})/(150 \text{ kg}) = 2 \text{ m/s}^2$.

b)   Because M and m are in direct contact, each is pushing on the other with a certain force. Let F_2 be the force that M exerts on m. Then we must have $F_2 = ma$, so $F_2 = (50 \text{ kg})(2 \text{ m/s}^2) = 100$ N.

c)   By Newton's Third Law, if the force that M exerts on m is F_2, then the force that m exerts on M must be $-F_2$. So, if we call "to the right" our positive direction, then the force that m exerts on M is -100 N. We can check that this is correct by looking at all the forces acting on M. We have **F** pushing to the right and $-F_2$ pushing to the left. The net force on M is therefore $F_{\text{net on } M} = F + (-F_2) = (300 \text{ N}) + (-100 \text{ N}) = 200$ N. If this is correct, then $F_{\text{net on } M}$ should equal Ma. Since $M = 100$ kg and $a = 2 \text{ m/s}^2$, we get $Ma = 200$ N, which does match what we found for $F_{\text{net on } M}$. (In effect, what's happening here is that M is using 200 N of the 300 N force from **F** for its own motion and passing the remaining 100 N along to m, so that both move together with the same acceleration.)

Example 4-6: Two forces act on an object of mass $m = 5$ kg. One of the forces has a magnitude of 6 N, and the other force, perpendicular to the first, has a magnitude of 8 N. What's the acceleration of the object?

Solution: Forces are vectors, and when we find the net force on this object, we see that it's the hypotenuse of a 6-8-10 right triangle.

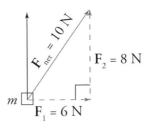

Since $F_{net} = 10$ N, the acceleration of the object will be $a = F_{net}/m = (10 \text{ N})/(5 \text{ kg}) = 2 \text{ m/s}^2$.

Example 4-7: The figure below shows all the forces acting on a 5 kg object. The magnitude of $\mathbf{F}_1$ is 50 N. If the acceleration of the object is 8 m/s², what's the magnitude of $\mathbf{F}_2$?

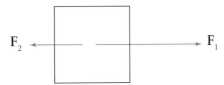

Solution: The net force on the block is just the sum of $\mathbf{F}_1$ and $\mathbf{F}_2$, so $\mathbf{F}_{net} = \mathbf{F}_1 + \mathbf{F}_2 = (+50 \text{ N}) + \mathbf{F}_2$, if we call "to the right" our positive direction. The net force must be $ma = (5 \text{ kg})(8 \text{ m/s}^2) = 40$ N. Since $(+50 \text{ N})$ + $\mathbf{F}_2$ must be 40 N, we know that $\mathbf{F}_2 = -10$ N; that is, $\mathbf{F}_2$ has magnitude 10 N (and points to the left).

Example 4-8: According to Newton's Third Law, every force is "accompanied by" an equal but opposite force. If this is true, shouldn't these forces cancel out to zero? How could we ever accelerate an object?

Solution: The answer does not involve the masses of the objects; Newton's Third Law says nothing about mass. The key is to remember what $\mathbf{F}_{net}$ means; it's the sum of all the forces that act *on* an object, not *by* the object. Let's say we have a pair of objects, 1 and 2, and an action–reaction pair of forces between them, and we wanted to find the acceleration of Object 2. We'd find all the forces that act on Object 2. One of these forces is $\mathbf{F}_{1\text{-on-}2}$. The reaction force, $\mathbf{F}_{2\text{-on-}1}$, is *not* included in $\mathbf{F}_{net\text{-on-}2}$ because it doesn't act on Object 2; it's a force *by* Object 2. So, the reason why the two forces in an action–reaction pair don't cancel each other is that we'd never add them in the first place because they don't act on the same object.

4.2 NEWTON'S LAW OF GRAVITATION

The mass of an object is a measure of its inertia, its resistance to acceleration. We'll now look at the related concept of an object's weight.

Although in everyday language the terms *mass* and *weight* are sometimes used interchangeably, in physics they have very different technical meanings. The **weight** of an object is the gravitational force exerted on it by the Earth (or by whatever planet it happens to be on or near). **Mass** is an intrinsic property of an object and does not change with location. Put a baseball in a rocket and send it to the Moon. The baseball's *weight* on the Moon is less than its weight here on Earth, but you'd have as much "baseball stuff" there as you would here; that is, the baseball's *mass* would *not* change.

Since weight is a force, we can use $\mathbf{F} = m\mathbf{a}$ to compute it. What acceleration would the gravitational force (which is what *weight* means) impose on an object? The gravitational acceleration, of course! Therefore, setting $\mathbf{a} = \mathbf{g}$, the equation $\mathbf{F} = m\mathbf{a}$ becomes

$$\mathbf{w} = m\mathbf{g}$$

This is the equation for the weight, $\mathbf{w}$, of an object of mass m. (Weight is often symbolized by $\mathbf{F}_{grav}$, rather than $\mathbf{w}$; we'll use both notations.) Note that mass and weight are proportional but not identical. Furthermore, mass is measured in kilograms, while weight is measured in newtons.

Example 4-9:

a) Find the weight of an object whose mass is 50 kg.
b) Find the mass of an object whose weight is 50 N.

Solution:

a) To find an object's weight, we multiply its mass by g. Using $g = 10$ m/s² (or, equivalently, $g = 10$ N/kg), we find that $w = mg = (50 \text{ kg})(10 \text{ N/kg}) = 500$ N.
b) To find an object's mass, we divide its weight by g. With $g = 10$ N/kg, we find that $m = w/g = (50 \text{ N})/(10 \text{ N/kg}) = 5$ kg.

Most of the time, we'll use the formula $w = mg$ to find the weight of an object whose mass is m. However, the value of g can change, and if we're not near the surface of the earth (where we know that g is approximately 10 m/s²) we may not know the value of g. In that case, we'll invoke another law discovered by Newton:

Newton's Law of Gravitation

Every object in the universe exerts a gravitational pull on every other object. The magnitude of this gravitational force is proportional to the product of the objects' masses and inversely proportional to the square of the distance between them. The constant of proportionality is denoted by G and known as Newton's universal gravitational constant.

$$F_{grav} = G\frac{Mm}{r^2}$$

distance between centers

The value of G is roughly 6.7×10^{-11} N·m^2/kg^2, but don't bother memorizing this constant. If you actually need the value on the OAT (which is unlikely), it will be provided. Unfortunately, sometimes it will be provided even when you don't need it.

One of the most important features of Newton's Law of Gravitation is that it's an **inverse-square law**. This means that the magnitude of the gravitational force is *inversely* proportional to the *square* of the distance between the centers of the objects. (Another important physical law, Coulomb's Law [for the electrostatic force between two charges], which we'll see later, is also an inverse-square law.)

Also notice that the forces illustrated in the box above form an action–reaction pair. Even if M and m are different, the gravitational force that M exerts on m has the same magnitude as the gravitational force that m exerts on M. (If the directions of the force vectors in the box above seem backward, remember that gravity is always a *pulling* force; therefore, in the figure above, $\mathbf{F}_{M\text{-on-}m}$ pulls to the left, toward M, while $\mathbf{F}_{m\text{-on-}M}$ pulls to the right, toward m.) Of course, the accelerations of the objects will have different magnitudes if the masses are different, as we discussed earlier when we studied Newton's Third Law.

Example 4-10: What will happen to the gravitational force between two objects if the distance between them is doubled? What if the distance is cut in half?

Solution: Since the gravitational force obeys an inverse-square law, if r increases by a factor of 2, then F_{grav} will *decrease* by a factor of $2^2 = 4$. On the other hand, if r decreases by a factor of 2, then F_{grav} will *increase* by a factor of $2^2 = 4$.

Notice that the two formulas given in this section, $w = mg$ and $F_{grav} = GMm/r^2$, are really formulas for the same thing. After all, weight *is* gravitational force. Therefore, we could set these expressions equal to each other:

$$mg = G\frac{Mm}{r^2}$$

Then, dividing both sides by m, we get

$$g = G\frac{M}{r^2}$$

This formula tells us how to find the value of the gravitational acceleration, g. On Earth, we know that $g \approx 10$ m/s². If we were to go to the top of a mountain, then the distance r to the center of the Earth would increase, but compared to the radius of the Earth, the increase would be very small. As a result, while the value of g *is* less at the top of a mountain than at the Earth's surface, the difference is small enough that it can usually be neglected. However, at the position of a satellite orbiting the Earth, for example, the distance to the center of the Earth has now increased dramatically (for example, many satellites have an orbit radius that's over 6.5 times the radius of the Earth), and the resulting decrease in g would definitely need to be taken into account.

This formula for g also shows us why g changes from planet (or Moon) to planet. For example, on Earth's Moon, the value of g is only about 1.6 m/s² (about a sixth of what it is on Earth) because the mass of the Moon is so much smaller than the mass of the Earth. It's true that the radius of the Moon is smaller than the radius of the Earth, which would, by itself, make g bigger, but M is *much* smaller, and this is why the value of g on the surface of the Moon is smaller than its value on the surface of the Earth. So, while big G is a universal gravitational constant, the value of little g depends on where you are.

Example 4-11: The radius of the Earth is approximately 6.4×10^6 m. What's the mass of the Earth?

Solution: We can use the formula $g = GM/r^2$ to solve for M:

$$M = \frac{gr^2}{G} = \frac{(10 \text{ m/s}^2)(6.4 \times 10^6 \text{ m})^2}{6.7 \times 10^{-11} \frac{\text{N} \cdot \text{m}^2}{\text{kg}^2}} \approx 6 \times 10^{24} \text{ kg}$$

Example 4-12: The mass of Mars is about 1/10 the mass of Earth, and the radius of Mars is about half that of Earth. Is the value of g on the surface of Mars less than, greater than, or equal to the value of g on Earth?

Solution: We'll use the formula $g = GM/r^2$ to compare the two values of g:

$$\frac{g_{\text{Mars}}}{g_{\text{Earth}}} = \frac{G\dfrac{M_{\text{Mars}}}{r_{\text{Mars}}^2}}{G\dfrac{M_{\text{Earth}}}{r_{\text{Earth}}^2}} = \frac{M_{\text{Mars}}}{M_{\text{Earth}}} \cdot \left(\frac{r_{\text{Earth}}}{r_{\text{Mars}}}\right)^2 = \frac{1}{10} \cdot 2^2 = 0.4$$

Therefore, the value of g on Mars is only about 40% of its value here.

Example 4-13: A long, flat, frictionless table is set up on the surface of the Moon (where $g = 1.6$ m/s²). An object whose mass on Earth is 4 kg is also transported there.

a) What is the object's mass on the Moon?
b) What is the object's weight on the Moon?
c) If we drop this object from a height of $h = 20$ m, with what speed will it strike the lunar surface?
d) If we wish to push this object across the table to give it an acceleration of 3 m/s², how much force must we exert? Would this force be different if the table and object were back on Earth?

Solution:

a) The mass is the same, 4 kg.
b) The weight of the object on the Moon is $w = m \cdot g_{\text{Moon}} = (4$ kg$)(1.6$ m/s²$) = 6.4$ N. Notice that the object's weight on the Moon is different from its weight on Earth.
c) Calling *down* the positive direction and using Big Five #5 with $v_0 = 0$ and $a = g_{\text{Moon}} = 1.6$ m/s², we find that

$$v^2 = v_0^2 + 2ad \rightarrow v^2 = 2gh \rightarrow v = \sqrt{2gh} = \sqrt{2(1.6 \text{ m/s}^2)(20 \text{ m})} = 8 \text{ m/s}$$

d) Using $F = ma$, we get $F = (4$ kg$)(3$ m/s²$) = 12$ N. Since Newton's Second Law depends only on mass (not on weight, because there's no g in Newton's Second Law), we'd need this same force even if the object and table were back on Earth.

Example 4-14: A satellite is orbiting the Earth at an altitude equal to 3 times the Earth's radius. If the satellite weighs 144,000 N on the surface of the Earth, what is the gravitational force on the satellite while it's in orbit?

Solution: Let R be the radius of the Earth. If the satellite's *altitude*, h, is $3R$, then its distance *from the center* of the Earth is $R + h = R + 3R = 4R$. Therefore, the distance from the Earth's center has increased by a factor of 4, not 3. Since Newton's Law of Gravitation is an inverse-square law, the fact that r has increased by a factor of 4 means that F_{grav} has decreased by a factor of $4^2 = 16$. The gravitational force on the satellite while it's in orbit is therefore $\frac{1}{16}(144,000 \text{ N}) = 9,000 \text{ N}$.

4.3 FRICTION

4.3

Some of the examples in the preceding sections described a frictionless surface. Of course, there's no such thing as a truly frictionless surface, but when a problem uses a term like *frictionless*, it simply means that friction is so weak that it can be neglected. Having frictionless surfaces also made those examples easier, so we could become comfortable with Newton's laws while first learning to apply them. However, there are cases in which friction cannot be ignored, so we need to learn how to handle such situations.

When two materials are in contact, there's an electrical attraction between the atoms of one surface with those of the other; this attraction will make it difficult to slide one object relative to the other. In addition, if the surfaces aren't perfectly smooth, the roughness will also increase the force required to slide the objects against each other. **Friction** is the term we use for the combination of these effects. Fortunately, the forces due to all those intermolecular forces and to the interactions of surface irregularities can be expressed by a single equation.

The OAT will expect you to know about two big categories of friction; they're called **static friction** and **kinetic (or sliding) friction**.[1] When there's no relative motion between the surfaces that are in contact (that is, when there's no sliding), we have static friction; when there *is* relative motion between the surfaces (that is, when there *is* sliding), we have kinetic friction.

Now, in order to state the equations we'll use to figure out these frictional forces, we first need to discuss another contact force, the one known as the normal force.

Place a book on a flat table. Assuming that the book isn't too heavy and the tabletop isn't made of, say, tissue paper, the book will remain supported by the table. One force acting on the book is the downward gravitational force. If this were the only force acting on the book, then the book would fall through the table. Hence, there must be an upward force acting on the book that cancels out the book's weight. This supporting force, which acts perpendicular to the tabletop, is called the **normal force**. It's called the *normal* force because it is, by definition, perpendicular to the surface that exerts it. The word *normal* means *perpendicular*. We'll denote the normal force by $\mathbf{N}$ or by $\mathbf{F}_N$. [Don't confuse $\mathbf{N}$ (or its magnitude, N) with the abbreviation for the newton, N.] In the case of an object simply lying on a flat surface, the magnitude of the normal force is just equal to the object's weight. As a result, the book feels a downward force of magnitude $w = mg$ and an upward force of magnitude $N = mg$, so the net force on the book is 0.

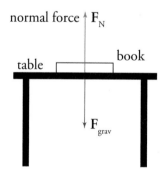

---

[1] Occasionally, the OAT may refer to **rolling resistance**. Rolling resistance is not technically friction; it is the force that resists an object's rolling motion. Do not confuse rolling resistance with kinetic friction; an object can roll without sliding (or skidding), and any friction at the contact point between the object and the surface will then be static, not kinetic.

4.3

Example 4-15: Do the normal force and the gravitational force described in the preceding paragraph form an action–reaction pair?

Solution: No. While these forces *are* equal but opposite, they do not form an action–reaction pair, because they act on the same object (namely, the book). The forces in an action–reaction pair always act on different objects. So, while it's true that the forces in an action–reaction pair are always equal but opposite, it is not true that any pair of equal but opposite forces must always form an action–reaction pair. The reaction force to $\mathbf{F}_{\text{table-on-book}}$, which is the normal force, is $\mathbf{F}_{\text{book-on-table}}$. The reaction force to $\mathbf{F}_{\text{Earth-on-book}}$, which is the weight of the book, is $\mathbf{F}_{\text{book-on-Earth}}$. The force $\mathbf{F}_{\text{table-on-book}}$ is not the reaction to $\mathbf{F}_{\text{Earth-on-book}}$.

For an object on a horizontal surface that feels no other downward forces, the normal force will be equal to the weight of the object. However, there are many cases in which the normal force isn't equal to the weight of the object. For example, suppose we place a book against a vertical wall and push on the book with a horizontal force **F**. Then the magnitude of the normal force exerted by the wall will be equal to F, which may certainly be different from the weight of the book. Here's another example (which we'll look at in more detail in the next section): if we place a book on an inclined plane (e.g., a ramp), then the normal force exerted by the ramp on the book will not be equal to the weight of the book. What we can say is the general definition of the normal force: *the normal force is the perpendicular component of the contact force exerted by a surface on an object.*

We had to discuss the normal force here, because the force of friction exerted by a surface on an object in contact is related to the normal force. In the case of sliding (kinetic) friction, the magnitude of the force of friction is directly proportional to the magnitude of the normal force. The constant of proportionality depends on what the surface is made of and what the object is made of; this constant is called the **coefficient of kinetic friction**, denoted by μ_k (the Greek letter *mu*, with subscript k), where the k denotes kinetic friction. For every pair of surfaces, the coefficient μ_k is an experimentally determined positive number with no units, and the greater its value, the greater the force of kinetic friction. For example, the value of μ_k for rubber-soled shoes on ice is only about 0.1, while for rubber-soled shoes on wood, the value of μ_k is much higher; it's about 0.7 for your sneakers, but could be greater than 1 if you walk around in rock-climbing shoes.

Notice carefully that this is *not* a vector equation. It is only an equation giving the *magnitude* of $\mathbf{F}_f$ in terms of the *magnitude* of $\mathbf{F}_N$.

Force of Kinetic Friction

$$F_f = \mu_k F_N$$

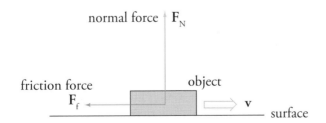

The magnitude of the force of kinetic friction is given by the equation $F_f = \mu_k F_N$. The direction of the force of kinetic friction is always parallel to the surface and in the opposite direction to the object's velocity (relative to the surface).

Example 4-16: A book of mass $m = 2$ kg slides across a flat tabletop. If the coefficient of kinetic friction between the book and table is 0.4, what's the magnitude of the force of kinetic friction on the book?

Solution: Because the magnitude of the normal force is $F_N = mg = (2 \text{ kg})(10 \text{ m/s}^2) = 20$ N, the magnitude of the force of kinetic friction is $F_f = \mu_k F_N = (0.4)(20 \text{ N}) = 8$ N.

The formula for static friction is similar to the one for kinetic friction, but there are two important differences. First, given a pair of surfaces, there's a **maximum coefficient of static friction** between them, μ_s (the subscript s now denotes static friction), and on the OAT, it's always greater than the coefficient of kinetic friction. This is equivalent to saying that, in general, static friction is capable of being stronger than kinetic friction. To illustrate this, imagine there's a heavy crate sitting on the floor and you want to push the crate across the room. You walk up to the crate and push on it, harder and harder until, finally, it "gives" and starts sliding. Once the crate is sliding, it's easier to keep it sliding than it was to get it started in the first place. The friction that resisted your initial push to get the crate moving was static friction. Because it was easier to keep it sliding than it was to get it started sliding, kinetic friction must be weaker than the maximum static friction force.

The second difference between the formula for kinetic friction and the one for static friction is that there's actually no general formula for the force of static friction. All we have is a formula for the *maximum* force of static friction. It's important that you understand this distinction. Let's go back to that heavy crate sitting on the floor. Let's say you know by previous experience that it'll take 400 N of force on your part to get that crate sliding. So, what if you push with a force of 100 N? Well, obviously, the crate won't move. Therefore, there must be another 100 N acting on the crate, opposite to your push, to make the net force on the crate zero. Okay, what if you now push on the crate with a force of 200 N? The crate still won't move, so there must now be another 200 N acting on the crate, opposite to your push, to make the net force on the crate zero. Whatever force you exert on the crate, as long as it's less than 400 N, will cause the force of static friction to cancel you out. Static friction is capable of supplying any necessary force, but only up to a certain maximum. That's why we can't write down a general formula for the force of static friction, only a formula for the maximum force of static friction. The formula looks just like the one above, except we replace μ_k by μ_s, and add the word "max" to denote that all this formula gives is the maximum force of static friction.

Maximum Force of Static Friction

$$F_{f,\text{max}} = \mu_s F_N$$

The maximum magnitude of the force of static friction is given by the equation $F_{f,\text{max}} = \mu_s F_N$. The direction of the force of static friction (maximum or not) is always parallel to the surface and in the opposite direction to the object's intended velocity. The magnitude of the force of static friction is whatever value, up to the maximum given by the equation, it takes exactly to cancel out the force(s) that are trying to make the object slide.

Example 4-17: A crate that weighs 1000 N rests on a horizontal floor. The coefficient of static friction between the crate and the floor is 0.4. If you push on the crate with a force of 250 N, what is the magnitude of the force of static friction?

Solution: The answer is not 400 N. The *maximum* force of static friction that the floor could exert on the crate is $F_{f, max} = \mu_s F_N = (0.4)(1000 \text{ N}) = 400$ N. However, if you exert a force of only 250 N on the crate, then static friction will only be 250 N. (Just imagine what would happen to the crate if you pushed on it with a force of 250 N and the floor pushed it back toward you with a force of 400 N!)

Example 4-18: You push a 50 kg block of wood across a flat concrete driveway, exerting a constant force of 300 N. If the coefficient of kinetic friction between the wood and concrete is 0.5, what will be the acceleration of the block?

Solution: The normal force acting on the block has magnitude $F_N = mg = (50 \text{ kg})(10 \text{ m/s}^2) = 500$ N. Therefore, the force of kinetic friction acting on the sliding block has magnitude $F_f = \mu_k F_N = (0.5)(500 \text{ N}) = 250$ N. This means that the net force acting on the block (and parallel to the driveway) is equal to $F - F_f = (300 \text{ N}) - (250 \text{ N}) = 50$ N. If $F_{net} = 50$ N and $m = 50$ kg, then $a = F_{net}/m = (50 \text{ N})/(50 \text{ kg}) = 1 \text{ m/s}^2$.

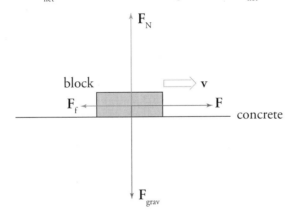

Example 4-19: Instead of pushing the block by a force that's parallel to the driveway, you wrap a rope around the block, sling the rope over your shoulder, and walk it across the driveway. If the rope makes an angle of 30° to the horizontal, and the tension in the rope is 300 N (the same force you exerted on the block in the last example), what will the block's acceleration be now?

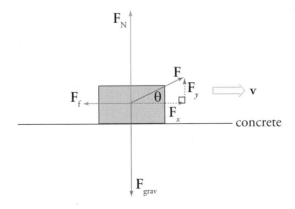

4.4

Solution: This is a tough question, but it uses a lot of the material we've covered so far. First, we'll need the normal force to find the friction force. The net vertical force on the block is 0 (because we're not lifting the block off the ground or watching it fall through the concrete). Therefore, $F_N + F_y = F_{grav}$, so $F_N = F_{grav} - F_y$. (Here's another example of the normal force not equaling the weight of the object.) Since $F_y = F \sin \theta = F \sin 30° = (300 \text{ N})(0.5) = 150 \text{ N}$, we have $F_N = (500 \text{ N}) - (150 \text{ N}) = 350 \text{ N}$. (Intuitively, the normal force is less than the weight of the block because the vertical component of the tension in the rope is "taking some of the pressure" off the surface.) Therefore, $F_f = \mu_k F_N = (0.5)(350 \text{ N}) = 175 \text{ N}$. Now, the horizontal force that you provide is $F_x = F \cos \theta = F \cos 30° \approx (300 \text{ N})(0.85) = 255 \text{ N}$. Therefore, the net force acting on the block, parallel to the driveway, is equal to $F_x - F_f = (255 \text{ N}) - (175 \text{ N}) = 80 \text{ N}$. If $F_{net} = 80 \text{ N}$ and $m = 50 \text{ kg}$, then $a = F_{net}/m = (80 \text{ N})/(50 \text{ kg}) = 1.6 \text{ m/s}^2$. (Notice that you get the block moving faster—even exerting the same force—by doing it this way!)

4.4 INCLINED PLANES

So far, we've had practice working problems where the object is moving along a flat, horizontal surface. However, the OAT will also expect you to handle questions in which the object is on a ramp, or, in fancier language, an **inclined plane**.

The figure below shows an object of mass m on an inclined plane; the angle the plane makes with the horizontal (the **incline angle**) is labeled θ. If we draw the vector representing the weight of the object, we notice that it can be written in terms of two components: one parallel to the ramp and one perpendicular to it. The diagram on the left shows that the magnitudes of the components of the object's weight, $\mathbf{w} = m\mathbf{g}$, are $mg \sin \theta$ (parallel to the ramp) and $mg \cos \theta$ (perpendicular to the ramp).

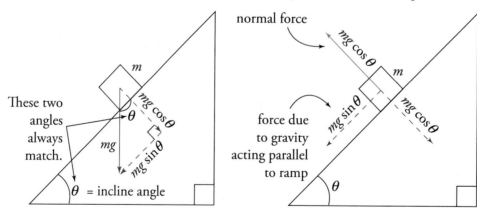

Therefore, as illustrated in the diagram on the right,

the force due to gravity acting parallel to the inclined plane $= mg \sin \theta$

where θ is measured between incline and horizontal. **You should memorize both of these facts.**

Incidentally, any time we see an angle in an OAT problem we'll probably be breaking a vector (say a force, a velocity, or an acceleration) into components. When we looked at projectile motion we broke the projectile's initial velocity into horizontal and vertical components; here, we're breaking the force of gravity into a component parallel to and one perpendicular to the surface of the incline. Why the difference? In general, the components you'll use will be vertical and horizontal, *unless* the object can only move along one possible line; in that case, the components to use will be the direction of (possible) travel (in this case, parallel to the incline), and the direction perpendicular to that.

Example 4-20: A block of mass $m = 4$ kg is placed at the top of a frictionless ramp of incline angle 30° and length 10 m.

a)   What is the block's acceleration down the ramp?
b)   How long will it take for the block to slide to the bottom?

Solution:

a)   Because the force due to gravity acting parallel to the ramp is $F = mg \sin \theta$, the acceleration of the block down the ramp will be

$$a = \frac{F}{m} = \frac{mg \sin \theta}{m} = g \sin \theta = \left(10 \text{ m/s}^2\right) \sin 30° = 5 \text{ m/s}^2$$

b)   Using Big Five #3 with $d = 10$ m, $v_0 = 0$, and $a = 5$ m/s², we find that

$$d = v_0 t + \frac{1}{2} at^2 = \frac{1}{2} at^2 \rightarrow t = \sqrt{\frac{2d}{a}} = \sqrt{\frac{2(10 \text{ m})}{5 \text{ m/s}^2}} = 2 \text{ s}$$

Notice that the block's mass was irrelevant to both of these questions. That's because all of the forces were directly proportional to mass, but so was the object's inertia; in effect, mass cancelled out of both sides of $F = ma$. This is common in problems in which the forces on an object are all functions of gravity.

Example 4-21: A block of mass m slides down a ramp of incline angle 60°. If the coefficient of kinetic friction between the block and the surface of the ramp is 0.2, what's the block's acceleration down the ramp?

Solution: There are now two forces acting parallel to the ramp: $mg \sin \theta$ (directed downward along the ramp) and F_f, the force of kinetic friction (directed upward along the ramp). Therefore, the net force down the ramp is $F_{net} = mg \sin \theta - F_f$. To find F_f, we multiply F_N by μ_k. Since $F_N = mg \cos \theta$, we have

$$F_{net} = mg \sin \theta - \mu_k mg \cos \theta$$

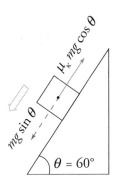

Dividing F_{net} by m gives us a:

$$a = \frac{F_{net}}{m} = \frac{mg \sin\theta - \mu_k mg \cos\theta}{m} = g(\sin\theta - \mu_k \cos\theta)$$

Putting in the numbers, we get

$$a = (10 \text{ m/s}^2)(\sin 60° - 0.2\cos 60°) \approx (10 \text{ m/s}^2)(0.85 - 0.2 \cdot \tfrac{1}{2}) = 7.5 \text{ m/s}^2$$

Example 4-22: A block of mass m is placed on a ramp of incline angle θ. If the block doesn't slide down, find the relationship between μ_s (the coefficient of static friction) and θ.

Solution: If the block doesn't slide, then static friction is strong enough to withstand the pull of gravity acting downward parallel to the ramp. This means that the *maximum* force of static friction must be greater than or equal to $mg \sin\theta$. Since $F_{f(static), max} = \mu_s F_N$, and $F_N = mg \cos\theta$, we have $F_{f(static), max} = \mu_s mg \cos\theta$. Therefore,

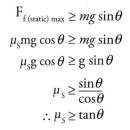

$$F_{f(static) max} \geq mg \sin\theta$$

$$\mu_s mg \cos\theta \geq mg \sin\theta$$

$$\mu_s g \cos\theta \geq g \sin\theta$$

$$\mu_s \geq \frac{\sin\theta}{\cos\theta}$$

$$\therefore \mu_s \geq \tan\theta$$

4.5 PULLEYS

A **pulley** is a device that changes the direction of the **tension** (the force exerted by a stretched string, cord, or rope) that pulls on the object that the string is attached to. (We'll use $\mathbf{F_T}$ or $\mathbf{T}$ to denote a tension force.) For example, in the picture below, if we pull *down* on the string on the right with a force of magnitude F_T, then the tension force on the left side of the pulley will pull *up* on the block with the same magnitude of force, F_T.

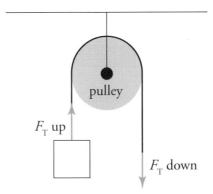

Pulleys can also be used to decrease the force necessary to lift an object. For example, consider the pulley system illustrated on the left below. If we pull down on the string on the right with a force of magnitude F_T, then we'll create a tension force of magnitude F_T throughout the entire string. As a result, there will be *two* tension forces, each of magnitude F_T, pulling up to lift the block (and the bottom pulley, too, but we assume that the pulleys are massless; that is, the mass of any pulley is small enough that it can be ignored). Therefore, we only need to exert half as much force to lift the block! This simple observation, that a pulley system (with massless, frictionless pulleys) causes a constant tension to exist through the entire string, which can lead to multiple tension forces pulling on an object, is the key to many OAT problems on pulleys.

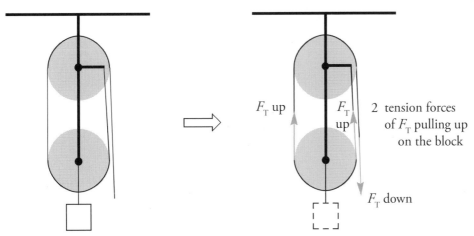

Pulley systems like this multiply our force by however many strings are pulling on the object.

Notice carefully that the tension force is applied wherever a string (or rope, or cable, or whatever) comes in contact with a pulley, which means that there will often be *two* tension forces on a single pulley, one on each side. You can see this in the right-hand diagram just above this text.

Example 4-23: In the figure below, how much force would we need to exert on the free end of the cord in order to lift the plank (mass $M = 300$ kg) with constant velocity? (Ignore the masses of the pulleys.)

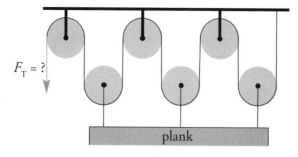

Solution: As a result of our pulling downward, there will be 6 tension forces pulling up on the plank:

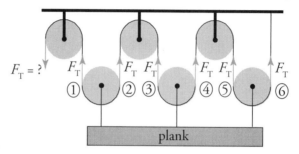

In order to lift with constant velocity (acceleration = zero), we require the net force on the plank to be zero. Therefore, the total of all the tension forces pulling up, $6F_T$, must balance the weight of the plank downward, Mg. This gives us

$$6F_T = Mg \rightarrow F_T = \frac{Mg}{6} = \frac{(300 \text{ kg})(10 \text{ N/kg})}{6} = 500 \text{ N}$$

Example 4-24: Two blocks are connected by a cord that hangs over a pulley. One block has a mass, M, of 10 kg, and the other block has a mass, m, of 5 kg. What will be the magnitude of the acceleration of the system of blocks once they are released from rest?

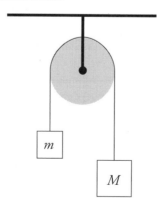

Solution: We'll solve this by a step-by-step approach using a **force diagram**. To apply Newton's Second Law, $F_{net} = ma$, to any problem, we follow these steps:

Step 1: Draw all the forces that act *on* the object. (That is, draw the force diagram.)
Step 2: Choose a direction to call *positive* (simply take the direction of the object's motion to be positive; it's almost always the easiest, most natural decision).
Step 3: Find F_{net} and set it equal to ma.

We have effectively done these steps in the solutions to the examples we have seen already, but now that we have a situation involving two accelerating objects, it is even more important to make sure that we have a systematic plan of attack. When you have more than one object to worry about, just make sure that the Step-2 decision you make for one object is compatible with the Step-2 decision you make for the other one(s). On the left below are the force diagrams for the blocks on the pulley. Notice that we call *up* the positive direction for m (because that's where it's going), and we call *down* the positive direction for M (because that's where *it's* going); these decisions are compatible, because when m moves in its positive direction, so does M.

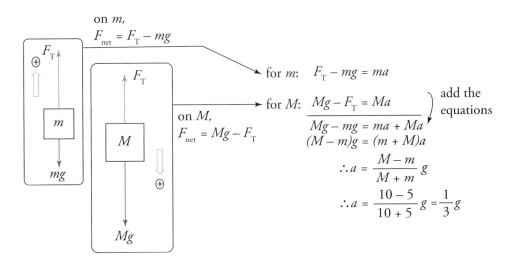

for m: $F_T - mg = ma$

for M: $Mg - F_T = Ma$ } add the equations

$$Mg - mg = ma + Ma$$
$$(M - m)g = (m + M)a$$
$$\therefore a = \frac{M - m}{M + m} g$$
$$\therefore a = \frac{10 - 5}{10 + 5} g = \frac{1}{3} g$$

Because *up* is the positive direction for little m, the force F_T on m is positive and the force mg is negative; therefore, for little m, we have $F_{net} = F_T + (-mg) = F_T - mg$. Since *down* is the positive direction for big M, the force Mg on M is positive and the force F_T is negative; therefore, for big M, we have $F_{net} = Mg + (-F_T) = Mg - F_T$. On the right above, we've written down $F_{net} = \text{mass} \times \text{acceleration}$ for each block. There are two equations, but we have two unknowns (F_T and a), so we *need* two equations. To solve the equations, the trick is simply to *add the equations*. Notice that this makes the F_T's drop out, so all we're left with is one unknown, a, which we can solve for immediately. The calculation shown above gives $a = g/3$, so we get $a = 3.3 \text{ m/s}^2$.

If the question had asked for the tension in the cord, we could now use the value we found for a and plug it back into either of our two equations (we'd get the same answer no matter which one we used). Using $F_T - mg = ma$, we'd find that

$$F_T = ma + mg = m(a + g) = m(\tfrac{1}{3}g + g) = \tfrac{4}{3}mg = \tfrac{4}{3}(5 \text{ kg})(10 \text{ N/kg}) = 67 \text{ N}$$

Example 4-25: In the figure below, the block of mass m slides up a frictionless inclined plane, pulled by another block of mass M that is falling. If $\theta = 30°$, $m = 20$ kg, and $M = 40$ kg, what's the acceleration of the block on the ramp?

4.5

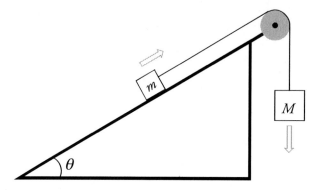

Solution: On the left below are the force diagrams for the blocks. Notice that we call *up the ramp* the positive direction for m (because that's where it's going), and we call *down* the positive direction for M (because that's where *it's* going); these decisions are compatible, because when m moves in its positive direction, so does M.

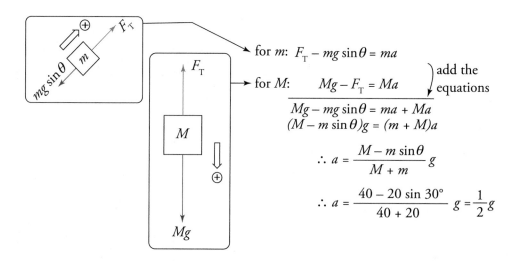

for m: $\quad F_T - mg\sin\theta = ma$

for M: $\qquad Mg - F_T = Ma$ $\quad$ } add the equations

$$Mg - mg\sin\theta = ma + Ma$$
$$(M - m\sin\theta)g = (m + M)a$$

$$\therefore a = \frac{M - m\sin\theta}{M + m}g$$

$$\therefore a = \frac{40 - 20\sin 30°}{40 + 20}g = \frac{1}{2}g$$

Because *up the ramp* is the positive direction for little m, the force F_T on m is positive and the force due to gravity along the ramp, $mg\sin\theta$, is negative; therefore, for little m, we have $F_{net} = F_T + (-mg\sin\theta) = F_T - mg\sin\theta$. Since *down* is the positive direction for big M, the force Mg on M is positive and the force F_T is negative; therefore, for big M, we have $F_{net} = Mg + (-F_T) = Mg - F_T$. On the right above, we've written down $F_{net} = $ mass × acceleration for each block. As in the preceding example, there are two equations (and two unknowns, F_T and a). Again using the trick of adding the equations, the F_T's drop out, and all we're left with is one unknown, a, to solve for. The calculation shown above gives $a = g/2$, so we get $a = 5$ m/s².

Summary of Formulas

Newton's Laws:

First law: $\mathbf{F}_{net} = 0 \Leftrightarrow v = \text{constant}$

Second law: $\mathbf{F}_{net} = ma$

Third law: $\mathbf{F}_{1\text{-on-}2} = -\mathbf{F}_{2\text{-on-}1}$

Weight: $\mathbf{w} = m\mathbf{g}$

Gravitational force: $F_{grav} = G\dfrac{Mm}{r^2}$ given that $w = F_{grav}$, we get $g = G\dfrac{M}{r^2}$.

Kinetic friction: $F_f = \mu_k F_N$

Static friction: $F_{f,max} = \mu_s F_N$

$$\mu_{s,\,max} > \mu_k$$

Direction of friction is opposite to the direction of motion (or intended direction of motion).

Force due to gravity acting parallel to inclined plane: $mg \sin \theta$

Force due to gravity acting perpendicular to inclined plane: $mg \cos \theta$, where θ is measured between incline and horizontal.

Chapter 5
Statics and Dynamics II

5.1 CENTER OF MASS

In the examples we looked at in the preceding chapter, objects were treated as though they were each a single particle. In fact, in the step-by-step solution to one of the pulley problems, we drew a force diagram showing all the forces acting on the objects in the system. To make that step go faster, we sometimes just represent each object by a dot and draw the force arrows on the dot. For example, the force diagram in the solution to Example 4-24 could have been drawn like this:

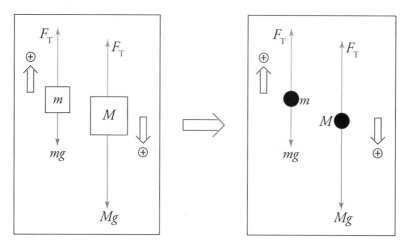

Each dot really denotes the *center of mass* of the object, which we'll now describe and define.

Imagine the following series of experiments. You walk into a large room with a friend, a hammer, and a glow-in-the-dark (phosphorescent) sticker. After shining light on the sticker (so that it will glow), stick it on the metal head of the hammer. Hand the hammer to your friend, stand back, and turn off the light. Ask your friend to flip and toss the hammer across the room so that you can watch its trajectory. You'll see only the glow-in-the-dark sticker, and it will, in general, trace out some complicated loopy path as the hammer tumbles and flies through the air.

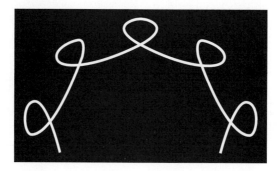

Repeat the experiment with the sticker attached to the end of the handle of the hammer. Once again, when your friend flips and tosses the hammer across the room so that you can watch it face on, you'll see only the glow-in-the-dark sticker, and it'll trace out another complicated loopy path.

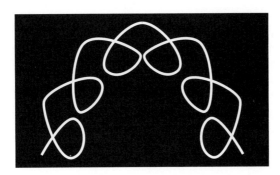

Now let's try this one more time, but rather than attaching the sticker at some random spot on the hammer, first find the point where the hammer just balances on the tip of your finger. Put the sticker on that spot and hand the hammer to your friend. Turn off the light, and watch as the hammer is tossed across the room. This time you'll see the sticker trace out a nice parabola, no loops.

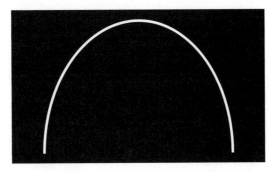

Apparently there was something special about the final location of the sticker. Most points on the hammer traced out complicated loopy trajectories, but this final point traced out a simple parabolic path, just as a single particle would. It is this one point that behaves as if the object (whether it's a block or a hammer or whatever) was a single particle. This special point is the **center of mass**. Another way of looking at it is to say that the center of mass is the point at which we could consider all the mass of the object to be concentrated. It's the dot in our simplified force diagrams.

For a simple object such as a sphere, block, or cylinder, whose density is constant (that is, for an object that's *homogeneous*), the center of mass is where you'd expect it to be—at its geometric center.

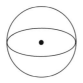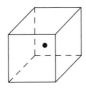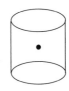

Note that in some cases, the center of mass isn't even located within the body of the object:

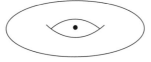

For a nonhomogeneous object, such as a hammer, whose density *does* vary from point to point, there's no single-step way mathematically to calculate the location of the center of mass.

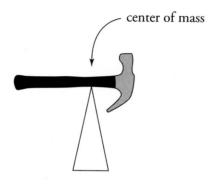

center of mass

However, there is a simpler type of problem on which the OAT *will* expect you to locate the center of mass. The situation involves a series of masses arranged in a line. For example, imagine that you had a stick with several blocks hanging from it. Where should you attach a string to the stick so that this mobile would balance?

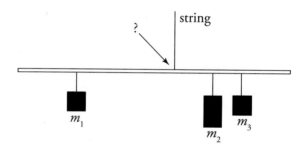

For a problem like this, in which each individual mass can be considered to be at a single point in space, here's the formula for the location of the center of mass:

Center of Mass for Point Masses

$$x_{CM} = \frac{m_1 x_1 + m_2 x_2 + m_3 x_3 \ldots}{m_1 + m_2 + m_3 \ldots}$$

(The location of the center of mass is often denoted by $\bar{x}$ as well. We'll use both notations.) To use this formula, follow these steps:

Step 1: Choose an origin (a reference point to call $x = 0$). The locations of the objects will be measured relative to this point. Often the easiest point to use will be at the location of the left-hand mass, but any point is fine; if a coordinate system is given in the problem, use it.

Step 2: Determine the locations (x_1, x_2, x_3, etc.) of the objects.

Step 3: Multiply each mass by its location ($m_1 x_1$, $m_2 x_2$, $m_3 x_3$, etc.) then add.

Step 4: Divide by the total mass ($m_1 + m_2 + m_3 + \ldots$).

Example 5-1: In the figure below, three blocks hang below a massless meter stick. Block m_1 hangs from the *20 cm* mark, block m_2 hangs from the *70 cm* mark, and block m_3 hangs from the *80 cm* mark. If m_1 = 2 kg, m_2 = 5 kg, and m_2 = 3 kg, at what mark on the meter stick should a string be attached so that this system would hang horizontally?

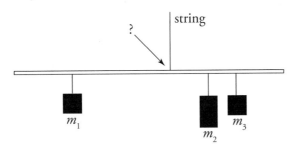

Solution: The first step is to choose an origin, a reference point to call $x = 0$. We are free to choose our zero mark anywhere we want, but the simplest choice here is the one implicitly mentioned in the question itself. The question wants to know at what mark on the meter stick we should attach the string; in other words, how far from the left end of the meter stick should we attach the string? Since the question asks essentially, "How far from the *left end*...?" the best place to choose our zero mark is at the *left end*. We now can write $x_1 = 20$ cm, $x_2 = 70$ cm, and $x_3 = 80$ cm. Using the formula above, we find that

$$x_{CM} = \frac{m_1 x_1 + m_2 x_2 + m_3 x_3}{m_1 + m_2 + m_3}$$

$$= \frac{(2\text{ kg})(20\text{ cm}) + (5\text{ kg})(70\text{ cm}) + (3\text{ kg})(80\text{ cm})}{(2\text{ kg}) + (5\text{ kg}) + (3\text{ kg})}$$

$$= \frac{630\text{ kg} \times \text{cm}}{10\text{ kg}}$$

$$\therefore x_{CM} = 63\text{ cm}$$

What if we had instead chosen the center of the meter stick (the *50 cm* mark) to be our origin? In that case, we would have found $x_1 = -30$ cm (because m_1 hangs from the *20 cm* mark, and *20 cm* is 30 cm to the *left*—hence the minus sign—of *50 cm*), $x_2 = 20$ cm, and $x_3 = 30$ cm. The formula would have told us that

$$x_{CM} = \frac{m_1 x_1 + m_2 x_2 + m_3 x_3}{m_1 + m_2 + m_3}$$

$$= \frac{(2\text{ kg})(-30\text{ cm}) + (5\text{ kg})(20\text{ cm}) + (3\text{ kg})(30\text{ cm})}{(2\text{ kg}) + (5\text{ kg}) + (3\text{ kg})}$$

$$= \frac{130\text{ kg} \cdot \text{cm}}{10\text{ kg}}$$

$$\therefore x_{CM} = 13\text{ cm}$$

Well, 13 cm to the *right* (because x_{CM} is *positive*) of the *50 cm* mark is the *63 cm* mark, the same answer we found before.

Example 5-2: In the figure below, three blocks hang below a uniform (homogeneous) meter stick of mass 3 kg. Block m_1 hangs from the *20 cm* mark, block m_2 hangs from the *70 cm* mark, and block m_3 hangs from the *80 cm* mark. If m_1 = 2 kg, m_2 = 5 kg, and m_3 = 3 kg, at what mark on the meter stick should a string be attached so that this system would hang without tipping?

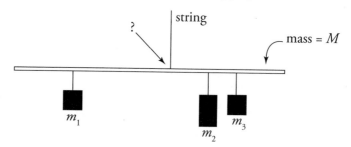

Solution: Does the mass of the stick (even if the stick is homogeneous) need to be taken into account? Well, let's see. If we were to include the mass of the stick (let's call it M) in the formula for the center of mass, it would seem that we'd just add it in the denominator, but what do we do in the numerator? What x would we multiply M by? The answer is: the stick's own center of mass! Since the stick is homogeneous, its center of mass (by itself) would be at its geometric center—that is, at the *50 cm* mark. So, with M = 3 kg and X = 50 cm, we'd find that

$$x_{CM} = \frac{m_1x_1 + m_2x_2 + m_3x_3 + MX}{m_1 + m_2 + m_3 + M}$$

$$= \frac{(2 \text{ kg})(20 \text{ cm}) + (5 \text{ kg})(70 \text{ cm}) + (3 \text{ kg})(80 \text{ cm}) + (3 \text{ kg})(50 \text{ cm})}{(2 \text{ kg}) + (5 \text{ kg}) + (3 \text{ kg}) + (3 \text{ kg})}$$

$$= \frac{780 \text{ kg} \cdot \text{cm}}{13 \text{ kg}}$$

$$\therefore x_{CM} = 60 \text{ cm}$$

Notice that this is a different location from what we found if the stick's mass could be neglected. Therefore, the mass of the stick *does* need to be included, even if it's homogeneous.

What if we had instead chosen the center of the meter stick (the *50 cm* mark) to be our origin? In that case, we would have had X = 0 for the location of M, and the formula would have told us that

$$x_{CM} = \frac{m_1x_1 + m_2x_2 + m_3x_3 + MX}{m_1 + m_2 + m_3 + M}$$

$$= \frac{(2 \text{ kg})(-30 \text{ cm}) + (5 \text{ kg})(20 \text{ cm}) + (3 \text{ kg})(30 \text{ cm}) + (3 \text{ kg})(0 \text{ cm})}{(2 \text{ kg}) + (5 \text{ kg}) + (3 \text{ kg}) + (3 \text{ kg})}$$

$$= \frac{130 \text{ kg} \cdot \text{cm}}{13 \text{ kg}}$$

$$\therefore x_{CM} = 10 \text{ cm}$$

Well, 10 cm to the right of the *50 cm* mark is the *60 cm* mark; the same answer we found before.

Example 5-3: An ammonia molecule (NH_3) contains 3 hydrogen atoms that are positioned at the vertices of an equilateral triangle. The nitrogen atom lies 38 pm (1 pm = 1 picometer = 10^{-12} m) directly above the center of this triangle. If the N:H mass ratio is 14:1, how far below the N atom is the center of mass of the molecule?

Solution: The objects in this system (the four atoms) are not arranged in a line, so how can we hope to determine the center of mass? The key to the answer is to realize that we don't need to include all four of these objects in a single calculation; we can divide the problem into stages. Since the three H atoms have equal masses and are symmetrically arranged at the corners of an equilateral triangle, the center of mass of just these 3 H's is at their geometric center: namely, the center of the triangle. Therefore, by definition of center of mass, the 3 H atoms behave as if all their mass were concentrated at the center of the triangle. This now turns the problem into computing the center of mass of 2 objects (which obviously lie on a line): the 3 H atoms at the center of the triangle and the N atom:

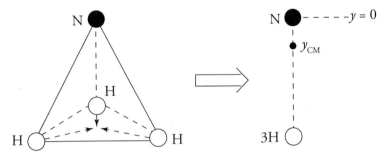

Because the question asks for the center of mass of the molecule relative to the N atom, we'll let the position of the N atom be our zero mark. (It's labeled y in the diagram on the right simply because the way the system is drawn, the objects are arranged along a *vertical* line.) The formula now gives us

$$y_{CM} = \frac{m_N y_N + m_{3H} y_{3H}}{m_N + m_{3H}}$$

$$= \frac{(14)(0 \text{ cm}) + (3 \cdot 1)(38 \text{ pm})}{(14) + (3 \cdot 1)}$$

$$= \frac{114 \text{ pm}}{17}$$

$$\therefore y_{CM} \approx 7 \text{ pm}$$

Therefore, the center of mass of the NH_3 molecule is 7/38, or about 1/6 of the way down from the nitrogen atom toward the plane of the hydrogens. Because the nitrogen atom is more massive than the hydrogens, we expect the center of mass to not be at the geometric center but, rather, much closer to the nitrogen atom. (This is just like the balancing point of the hammer: since the metal head is much heavier [because it's denser] than the rest of the hammer, we expect the hammer's center of mass to be not at the geometric center, but, instead, closer to the heavier end.)

You may have noticed in Example 5-2 that we applied the point mass formula to a system that didn't include only point masses: the stick's mass was spread along its entire length. What we did in that problem is what we can *always* do with a collection of homogenous (i.e., constant density) masses: First, find the center of mass of each piece; second, apply the point mass formula, assuming that each piece's mass is concentrated at its own center of mass.

It's possible (though unlikely) that on the OAT you'll have to find the center of mass of a two-dimensional collection of masses. In Example 5-3 on the previous page, we were able to simplify the problem to reduce it to a single dimension, but that might not always be the case. If you can't simplify the problem in this way, do what we always do with multidimensional problems: break it into components, and consider the components separately. In other words, first find the center of mass in, say, the x-direction, using only the x-components of position; then do the same in the y-direction.

Center of Gravity

If the gravitational field is uniform throughout a system, then the center of gravity is the same as the center of mass. The **center of gravity (CG)** is the point at which the total gravitational force on the system can be considered to act. The formula for calculating the center of gravity of a collection of objects arranged in a line looks just like the formula for calculating the center of mass, except the object's masses are replaced by their *weights* (that is, the *m*'s are replaced by *w*'s):

Center of Gravity

$$x_{CG} = \frac{w_1 x_1 + w_2 x_2 + w_3 x_3 \ldots}{w_1 + w_2 + w_3 \ldots}$$

It's now easy to see why the center of gravity is the same as the center of mass if g is constant, because the g's cancel:

$$x_{CG} = \frac{w_1 x_1 + w_2 x_2 + w_3 x_3 \ldots}{w_1 + w_2 + w_3 \ldots}$$
$$= \frac{(m_1 g) x_1 + (m_2 g) x_2 + (m_3 g) x_3 \ldots}{m_1 g + m_2 g + m_3 g \ldots}$$
$$= \frac{g(m_1 x_1 + m_2 x_2 + m_3 x_3 \ldots)}{g(m_1 + m_2 + m_3 \ldots)}$$
$$= \frac{m_1 x_1 + m_2 x_2 + m_3 x_3 \ldots}{m_1 + m_2 + m_3 \ldots}$$
$$\therefore x_{CG} = x_{CM}$$

Example 5-4: A long homogeneous plank of weight 30 N supports two blocks: one of weight 120 N that is 8 m to the left of the plank's midpoint, and another of weight 40 N that is 5 m to the right of the plank's midpoint. Where's the center of gravity of this system?

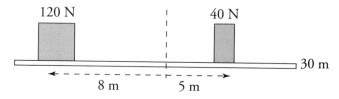

Solution: Choosing the midpoint of the plank to be $x = 0$, we have

$$x_{CG} = \frac{w_1 x_1 + w_2 x_2 + WX}{w_1 + w_2 + W}$$

$$= \frac{(120\ \text{N})(-8\ \text{m}) + (40\ \text{N})(5\ \text{m}) + (30\ \text{N})(0\ \text{m})}{(120\ \text{N}) + (40\ \text{N}) + (30\ \text{N})}$$

$$= \frac{-760\ \text{N·m}}{190\ \text{N}}$$

$$\therefore x_{CG} = -4\ \text{m}$$

Therefore, the center of gravity (as well as the center of mass) is 4 m to the left of the plank's midpoint.

On the OAT, you can almost always assume that as in the example above, the center of mass is the same as the center of gravity. The only exception would be if the gravitational field was specifically defined as being nonuniform within the space of the object, and this would be very rare on the OAT.

5.2 UNIFORM CIRCULAR MOTION

So far, we've analyzed motion that takes place along a straight line (horizontal, vertical, or slanted) or along a parabola. The OAT will also require that you know how to analyze an object that moves in a circular path.

The title of this section is Uniform Circular Motion (often abbreviated UCM). What does *uniform* mean here? When we talk about uniform acceleration, we mean constant acceleration; uniform density means constant density; *uniform* is a term used in physics to denote something that remains constant. What property of an object undergoing uniform circular motion is constant? The radius of its path is constant, but that's already in the definition of *circular*, so it must be something else.

> An object moving in a circular path is said to execute
>
> **uniform circular motion**
>
> if its *speed* is constant.

Notice right away that this does *not* mean the object's *velocity* is constant. Velocity is a vector: it has both speed and direction. If an object is moving in a circular path, then it's constantly turning, so its direction is constantly changing. A changing direction, even at constant speed, automatically means a changing velocity. An object's velocity vector is always tangent to its path, regardless of the shape of the path (parabola, circle, figure-8, or whatever) so in the figure below, you can see that the object will have a different velocity vector at every point on the circle, even though the magnitudes of these vectors are all the same.

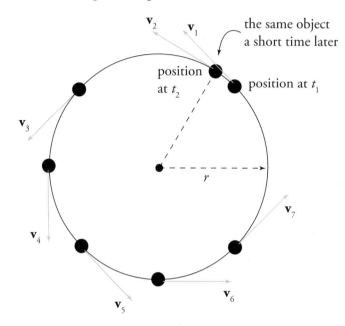

The first thing that should come to mind when you see an object's velocity changing is that the object is experiencing acceleration. The acceleration of an object undergoing uniform circular motion is not affecting the *speed* of the object; this acceleration is only changing the direction of the velocity in order to keep the object moving in a circle.

In the figure below, the velocity vectors of the object are drawn at two close points in its path; they're labeled v_1 and v_2. By definition, the direction of the acceleration is the same as the direction of the velocity change (remember the definition: $a = \Delta v / \Delta t$). So, the acceleration of the object has the same direction as $\Delta v = v_2 - v_1$. Notice that $v_2 - v_1$, which is $v_2 + (-v_1)$, points toward the center of the circle. Therefore, the acceleration of the object always points toward the center of the circle. (This will be true no matter where on the circle we look.)

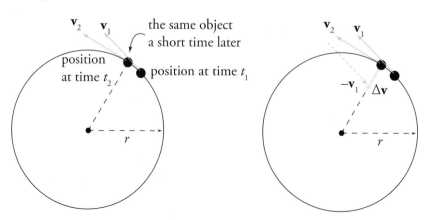

The acceleration of an object undergoing uniform circular motion always points toward the center of the circle. The term **centripetal** (from the Latin, meaning *to seek the center*) is therefore used to describe the acceleration of an object undergoing UCM. We'll denote centripetal acceleration by $\mathbf{a}_c$.

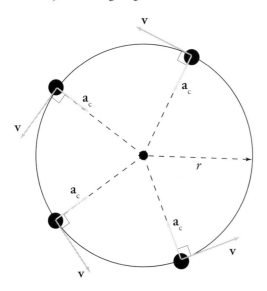

Since $\mathbf{v}$ is always tangent to the circle, and $\mathbf{a}_c$ always points to the center of the circle, $\mathbf{v}$ and $\mathbf{a}_c$ are always perpendicular to each other at any position of the object.

(*Note*: In the figure above, all the velocity vectors are different—because they point in different directions—so they really shouldn't all be labeled by the same **v**. The same is true for the centripetal acceleration vectors. However, adding subscripts to distinguish all the **v** vectors and all the $\mathbf{a}_c$ vectors would have made the picture look too confusing.)

We now know the *direction* of the centripetal acceleration at any point on the circle; what is its *magnitude*? If v is the speed of the object and r is the radius of the circular path, then the magnitude of the centripetal acceleration, a_c, is v^2/r.

Magnitude of Centripetal Acceleration

$$a_c = \frac{v^2}{r}$$

If an object is accelerating, then it must be feeling a force (after all, $F_{net} = ma$, so you can't have an acceleration without a force). Since $\mathbf{F}_{net}$ and $\mathbf{a}$ always point in the same direction, no matter what the path of the object, the net force on an object undergoing UCM must, like $\mathbf{a}$, point toward the center. So, guess what we call it? **Centripetal force** (denoted $\mathbf{F}_c$). This is the *net* force directed toward the center that acts on an object to make it execute uniform circular motion. And since $F_{net} = ma$, we'll have $\mathbf{F}_c = m\mathbf{a}_c$ and $F_c = ma_c$, so the magnitude of the centripetal force is mv^2/r, where m is the mass of the object that's moving around the circle.

Magnitude of Centripetal Force

$$F_c = ma_c = \frac{mv^2}{r}$$

Example 5-5: An object of mass 3 kg moves at a constant speed of 4 m/s in a circular path of radius 0.5 m. What is the magnitude of its acceleration? What is the magnitude of the net force on the object?

Solution: An object moving in a circular path at constant speed is undergoing uniform circular motion. Although its speed is constant, the object is always accelerating, because its direction is constantly changing. The acceleration of the object is the centripetal acceleration,

$$a_c = \frac{v^2}{r} = \frac{(4 \text{ m/s})^2}{0.5 \text{ m}} = 32 \text{ m/s}^2$$

From Newton's Second Law, we can now determine the magnitude of the net force the object feels:

$$F_c = ma_c = (3 \text{ kg})(32 \text{ m/s}^2) = 96 \text{ N}$$

Example 5-6: If an object undergoing uniform circular motion is being acted upon by a constant force toward the center, why doesn't the object fall into the center?

Solution: Actually, it *is* falling toward the center, but because of its speed, the object remains in a circular orbit around the center. Remember that the direction of **v** is not necessarily the same as the direction of **F**_net. So, just because **F**_net points toward the center does not mean that **v** must point toward the center. It's the direction of the *acceleration*, not the velocity, that always matches the direction of **F**_net. Let's look at the motion of the object at a certain point in its circular path:

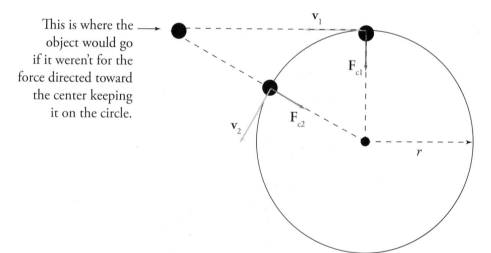

This is where the object would go if it weren't for the force directed toward the center keeping it on the circle.

In this figure, the net force on the object at Position 1 points downward (toward the center of the circle). Therefore, it's telling v_1 to move downward a little, so that at the next moment, at Position 2, the velocity will point downward slightly. Notice that this is just what we want in order to keep the object traveling in a circle! If it weren't for this force pointing toward the center (that is, if the centripetal force were suddenly removed), then the object's velocity wouldn't change. It would not continue to move in a circle but would instead fly off in a straight line, tangent to the circle at the point where the force was removed.

Example 5-7: How would the net force on an object undergoing uniform circular motion have to change if the object's speed doubled?

Solution: Centripetal force, mv^2/r, is proportional to the *square* of the speed. So, if the object's speed increased by a factor of 2, then the magnitude of $\mathbf{F}_c$ would have to increase by a factor of $2^2 = 4$.

Solving circular motion problems often involves something more than simply using the formulas $a_c = v^2/r$ or $F_c = mv^2/r$. The key to solving such problems is to answer this question:

What provides the centripetal force?

In other words, what force(s) act in the dimension toward the center of the circle?

Centripetal force is not some new kind of force like gravity or tension. It's simply the name for the net force directed toward the center of the circular path. The vector sum of forces such as gravity and tension is what gets *called* centripetal force, when those forces, or components of them, are directed toward the center of the circle. When drawing a force diagram for an object undergoing UCM, here are a couple of tips:

1. Do not add a force called $\mathbf{F}_c$ in your picture; forces such as gravity, tension, normal force, etc. *do* go in your picture, but $\mathbf{F}_c$ doesn't. Remember, $\mathbf{F}_c$ is what the forces toward the center have to add up to.
2. Always call *toward the center* the positive direction. Any forces toward the center are then positive forces, and any forces directed away from the center are negative. You'll need this to find F_{net} and then set the result equal to F_c.

Example 5-8: The Moon orbits the Earth in a (nearly) circular path at (nearly) constant speed. If M is the mass of the Earth, m is the mass of the Moon, and r is the Moon's orbit radius, find an expression for the Moon's orbit speed.

Solution: We begin by answering the question, *What provides the centripetal force?* The answer is the gravitational pull by the Earth. We now simply translate our answer into an equation, like this:

$$\underbrace{\text{gravitational pull}} \qquad \text{provides} \qquad \underbrace{\text{the centripetal force}}$$

$$F_{grav} \qquad\qquad = \qquad\qquad m\frac{v^2}{r}$$

Since we know $F_{grav} = GMm/r^2$, we get

$$F_{grav} = F_c \;\rightarrow\; G\frac{Mm}{r^2} = m\frac{v^2}{r} \;\rightarrow\; G\frac{M}{r} = v^2 \;\rightarrow\; \therefore v = \sqrt{G\frac{M}{r}}$$

Notice that the mass of the Moon, m, cancels out. So, any object orbiting at the same distance from the Earth as the Moon must move at the same speed as the Moon.

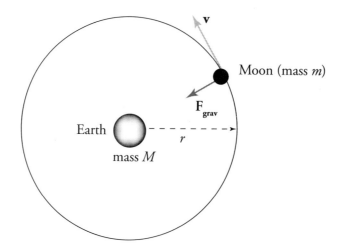

Example 5-9: A string is tied around a rock of mass 0.2 kg, and the rock is then whirled at a constant speed v in a horizontal circle of radius 0.4 m, as shown in the figure below. If $\sin \theta = 0.4$ and $\cos \theta = 0.9$, what's v?

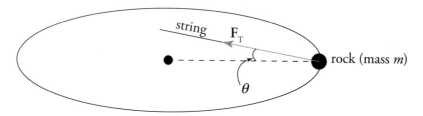

Solution: First, let's draw a bigger force diagram:

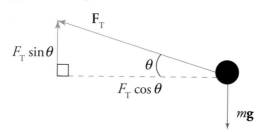

(This figure also shows why the end of the string is slightly above the center of the circle. The string has to point upward a little in order for there to be an upward component of the tension to cancel out the weight of the rock and allow the rock to revolve in a *horizontal* circle.) Because the rock is moving in a horizontal circle and not accelerating vertically, we know that the net vertical force must be zero. Therefore, the vertical component of the string's tension, $F_y = F_T \sin \theta$, must balance out the weight of the rock, mg:

$$F_T \sin \theta = mg$$

From this, we can figure out that

$$F_T = \frac{mg}{\sin\theta} = \frac{(0.2 \text{ kg})(10 \text{ N/kg})}{0.4} = 5 \text{ N}$$

Now, let's look at the circular motion: *What provides the centripetal force?* As the diagram shows, there's only one force directed toward the center of the circle (namely, the horizontal component of the tension, $F_x = F_T \cos\theta$), so this must be it:

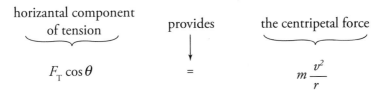

We now just plug in the value we found for F_T to get v:

$$F_T \cos\theta = m\frac{v^2}{r} \rightarrow v = \sqrt{\frac{rF_T \cos\theta}{m}} = \sqrt{\frac{(0.4 \text{ m})(5 \text{ N})(0.9)}{0.2 \text{ kg}}} = 3 \text{ m/s}$$

Example 5-10: A rope of length 60 cm is tied to the handle of a bucket (whose mass is 3 kg), and the bucket is then whirled in a vertical circle. At the bottom of its path, the tension in the rope is 50 N. What is the speed of the bucket at this point?

Solution: First, let's draw a diagram.

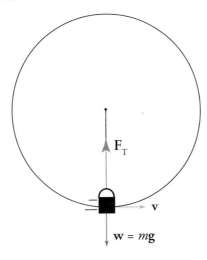

Because we call *toward the center* the positive direction when doing circular motion problems, we see that the tension, $\mathbf{F}_T$, is a positive force, and the bucket's weight, $\mathbf{w}$, is a negative force. (Because $\mathbf{w}$ points *away* from the center, we count it as negative.) Therefore, the net force on the bucket at this point is $F_T - w$. Because the net force directed toward the center is called the centripetal force, we'd write

$$F_T - w = F_c$$

5.2

Because $w = mg$ and $F_c = mv^2/r$, this equation becomes

$$F_T - mg = m\frac{v^2}{r}$$

We now just use this equation and the numbers we were given to figure out v, realizing that the radius of the circle is equal to the length of the rope (so $r = 0.6$ m):

$$v = \sqrt{\frac{r(F_T - mg)}{m}} = \sqrt{\frac{(0.6 \text{ m})[50 \text{ N} - (3 \text{ kg})(10 \text{ N/kg})]}{3 \text{ kg}}} = 2 \text{ m/s}$$

Example 5-11: For the situation described in the preceding example, what is the centripetal force on the bucket when the bucket is at the position shown below?

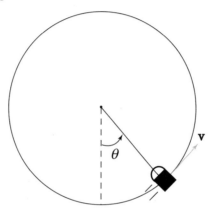

Solution: Here's the force diagram:

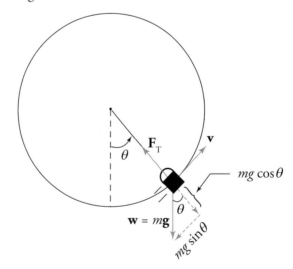

Because there's a force of F_T pointing toward the center and a force of $mg \cos \theta$ pointing *away* from the center, the net force toward the center of the circle (which is the centripetal force) is

$$\underset{\substack{net \\ toward\ center}}{F} = F_c = F_T - mg \cos \theta$$

Let's examine this situation a little more closely. Notice that at the position of the bucket shown, we also have a force component *tangent* to the circle ($mg \sin \theta$), which *opposes* the direction of the bucket's velocity. As a result, the bucket's speed will be reduced. Centripetal acceleration only makes an object turn so that it moves in a circular path; it does not change the speed. **Tangential** acceleration, on the other hand, *does* change the speed. Therefore, the bucket's speed will decrease as it rises to the top of the circle, and we wouldn't call the entire motion of the bucket "uniform." However, even if the speed of an object moving in a circle changes, there will always be a component of the net force that points toward the center of the circle; this is the centripetal force. The mathematical translation of the statement "the net force toward the center provides the centripetal force" becomes

$$F_T - mg \cos \theta = m \frac{v^2}{r} \rightarrow F_T = m \frac{v^2}{r} + mg \cos \theta$$

Because v decreases as the bucket rises (because of the downward tangential force, $mg \sin \theta$) and since $\cos \theta$ decreases as the bucket rises (because the angle θ increases from 0° to 180°), this final equation for F_T shows us that the tension in the rope will decrease as the bucket rises.

It's not often that we need to worry about both centripetal and tangential acceleration in an OAT problem, but the example above shows how to deal with it when we do encounter such a situation: ignore the tangential components of force and acceleration when calculating the centripetal force and acceleration. This is really just another example of the general principle: in OAT-level physics, you can always consider the components of motion separately.

Rotational Kinematics

Uniformly accelerated circular motion can be explored in terms of the same kinematics equations introduced in Chapter 3.2, i.e., the Big Five. However, the variables are relabeled as follows: θ (units of radians or rad) is the angular displacement or angle swept out as the object rotates, ω_0 (units of rad/s) is the initial angular speed or initial rotation rate, ω (units of rad/s) is the final angular speed, α (units of rad/s²) is the angular acceleration, and t is time in the usual sense. The linear quantities can be related to the angular quantities via the following equations

$$v = \omega r$$

$$a_t = \alpha r$$

where v and a_t are the magnitudes of the instantaneous velocity and acceleration of the object acting tangent to the circular path, respectively. It's worth noting the following unit conversions:

$$1\ rotation\ (rot) = 1\ revolution\ (rev) = 2\pi\ rad = 360°$$

The Big Five expressed in terms of uniformly accelerated circular motion are shown in the table below. Compare these equations to the Big Five shown in Chapter 3.2; they really are the same. As such, the approach to these rotational kinematics problems is the same as linear kinematics problems: the kinematic quantity that is neither given nor asked for in the question, and hence is missing, indicates which equation should be used to work the problem.

1. $\theta = \dfrac{1}{2}(\omega_0 + \omega)t$ missing α

2. $\omega = \omega_0 + \alpha t$ missing θ

3. $\theta = \omega_0 t + \dfrac{1}{2}\alpha t^2$ missing ω

4. $\theta = \omega t - \dfrac{1}{2}\alpha t^2$ missing ω_0

5. $\omega^2 = \omega_0^2 + 2\alpha\theta$ missing t

5.3 TORQUE

We can tie a rope to a bucket and make it move in a circular path, but how would we make the bucket itself spin? One way would be to grab the handle and then rotate our hand, or we could place our hands on opposite sides of the bucket and then, by moving our hands in opposite directions, rotate the bucket. In order to make an object's center of mass accelerate, we need to exert a force. In order to make an object *spin*, we need to exert a *torque*.

Torque is the measure of a force's effectiveness at making an object spin or rotate. (More precisely, it's the measure of a force's effectiveness at making an object *accelerate* rotationally.) If an object is initially at rest, and then it starts to spin, something must have exerted a torque. And if an object is already spinning, something would have to exert a torque to get it to stop spinning. In this section, we'll begin by looking at two different (but entirely equivalent) ways of figuring out torque.

All systems that can spin or rotate have a "center" of turning. This is the point that does not move while the remainder of the object is rotating, effectively becoming the center of the circle. There are many terms used to describe this point, including **pivot point** and **fulcrum**.

Let's say we want to tighten a bolt with a wrench. The figure below illustrates the situation.

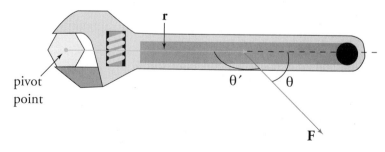

If we applied the force **F** to the wrench, would we make the wrench and the bolt rotate? Yes, because this force **F** has *torque*. (Notice: Torque is not a force; it's a property of a force.) To say how *much* torque **F** provides, we need a couple of preliminary definitions. First, the vector from the center of rotation (the **pivot point**) to the point of application of the force is called the **radius vector, r**. The angle between the vectors **r** and **F** is called θ. Now notice in the figure above that the angle between the vectors **r** and **F** at the point where they actually meet is denoted by θ'. This is because the angle between two vectors is actually the angle they make *when they start at the same point*. But in the figure, the vector **r** starts at the pivot point (which is where **r** always starts), and **F** starts at the *end* of **r** (which is where **F** always starts). One way to find the correct angle between these vectors is to imagine sliding **r** over so that it does start where **F** starts; the dashed line in the figure shows the line along which such a translated **r** vector would lie and the resulting correct angle θ. However, all this fuss about which angle is the correct one doesn't really matter, as you'll soon see.

The amount of torque a force **F** provides depends on three things: the magnitude of **F**, the length of **r**, and the angle θ.

Torque

$$\tau = rF \sin\theta$$

(The letter we use for torque is τ, the Greek letter *tau*.) From this equation, we can immediately figure out the unit of torque:

$$[\tau] = [r][F] = \text{m·N} = \text{N·m}$$

There's no special name for this unit; it's just a newton-meter.[1]

For example, let's say that $F = 20$ N, $r = 10$ cm, and $\theta = 30°$. Then the torque provided by this force would be $\tau = rF \sin\theta = (0.1 \text{ m})(20 \text{ N}) \sin 30° = 1$ N·m. Notice that if we had instead used θ', we would have gotten the same answer, since $\theta' = 150°$ and $\sin 150° = \sin 30°$. This is why we don't have to worry about which angle, θ or θ', is the true angle between **r** and **F** when we calculate torque, because **r** and **F** will always be *supplements* (they'll add up to 180°) and the sine of an angle is always equal to the sine of its supplement. Therefore, $\tau = rF \sin\theta = rF \sin\theta'$.

Look at this force on the wrench:

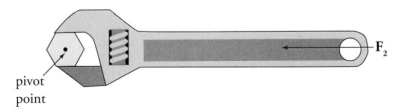

pivot
point

---

[1] In Chapter 6 we'll encounter another newton-meter and rename it the joule. What's the difference? Torque has a direction, like a vector (though technically it's what's called a pseudovector), while the joule, a unit of energy, is a scalar. For the OAT, there's no need to worry about this; just calculate torque in newton-meters, and then label it clockwise or counterclockwise.

Our intuition tells us that this force would not make the wrench (or bolt) rotate. Therefore, we expect that this force has zero torque. Using the definition, we can see that this is true. If we were to draw the **r** vector from the pivot to the point where F_2 is applied, we'd see that the value of $\sin\theta$ is 0, so $\tau_2 = 0$. Forces with no torque (like this one) cannot increase (or decrease) the rotational speed of an object.

How about this force on the wrench?

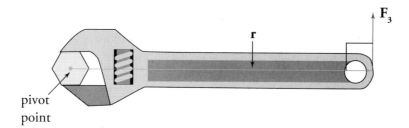

The force F_3 is perpendicular to its **r** vector, so $\theta = 90°$ and $\sin\theta = 1$, its maximum value. Therefore, when r $\perp$ F, we get the maximum torque for a given r and F, and the equation for torque gives us simply $\tau_3 = rF_3$. (This situation is very common, by the way.)

$$\text{If } r \perp F, \text{ then } \tau = rF.$$

The force F_3 above would produce counterclockwise rotation, so we say that it produces a **counterclockwise (CCW)** torque. The force F_4 below would produce clockwise rotation, so we say it produces a **clockwise (CW)** torque.

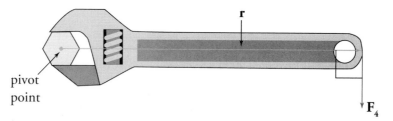

If $F_3 = F_4$, then these forces produce the same amount of torque, but one is clockwise and the other is counterclockwise. If we want to distinguish between them mathematically, we can say that $\tau_3 = +rF_3$ and $\tau_4 = -rF_4$, since it's customary to specify CCW rotation as positive and CW as negative.

The other method for calculating torque, which gives the same answer as the method we've just described, is based on the *lever arm* of a force. Let's look again at the first picture of our wrench:

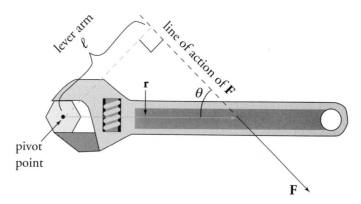

This time, however, rather than measuring the distance from the pivot to the *point* where the force is applied (the length r), we'll measure the shortest distance from the pivot to the *line* along which $\mathbf{F}$ is applied. This distance, which is always perpendicular to the line of action of F, is called the **lever arm** of F, written as ℓ or l.

Once we know the lever arm, ℓ, the definition of the torque of $\mathbf{F}$ is then simply $\tau = \ell F$.

Torque

$$\tau = \ell F$$

To see that this gives the same value for the torque as the formula $\tau = rF \sin \theta$, just notice that in the picture on the preceding page (bottom), the lever arm, ℓ, is the side opposite the angle θ in a right triangle whose hypotenuse is r; therefore, $\ell = r \sin \theta$. So, $\tau = \ell F$ is the same as $\tau = (r \sin \theta)F$. Because you can use either formula for calculating the torque, use whichever one is more convenient in a particular problem. In general, it's convenient to use the lever arm method if the length of the lever arm is obvious from the situation; otherwise, use $\tau = rF \sin \theta$.

For the force $\mathbf{F}_5$ shown below, our intuition tells us that this force would not make the wrench (or bolt) rotate. Therefore, we expect that this force has zero torque. Using the definition of lever arm, we can see that this is true. The line of action of $\mathbf{F}_5$ passes right through the pivot point, so the level arm of the force is zero, and $\tau_5 = \ell_5 F_5 = (0)F_5 = 0$.

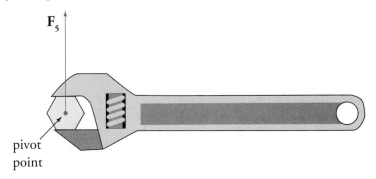

In general, if a force acts at the pivot or along a line through the pivot, then its torque is zero.

Example 5-12: A square metal plate (of side length s) rests on a flat table, and we exert a force $\mathbf{F}$ at one corner, parallel to one of the sides, as shown below. What is the torque of this force? (Use the center of the plate as the pivot point.)

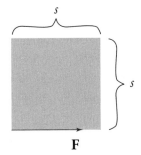

Solution: We'll calculate the torque of **F** by two different methods: first using the formula $\tau = rF \sin \theta$, and then using the formula $\tau = \ell F$.

Method 1. We draw in the **r** vector, which points from the pivot to the point where the force is applied. The angle between **r** and **F** can be taken to be $\theta = 45°$. If s is the length of each side of the square, then the length of **r** is $\frac{1}{2} s \sqrt{2}$ (because r is the hypotenuse of a 45°-45° right triangle, it's $\sqrt{2}$ times the length of each leg).

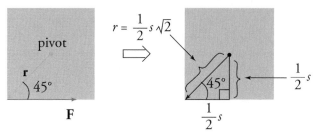

This gives $\tau = rF \sin \theta = \left(\frac{1}{2} s \sqrt{2}\right)(F) \sin 45° = \left(\frac{1}{2} s \sqrt{2}\right)(F)\left(\frac{\sqrt{2}}{2}\right) = \frac{1}{2} sF$.

Method 2. The line of action of the force **F** is simply the bottom side of the square. The perpendicular distance from the pivot to the side of the square is half the length of the square, $\frac{1}{2} s$, so this is the lever arm, ℓ.

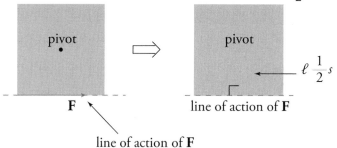

Therefore, $\tau = \ell F = \frac{1}{2} sF$

In this situation, the formula using the lever arm is the easier way to calculate the torque. That's because you can look at the diagram and see the length of the lever arm right away. If you find yourself having to *calculate* the length of the lever arm, you probably should just be using $\tau = rF \sin \theta$.

Example 5-13: Two children are sitting on a homogeneous seesaw that pivots at its center. One child has a mass m of 20 kg, and the other child has a mass M of 30 kg. If the child of mass M sits 1 m to the left of center, how far to the right of center must the child of mass m sit in order to keep the seesaw level?

Solution: In the figure just below, we draw the force vectors acting on the seesaw; these are the weights of the children.

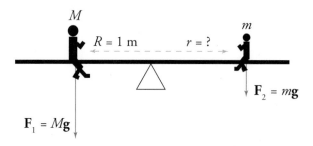

In order for the seesaw to balance, each child must produce the same amount of torque. The weight of the child on the left produces a torque that would cause counterclockwise rotation, so we'll call it a counter-clockwise (CCW) torque. The weight of the child on the right would cause clockwise rotation, so we'll call it a clockwise (CW) torque. If the torques have the same magnitude, the net torque will be zero and the seesaw will remain level.

Because $\mathbf{F}_1$ is perpendicular to $\mathbf{R}$, the CCW torque exerted by the child of mass M is

$$\tau_{CCW} = RF_1 = R \cdot Mg$$

and because $\mathbf{F}_2$ is perpendicular to $\mathbf{r}$, the CW torque exerted by the child of mass m is

$$\tau_{CW} = rF_2 = r \cdot mg$$

Setting these equal to each other (to balance the torques) will give us r:

$$\tau_{CW} = \tau_{CCW}$$
$$r \cdot mg = R \cdot Mg$$
$$r = R\frac{M}{m}$$
$$= (1 \text{ m})\frac{30 \text{ kg}}{20 \text{ kg}}$$
$$\therefore r = 1.5 \text{ m}$$

Notice that the weight of the seesaw itself exerts no torque. Since the seesaw is homogeneous, its center of gravity is at its center, which is where the pivot is; if a force acts *at* the pivot, then its r is zero, so the torque of the force is zero.

If you're thinking we could just have solved for the distance at which the center of mass of the system was at the fulcrum (pivot point) of the seesaw, you're right; we get the same answer either way.

Example 5-14: In the figure below, three blocks hang below a massless meter stick. Block m_1 hangs from the *20 cm* mark, block m_2 hangs from the *70 cm* mark, and block m_3 hangs from the *80 cm* mark. If $m_1 = 2$ kg, $m_2 = 5$ kg, and $m_3 = 3$ kg, at what mark on the meter stick should a string be attached so that this system would hang horizontally?

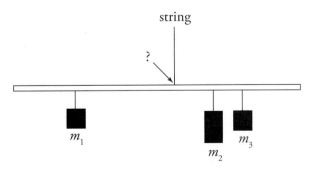

Solution: Look familiar? This is the same example we solved in the Center of Mass section. Let's see how we can answer this same question by balancing the torques. Let the pivot be the point where the string is attached to the stick. (Consider that the string is attached at the x cm mark, so that it's x cm from the left end of the stick.) Then the weight of mass m_1 produces a counterclockwise torque (τ_1), and the weights of m_2 and of m_3 each produce a clockwise torque (τ_2 and τ_3). If the counterclockwise torque (τ_1) balances the total clockwise torque ($\tau_2 + \tau_3$), the stick will remain level.

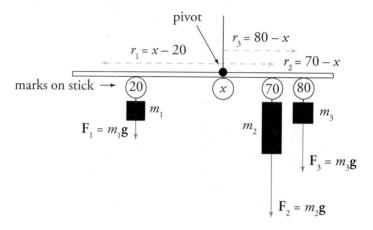

For each force, we need to find its corresponding r. For $\mathbf{F}_1$, we have $r_1 = (x - 20)$ cm; for $\mathbf{F}_2$, we have $r_2 = (70 - x)$ cm; and for $\mathbf{F}_3$, we have $r_3 = (80 - x)$ cm. The equation that balances the torques is

$$\tau_{CCW} = \tau_{CW}$$
$$r_1 \cdot m_1 g = r_2 \cdot m_2 g + r_3 \cdot m_3 g$$
$$r_1 m_1 = r_2 m_2 + r_3 m_3$$
$$(x - 20)(2 \text{ kg}) = (70 - x)(5 \text{ kg}) + (80 - x)(3 \text{ kg})$$
$$\therefore x = 63 \text{ cm}$$

This is the same answer we found before. (By the way, the torque exerted by the tension in the string is equal to zero [which is why we ignored it] because the tension acts *at* the pivot.)

Example 5-15: A homogeneous rectangular sheet of metal lies on a flat table and is able to rotate around an axis through its center, perpendicular to the table. Four forces, all of the same magnitude, are exerted on the sheet as shown below:

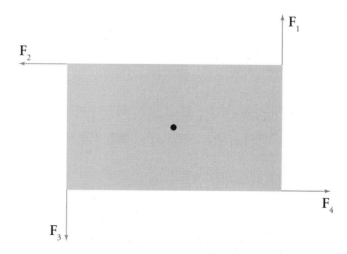

Which one of the following statements is true?

   A. The net force is zero, but the net torque is not.
   B. The net torque is zero, but the net force is not.
   C. Neither the net force nor the net torque is zero.
   D. Both the net force and the net torque equal zero.

Solution: There are two vertical forces that point in opposite directions (so they cancel), and two horizontal forces that point in opposite directions (so *they* cancel). Therefore, the net force, $F_{net} = F_1 + F_2 + F_3 + F_4$, is zero. Eliminate (B) and (C).

Now for the torques. In the figure below, each force has its corresponding lever arm. Notice that each force produces a counterclockwise (CCW) torque. As a result, the total, or net, torque cannot be zero. (The net torque is zero only when the total counterclockwise torque balances the total clockwise torque.) Therefore, the answer is (A).

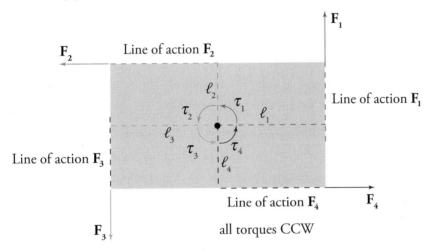

5.4 EQUILIBRIUM

As it's used in physics, the term **equilibrium** means *zero acceleration*. Notice that this does not mean zero velocity. As long as the velocity of the system remains constant (no change in speed or direction), then we can say that the system is in equilibrium. If the velocity happens to be zero, then we say the system is in **static** equilibrium.

There are actually two kinds of equilibrium, because there are two kinds of acceleration. There's *translational* equilibrium and *rotational* equilibrium. A system is said to be in **translational equilibrium** if the forces cancel; if $F_{net} = 0$, then the translational acceleration (*a*) is zero. A system is in **rotational equilibrium** if the torques cancel; if $\tau_{net} = 0$, then the rotational acceleration (denoted by α, the Greek letter *alpha*) is zero. If the term *equilibrium* is used without specifying which type, then it's assumed that the system is in *both* translational and rotational equilibrium.

Example 5-13 (the children on the seesaw) and Example 5-14 (the blocks balancing on the stick) both involved systems in equilibrium. In each case, we balanced the torques to ensure rotational equilibrium. We didn't explicitly analyze the translational equilibrium, but in the example of the children on the seesaw, the normal force exerted upward by the pivot balanced the total weight of the children, and in the example of the blocks hanging from the stick, the upward tension in the supporting string balanced the total weight of the blocks.

We'll now look at a couple of other examples of systems in equilibrium.

Example 5-16: A barber pole of mass 10 kg hangs from the end of a homogeneous rod of mass 40 kg that sticks out horizontally from the side of a vertical wall. The end of the rod, where the barber pole is attached, is connected to the upper part of the wall by a taut cable. For the angle θ, it is known that $\sin \theta = 0.6$ and $\cos \theta = 0.8$.

a)   What's the tension in the cable?
b)   What force is exerted by the wall on the rod?

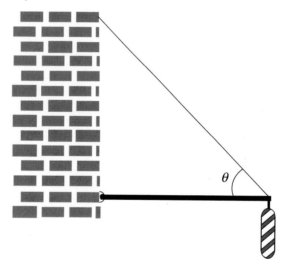

Solution:

a)   First, let's draw a diagram of all the forces acting on the rod.

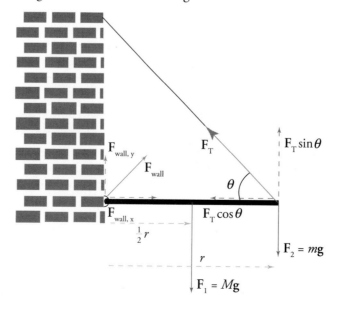

Notice that because the rod is in contact with the wall, the wall is exerting a force on the rod. However, at the start of the problem, we have no way of knowing what this force looks like (in other words, what either its magnitude or its direction are), so we break the force F_{wall} into a horizontal component and a vertical component. We do the same with the tension force, F_T, (which must act along the direction of the cable), and we can write these components as $F_{T,x} = F_T \cos \theta$ and $F_{T,y} = F_T \sin \theta$.

The system is in static equilibrium, so there must be no net torque and no net force. If we try to balance out all the forces, we find that we have too many unknowns. To balance the vertical forces, we'd write $F_{wall,y} + F_T \sin \theta = Mg + mg$, and to balance the horizontal forces, we'd write $F_{wall,x} = F_T \cos \theta$. We have three unknown ($F_{wall,x}$, $F_{wall,y}$, and F_T) but only two equations.

The trick is to balance the *torques* first and to choose our pivot to be the point of contact between the rod and wall. Notice that the torques of the components and the force exerted by the wall will both be zero (because they're applied *at* the pivot), so they won't even appear in the equation. As a result, our "balance-the-torques" equation will have just one unknown, F_T. That's why we chose to put the pivot point at the wall end of the rod: there are two unknown force components there, and only one at the other end.

So, with our pivot so chosen, we have three forces exerting torque: $\mathbf{F}_{T,y}$ produces a counterclockwise torque, and each of the weight vectors, $M\mathbf{g}$ and $m\mathbf{g}$, produces a clockwise torque. These torques balance to keep the rod level.

$$\tau_{CCW} = \tau_{CW}$$
$$r \cdot F_T \sin \theta = \tfrac{1}{2} r \cdot Mg + r \cdot mg$$
$$F_T \sin \theta = \tfrac{1}{2} Mg + mg$$
$$F_T = \frac{(\tfrac{1}{2}M + m)g}{\sin \theta}$$
$$= \frac{(\tfrac{1}{2} \cdot 40 \text{ kg} + 10 \text{ kg})(10 \text{ N/kg})}{0.6}$$
$$\therefore F_T = 500 \text{ N}$$

b)   Now that we've answered part (a) and found F_T, the tension in the cable, we can now find $F_{wall,x}$ and $F_{wall,y}$. We use the "balance-the-horizontal-forces" equation, $F_{wall,x} = F_T \cos \theta$, to get

$$F_{wall,x} = F_T \cos \theta = (500 \text{ N})(0.8) = 400 \text{ N}$$

Then we use the "balance-the-vertical-forces" equation to find $F_{wall,y}$:

$$F_{wall,y} + F_T \sin \theta = Mg + mg$$
$$F_{wall,y} = Mg + mg - F_T \sin \theta$$
$$= (40 \text{ kg})(10 \text{ N/kg}) + (10 \text{ kg})(10 \text{ N/kg}) - (500 \text{ N})(0.6)$$
$$\therefore F_{wall,y} = 200 \text{ N}$$

Finally, the magnitude of the force exerted by the wall on the rod can be found using the Pythagorean Theorem:

$$\left(F_{wall}\right)^2 = \left(F_{wall,x}\right)^2 + \left(F_{wall,y}\right)^2 \rightarrow F_{wall} = \sqrt{\left(F_{wall,x}\right)^2 + \left(F_{wall,y}\right)^2} \rightarrow F_{wall} = \sqrt{(400\,\text{N})^2 + (200\,\text{N})^2} \approx 447\,\text{N}$$

Whew! Let's now look at a problem that's more OAT-like in terms of the amount of calculation:

Example 5-17: In the figure below, a block of mass 40 kg is held in place by two ropes exerting equal tension forces. If $\cos\theta = 2/3$, what's the tension in each rope?

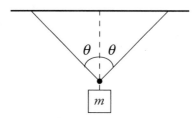

Solution: At the point where the mass is attached to the two ropes, we balance the forces. The horizontal forces automatically balance (we have $F_T \sin\theta$ pointing to the left and $F_T \sin\theta$ pointing to the right). For the vertical forces, we notice that there's the vertical component of the tension in the left-hand rope plus the vertical component of the tension in the right-hand rope ($F_T \cos\theta + F_T \cos\theta = 2F_T \cos\theta$), to balance out the weight of the block, mg. This gives us:

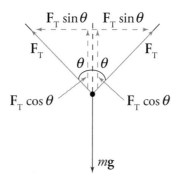

$$2F_T \cos\theta = mg$$

$$F_T = \frac{mg}{2\cos\theta}$$

$$= \frac{(40\,\text{kg})(10\,\text{N/kg})}{2\left(\frac{2}{3}\right)}$$

$$\therefore F_T = 300\,\text{N}$$

Summary of Formulas

Center of mass: $\quad x_{CM} = \dfrac{m_1 x_1 + m_2 x_2 + m_3 x_3 + \ldots}{m_1 + m_2 + m_3 + \ldots}$

Center of gravity: $\quad x_{CG} = \dfrac{w_1 x_1 + w_2 x_2 + w_3 x_3 + \ldots}{w_1 + w_2 + w_3 + \ldots}$

in uniform gravitational field (g constant), $x_{CM} = x_{CG}$

Centripetal acceleration: $\quad a_c = \dfrac{v^2}{r}$ (directed toward center of circle)

Centripetal force: $\quad F_c = ma_c = \dfrac{mv^2}{r}$

$$F_c = F_{\text{net towards center}}$$

Rotational Kinematics:

1. $\theta = \dfrac{1}{2}\left(\omega_0 + \omega\right)t$

2. $\omega = \omega_0 + \alpha t$

3. $\theta = \omega_0 t + \dfrac{1}{2}\alpha t^2$

4. $\theta = \omega t - \dfrac{1}{2}\alpha t^2$

5. $\omega^2 = \omega_0^2 + 2\alpha\theta$

6. $v = \omega r$

7. $a_t = \alpha r$

1 *rotation* (rot) = 1 *revolution* (rev) = 2π *rad* = 360°

Torque: $\qquad \tau = rF \sin\theta$ [θ = angle between **r** and **F**]

$\qquad\qquad \tau = \ell F$ [ℓ = lever arm of force]

Equilibrium: $\quad F_{net} = 0$ [translational equilibrium]

$\qquad\qquad \tau_{net} = 0$ [rotational equilibrium]

$\qquad\qquad$ static equilibrium means:

$\qquad\qquad\quad F_{net} = 0$

$\qquad\qquad\quad \tau_{net} = 0$

$\qquad\qquad\quad \mathbf{v} = 0$

Chapter 6
Energy and Momentum

6.1 WORK

Imagine a constant force **F** pushing a crate through a displacement **d**, as shown below:

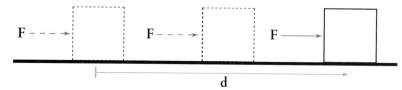

(Notice that the force **F** here doesn't just act momentarily at the initial position of the crate, with the crate then sliding across the floor with **F** removed; the force **F** is assumed to act constantly over the entire displacement.) We say that the **work** done by **F** is the product of F and d: Work $W = Fd$.

For example, if the magnitude of **F** is 20 N and the magnitude of **d** is 5 m, then the work done by the force **F** in the situation pictured above is (20 N)(5 m) = 100 N·m. When it's used to measure work, the newton-meter (N·m) is renamed the **joule**, abbreviated J. Therefore, we have $W = 100$ J.

The situation pictured above is quite special, however, because the vectors **F** and **d** point in the same direction. What if **F** and **d** do not point in the same direction? For example, what if we tie one end of a rope around the crate, sling the other end over our shoulder and pull the crate across the floor? Then our force **F** (which is actually the tension in the rope) will be at an angle to the displacement:

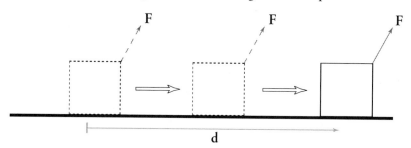

In this case, the work done by **F** is not the product of F and d. It's only the component of the force in the direction of **d** that does work. If θ is the angle between **F** and **d**, then the component of **F** that's parallel to **d** has magnitude $F \cos \theta$. Therefore, the work done by **F** is $(F \cos \theta)(d)$.

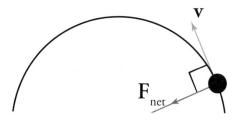

Work by a Constant Force, F

$$W = Fd \cos\theta$$

where θ = angle between **F** and **d**

Notice that the formula $W = Fd \cos \theta$ includes the formula $W = Fd$ as a special case. After all, if $\mathbf{F}$ and $\mathbf{d}$ do point in the same direction, then $\theta = 0$, and $\cos \theta = \cos 0 = 1$, so $Fd \cos \theta$ becomes Fd. Therefore, the formula $W = Fd \cos \theta$ covers all cases of a constant force $\mathbf{F}$ acting through a displacement $\mathbf{d}$.

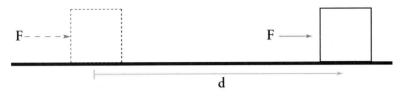

Example 6-1: In the situation pictured above, assume the mass of the crate, m, is 20 kg and the coefficient of kinetic friction between the crate and the floor is 0.4. If $F = 100$ N and $d = 6$ m,

a) How much work is done by $\mathbf{F}$?
b) How much work is done by the normal force?
c) How much work is done by gravity?
d) How much work is done by the force of friction?
e) What is the total work done on the crate?

Solution:

a) Because $\mathbf{F}$ is parallel to $\mathbf{d}$, the work done by $\mathbf{F}$ is simply $Fd = (100 \text{ N})(6 \text{ m}) = 600$ J.
b) The normal force is perpendicular to the floor, and to $\mathbf{d}$. Since the angle between $\mathbf{F}_N$ and $\mathbf{d}$ is $\theta = 90°$, and $\cos 90° = 0$, the work done by $\mathbf{F}_N$ is zero.
c) The gravitational force is also perpendicular to the floor, and to $\mathbf{d}$. Because the angle between $\mathbf{F}_{grav}$ and $\mathbf{d}$ is $\theta = 90°$, and $\cos 90° = 0$, the work done by $\mathbf{F}_{grav}$ is zero too.
d) First, since $F_N = mg = (20 \text{ kg})(10 \text{ N/kg}) = 200$ N, we have $F_f = \mu_k F_N = (0.4)(200 \text{ N}) = 80$ N. However, the direction of the vector $\mathbf{F}_f$ is opposite to the direction of $\mathbf{d}$, so the angle between $\mathbf{F}_f$ and $\mathbf{d}$ is $\theta = 180°$. Because $\cos 180° = -1$, the work done by the friction force is $(80 \text{ N})(6 \text{ m})(-1) = -480$ J.
e) To find the total work done on the crate, we just add up the work done by each of the forces that acts on the crate. In this case, then, we'd have

$$W_{total} = W_{by \, F} + W_{by \, F_N} + W_{by \, F_{grav}} + W_{by \, F_f} = (600 \text{ J}) + (0 \text{ J}) + (0 \text{ J}) + (-480 \text{ J}) = 120 \text{ J}$$

Here are a couple of things to notice about Example 6-1:

1) Although work depends on two vectors for its definition (namely, $\mathbf{F}$ and $\mathbf{d}$), work itself is *not* a vector. *Work is a scalar.* W may be positive, negative, or zero, but work has no direction.
2) In this example, there were four forces acting on the crate: the pushing force $\mathbf{F}$, gravity, the normal force, and friction. Each force does its own amount of work, which is why each part had to specify for which force we wanted the work. Only in the last part, where the total work is desired, can we omit the specific force we're looking at (because we're considering them all).

Example 6-2: In the situation described in Example 6-1, what is the net force on the crate? How much work is done by F_{net}?

Solution: The normal force cancels out the gravitational force, so the net force on the crate is just $\mathbf{F} + \mathbf{F}_f = (100 \text{ N}) + (-80 \text{ N}) = +20 \text{ N}$, where the + indicates that $\mathbf{F}_{net}$ points to the right. Now, since $\mathbf{F}_{net}$ is parallel to $\mathbf{d}$, the work done by $\mathbf{F}_{net}$ is just the product, $F_{net}d = (20 \text{ N})(6 \text{ m}) = 120 \text{ J}$. Notice that this is the same as the total amount of work done on the crate, as we figured out in part (e) of Example 6-1. This wasn't a coincidence. The total work done (found by adding up the values of the work done by each force separately) is always equal to the work done by the net force.

Remember that work is a scalar and it can be positive, zero, or negative. Now here's how to know *when* W will be positive, zero, or negative. Because $W = Fd \cos \theta$, and F and d are magnitudes (which means they're positive), the sign of W depends entirely on the sign of $\cos \theta$.

The diagrams below show the three cases.

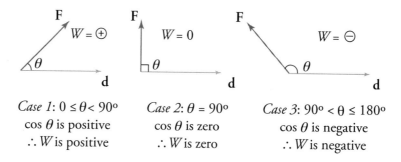

Case 1: $0 \leq \theta < 90°$
$\cos \theta$ is positive
$\therefore W$ is positive

Case 2: $\theta = 90°$
$\cos \theta$ is zero
$\therefore W$ is zero

Case 3: $90° < \theta \leq 180°$
$\cos \theta$ is negative
$\therefore W$ is negative

In Case 1, the angle between $\mathbf{F}$ and $\mathbf{d}$ is less than 90° (an acute angle); since the cosine of such an angle is positive, the work done by this force will be positive.

In Case 2, the angle between $\mathbf{F}$ and $\mathbf{d}$ is 90°; since the cosine of 90° is zero, the work done by this force will be zero.

In Case 3, the angle between $\mathbf{F}$ and $\mathbf{d}$ is greater than 90° (an obtuse angle); since the cosine of such an angle is negative, the work done by this force will be negative.

Example 6-1 illustrated all three cases. The force that pushed the crate across the floor did positive work; gravity and the normal force did zero work; and sliding friction did negative work.

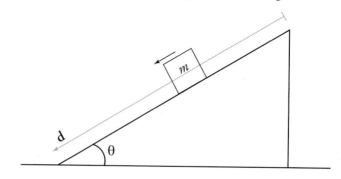

Example 6-3: In the situation pictured on the previous page, assume the mass of the block, m, is 20 kg and the coefficient of kinetic friction between the block and the ramp is 0.4. If d = 10 m and θ = 30°,

    a) How much work is done by the normal force?
    b) How much work is done by the force of friction?
    c) How much work is done by gravity?
    d) What is the total work done on the block?

Solution:

    a) The normal force is perpendicular to the ramp, and to **d**. Since the angle between $\mathbf{F}_N$ and **d** is θ = 90°, and cos 90° = 0, the work done by $\mathbf{F}_N$ is zero. Forces acting perpendicular to the direction of travel always do zero work.

    b) First, we know that since the block is on a ramp, we'll have $F_N = mg$ cos θ, where θ is the incline angle of the ramp. The magnitude of $\mathbf{F}_f$, the force of kinetic friction, is $\mu_k F_N$, so we get F_f = (0.4)(20 kg)(10 N/kg) cos 30°, which is approximately (0.4)(200 N)(0.85) = 68 N. Now, since the vectors $\mathbf{F}_f$ and **d** point in opposite directions (because **d** points down the ramp and $\mathbf{F}_f$ points up the ramp), the work done by $\mathbf{F}_f$ will be $-F_f d$ = –(68 N)(10 m) = –680 J.

    c) There are two ways we can answer this part. One way is to remember that the force due to gravity acting parallel to the ramp is mg sin θ, where θ is the incline angle. Since this component of the gravitational force is parallel to **d**, we can simply multiply mg sin θ by d to find the work done by gravity: W = $(mg$ sin $\theta)(d)$ = (20 kg)(10 N/kg)(sin 30°)(10 m) = 1000 J. Here's another way: the force $\mathbf{F}_{grav} = m\mathbf{g}$ points straight down, and the angle between $\mathbf{F}_{grav}$ and **d** is β, where β is the angle shown below. It's the complement of the incline angle θ; that is, $\beta = 90° - \theta$.

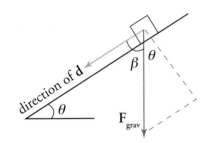

Since θ = 30°, we have β = 60°. Therefore, the work done by $\mathbf{F}_{grav}$ is $F_{grav} d$ cos β = mgd cos β = (20 kg)(10 N/kg)(10 m) (cos 60°) = 1000 J. You need to be very careful here; the formula for work reads, "$W = Fd$ cos θ," but the θ in this formula is *not* the same as the θ labeled in the figure. The angle in the formula for W is the angle between **F** and **d**, and this is not the same as the incline angle.

    d) To find the total work done on the block, we just add up the work done by each of the forces that acts on the block. In this case, then, we'd have

$$W_{total} = W_{by\ F_N} + W_{by\ F_f} + W_{by\ F_{grav}} = (0\,J) + (-680\,J) + (1000\,J) = 320\,J$$

6.2 POWER

Power measures how fast work gets done. For example, if a force does 100 J of work in 20 seconds, then work is being done at a *rate* of

$$\frac{100 \text{ J}}{20 \text{ s}} = 5 \text{ J/s}$$

This is the power.

We use the letter P to denote power, and from the sample calculation above, we can see that the unit of power is the joule-per-second. This unit has its own name: the **watt**, abbreviated W. Therefore, power is measured in watts: $[P] = \text{J/s} = \text{W}$. (Don't confuse the abbreviation for the watt, W, with the usual variable used for work, W.)

The term *watt* makes most of us think of light bulbs, but the watt is used to measure the power of anything, not just light bulbs. After all, should the unit *horsepower* make us think that only horses can provide power? By the way, 1 hp (1 horsepower) is equal to about 750 W.

The sample calculation above also shows us how we should define P in general:

Power

$$P = \frac{\text{work}}{\text{time}} = \frac{W}{t}$$

What if 100 J of work is done over a time interval of just 2 seconds? Then the power would be 50 W; it's easy to see that the faster work gets done, the greater the power.

A handy formula that you can also use to calculate P uses the fact that $v = d/t$:

$$P = \frac{W}{t} = \frac{Fd}{t} = F\frac{d}{t} = Fv \rightarrow P = Fv$$

(We're assuming here that **F** is parallel to **d**, so that $W = Fd$, and that the object's speed, v, is constant.) To see how this formula would be used, let's answer this question: How much power must be provided to a toy rocket of mass 50 kg to keep it moving upward at a constant speed of 40 m/s? Ignoring air resistance, the engine thrust must provide an upward force that's equal to the weight of the rocket: $F = mg = (50 \text{ kg})(10 \text{ N/kg}) = 500 \text{ N}$. Therefore, $P = Fv = (500 \text{ N})(40 \text{ m/s}) = 20,000 \text{ W} = 20 \text{ kW}$.

From the definition of power, we can see that

$$W = Pt$$

This equation is used as often on the OAT as the definition $P = W/t$. For example, if a machine has a power output of 200 W, how much work can it do in 1 hour? Multiplying power by time (and remembering to change 1 hour into $(60)(60) = 3600$ seconds) gives the work:

$$W = Pt = (200\,\text{W})(3600\,\text{s}) = 720,000\,\text{J} = 720\,\text{kJ}$$

Example 6-4: A force of magnitude 40 N pushes on an object of mass 8 kg through a displacement of 5 m for 10 seconds. What's the power provided by this force?

Solution: Power is equal to work divided by time, so

$$P = \frac{W}{t} = \frac{Fd}{t} = \frac{(40\,\text{N})(5\,\text{m})}{10\,\text{s}} = 20\,\text{W}$$

Example 6-5: You're lifting bricks, each with a mass of 2 kg, from the floor up to a shelf that is 1.5 m high.

a) How much work do you perform lifting each brick?
b) If you can place 20 bricks on the shelf every minute, what is your power output?

Solution:

a) The force you must provide to lift a brick is equal to the weight of the brick, which is $mg = (2\,\text{kg})(10\,\text{N/kg}) = 20\,\text{N}$. Since this force must act over a distance of 1.5 m to lift it up to the shelf, the work required is $W = Fd = (20\,\text{N})(1.5\,\text{m}) = 30\,\text{J}$.

b) If you can place 20 bricks on the shelf every 60 seconds, then on average you're lifting one brick every 3 seconds. If the work performed in 3 seconds is 30 J—as we found in part (a)— then your power output is

$$P = \frac{W}{t} = \frac{30\,\text{J}}{3\,\text{s}} = 10\,\text{W}$$

Example 6-6: A car of mass 2000 kg accelerates from rest to a speed of 30 m/s in 9 seconds. Given that the engine does a total of 900,000 J of work, what is the average power output of the car's engine?

Solution: Since we're given the amount of work done and the time interval, we can find the average power output of the engine simply by dividing work by time:

$$P = \frac{W}{t} = \frac{900,000\,\text{J}}{9\,\text{s}} = 100,000\,\text{W} = 100\,\text{kW}$$

Notice that neither the mass of the car, nor its final speed, were needed to answer the question because the required information (work and time) were given.

Example 6-7: One month, your electric bill states that you used 500 kWh of electricity, at a cost of 8¢ per kWh. What is a kWh, and how much is your electric bill that month?

Solution: A kilowatt (kW) is a thousand watts; it's a unit of power. An hour (h) is a time interval. Therefore, a kilowatt-hour, kWh, obtained by multiplying power times time, Pt, has units of work. (1 kWh = (1000 W)(3600 s) = 3.6×10^6 J = 3.6 MJ.) The electric company performed 500 kWh of work pushing and pulling the electrons within the wires in your home to make electrical devices function, at a cost to you of (500 kWh)(8¢/kWh) = \$40.

6.3 KINETIC ENERGY

An intuitive way to describe **energy** is that it's the ability to do work. Objects that move have this ability, since they can crash into something and thus exert a force over a distance. Therefore, objects that move have energy; specifically, we say they have **kinetic energy**, the energy due to motion.

To figure out how much kinetic energy a moving object has, imagine that an object of mass m is initially at rest (and thus has no kinetic energy). To get it moving, we have to exert a force **F** on it, over some distance d. (Let's assume, to keep things simple, that **F** points in the same direction as **d**.) How fast will the object be moving as a result? The acceleration is a constant $a = F/m$, so, using Big Five #5, we get

$$v^2 = v_0^2 + 2ad \;\rightarrow\; v^2 = 2ad \;\rightarrow\; v^2 = 2\frac{F}{m}d$$

Therefore, the final speed, v, will be $\sqrt{2Fd/m}$.

Now let's do a little algebra and rewrite the last equation above like this:

$$Fd = \tfrac{1}{2}mv^2$$

We recognize the product Fd as the work done by the force. So, we did work on the object to get it moving, and now because it's moving, it has kinetic energy. How much kinetic energy? This last equation tells us that we should consider the amount of kinetic energy to be $\frac{1}{2}mv^2$.

Kinetic Energy

$$KE = \tfrac{1}{2}mv^2$$

In words, this definition says that the kinetic energy of an object whose mass is m and whose speed is v is equal to one-half m times the square of the speed. Since $\frac{1}{2}mv^2$ is equal to the work Fd, we see right away that the unit of KE should also be the joule. In addition, like work, kinetic energy is a scalar.

6.3

Example 6-8: An object of mass 10 kg moves with a velocity of 4 m/s to the north. What is its kinetic energy? What would happen to the kinetic energy if the speed of the object doubled?

Solution: Kinetic energy is a scalar that cares only about the speed of an object; the direction of the object's velocity is irrelevant. So we find that

$$KE = \tfrac{1}{2}mv^2 = \tfrac{1}{2}(10\,\text{kg})(4\ \text{m/s})^2 = 80\,\text{J}$$

Because KE is proportional to v^2, if v were to increase by a factor of 2 then KE would increase by a factor of $2^2 = 4$.

The Work-Energy Theorem

The use of Big Five #5 shown above (to motivate the definition $KE = \tfrac{1}{2}mv^2$) assumed that the initial speed of the object was zero. But what if the initial speed wasn't zero? Then we'd have

$$v^2 = v_0^2 + 2ad \rightarrow v^2 - v_0^2 = 2ad \rightarrow \quad v^2 - v_0^2 = 2\frac{F}{m}d$$

$$\tfrac{1}{2}m(v^2 - v_0^2) = Fd$$

$$Fd = \tfrac{1}{2}mv^2 - \tfrac{1}{2}mv_0^2$$

$$W = KE_{\text{final}} - KE_{\text{initial}}$$

In other words, the total work done on the object is equal to the change in its kinetic energy. This fact is important enough that it's given a name:

> **Work-Energy Theorem**
>
> $$W_{\text{total}} = \Delta KE$$

This formula gives you another way to calculate work. You don't even need to know the force or the displacement! If you know the change in an object's kinetic energy, then you automatically know the total amount of work that was done on it.

Look back at the set of three diagrams showing when the work done by a force is positive, zero, or negative. In Case 1, the force is pulling in roughly the same direction as the object's displacement (more formally, the force **F** has a component that's in the same direction as **d**). We can think of such a force as "helping" the object move, and therefore causing its speed to increase. Is this consistent with the Work-Energy Theorem? Yes. This was the case of positive work being done, and according to the Work-Energy Theorem, positive work would automatically imply a positive change in kinetic energy. If the kinetic energy increases, then the speed increases.

Proven Techniques

In Case 3, the force is pulling in roughly the opposite direction from the object's displacement (more formally, the force **F** has a component that's in the opposite direction from **d**). We can think of such a force as "hindering" the object's motion, and therefore causing its speed to decrease. This is also consistent with the Work-Energy Theorem because Case 3 was the case of negative work being done, and according to the Work-Energy Theorem, negative work automatically implies a negative change in kinetic energy. If the kinetic energy decreases, then the speed decreases.

Example 6-9: An object of mass 10 kg whose initial speed is 4 m/s is accelerated until it achieves a final speed of 9 m/s.

a) How much work was done on this object?
b) If the acceleration took place over a displacement **d** of magnitude 13 m, and the force **F** exerted on it was constant and parallel to **d**, what was F?

Solution:

a) Although neither **F** nor **d** is given, we can still figure out the work done by using the Work-Energy Theorem:

$$W_{total} = \Delta KE$$
$$= KE_{fi} - KE$$
$$= \tfrac{1}{2}mv^2 - \tfrac{1}{2}mv_0^2$$
$$= \tfrac{1}{2}m(v^2 - v_0^2)$$
$$= \tfrac{1}{2}(10 \text{ kg})\left[\left(9 \text{ m/s}\right)^2 - \left(4 \text{ m/s}\right)^2\right]$$
$$\therefore W = 325 \text{ J}$$

b) Because **F** is parallel to **d**, we know that $W = Fd$. We just found W in part (a), and since we now know d, we can find F:

$$W = Fd \rightarrow F = \frac{W}{d} = \frac{325 \text{ J}}{13 \text{ m}} = 25 \text{ N}$$

Example 6-10: An object of mass 10 kg is moving at a speed of 9 m/s. How much work must be done on this object in order to stop it?

Solution: Once again, we're asked to find W without being given **F** and **d**, so we use the Work-Energy Theorem. If we want to stop the object, we want to bring its final kinetic energy to zero. Therefore,

$$W = \Delta KE$$
$$= \tfrac{1}{2}mv^2 - \tfrac{1}{2}mv_0^2$$
$$= 0 - \tfrac{1}{2}mv_0^2$$
$$= -\tfrac{1}{2}(10 \text{ kg})(9 \text{ m/s})^2$$
$$\therefore W = -405 \text{ J}$$

The work that must be done on the object has to be negative, because only negative work causes a decrease in speed.

Example 6-11: An object of mass 3 kg is undergoing uniform circular motion. The object's speed is 4 m/s, and the radius of the path is 0.5 m.

a) What's the magnitude of the net force on the object?
b) How much work is done by the net force during each revolution of the object?

Solution:

a) The net force on an object undergoing uniform circular motion (UCM) is the centripetal force:

$$F_c = m\frac{v^2}{r} = (3\,\text{kg})\frac{(4\ \text{m/s})^2}{0.5\ \text{m}} = 96\,\text{N}$$

b) We can answer this part in two ways. The centripetal force points toward the center of the circular path, so it's always perpendicular to the object's velocity:

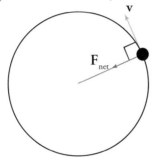

The work done by a force that's perpendicular to an object's motion is *zero* (remember Case 2 depicted in Section 6.1 (example 6-2): $\mathbf{F} \perp \mathbf{d}$ means $W = 0$).

Another way is to use the Work-Energy Theorem. Since the object's speed is constant, its kinetic energy is constant too. No change in kinetic energy means no work is being done.

Example 6-12: A box of mass 4 kg is initially at rest on a frictionless horizontal surface. A horizontal force **F** of magnitude 32 N is exerted on the object and then removed. If the speed of the object is then 2 m/s, over what distance did **F** act?

Solution: By the Work-Energy Theorem, the work done by **F** was

$$W = \Delta KE = KE_{fi} - KE = KE_f = \tfrac{1}{2}mv^2 = \tfrac{1}{2}(4\ \text{kg})(2\ \text{m/s})^2 = 8\ \text{J}$$

The question now is, "Given that **F** is parallel to **d** (so $W = Fd$), what's *d*?"

$$W = Fd \rightarrow d = \frac{W}{F} = \frac{8\,\text{J}}{32\,\text{N}} = 0.25\,\text{m}$$

Example 6-13: Consider the block described in Example 6-3. If the initial speed of the block was zero, what is the block's speed when it reaches the bottom of the ramp?

Solution: We figured out in part (d) of that example that the total work done on the block was 320 J. By the Work-Energy Theorem, we find that

$$W = \Delta KE = KE_f - KE_i = KE_f = \tfrac{1}{2}mv^2 \rightarrow v = \sqrt{\frac{2\ W_{total}}{m}} = \sqrt{\frac{2(320\ \text{J})}{20\,\text{kg}}} = \sqrt{32\ \text{m}^2/\text{s}^2} \approx 5.6\ \text{m/s}$$

Example 6-14: Consider the crate described in Example 6-1.

a)   If the initial speed of the crate was zero, what was the speed once the force **F** was removed after acting through the given displacement **d**?

b)   How far would the crate slide before coming to rest?

Solution:

a)   We figured out in part (e) of that example that the total work done on the crate was 120 J. The Work-Energy Theorem then tells us that

$$W = \Delta KE = KE_f - KE_i = KE_f = \tfrac{1}{2}mv^2 \rightarrow v = \sqrt{\frac{2\ W_{total}}{m}} = \sqrt{\frac{2(120\ \text{J})}{20\,\text{kg}}} = \sqrt{12\ \text{m}^2/\text{s}^2} \approx 3.5\ \text{m/s}$$

b)   Once the force **F** is removed, the only force acting on the crate that doesn't do zero work is friction. The work done by friction will be $-F_f d'$, where d' is the distance the crate will slide before coming to rest. By the Work-Energy Theorem, we have

$$W = \Delta KE = KE_f - KE_i = 0 - KE_i$$
$$-KE_i = -F_f d'$$
$$F_f d' = KE_i$$
$$d' = \frac{KE_i}{F_f}$$

Since the crate had 120 J of kinetic energy right when the force **F** was removed, and using the equation $F_f = \mu_k F_N = \mu_k mg$, we get

$$d' = \frac{KE_i}{F_f} = \frac{KE_i}{\mu_k mg} = \frac{120\ \text{J}}{(0.4)(20\ \text{kg})(10\ \text{N/kg})} = 1.5\,\text{m}$$

6.4 POTENTIAL ENERGY

In the preceding section, we defined kinetic energy as the energy an object has due to its motion. **Potential energy** is the energy an object has by virtue of its *position*. There are different "kinds" of potential energy because there are different kinds of forces. For example, in our study of OAT physics, we'll look at three types of potential energy: gravitational, electrical, and elastic. In this chapter, we'll study the first of these: *gravitational* potential energy.

Imagine a brick lying on the ground. Now, pick it up and place it on a shelf. You've just changed the position of the brick, and, since potential energy is the energy an object has by virtue of its position, you might expect that you've changed the brick's potential energy as well. You did. The brick's gravitational potential energy has been changed, because its position in a gravitational field has changed.

Now, let's be more specific. By *how much* did the brick's gravitational potential energy change? To find the answer, we need to look at the work done by the gravitational force (this is gravitational potential energy, after all). While the brick was being lifted, gravity did work on the brick. Let m be the mass of the brick, and let h be the height from the ground up to the shelf. The gravitational force on the brick is $\mathbf{F}_{\text{grav}} = m\mathbf{g}$, pointing downward; the displacement of the brick is h, upward.

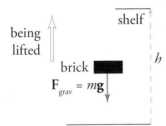

Because the force $\mathbf{F}_{\text{grav}}$ and the displacement $\mathbf{h}$ point in opposite directions, we know that the work done by $\mathbf{F}_{\text{grav}}$ will be the negative of F_{grav} times h: $W_{\text{by } F_{\text{grav}}} = -F_{\text{grav}}h = -mgh$. The change in gravitational potential energy is defined to be the opposite of the work done by the gravitational force:

$$\Delta PE_{\text{grav}} = -W_{\text{by } F_{\text{grav}}}$$

In this case, then, we have $\Delta PE_{\text{grav}} = -(-mgh) = mgh$. If the brick had *fallen* from the shelf to the floor, so that its height *decreased* by h, then we would have had $W_{\text{by } F_{\text{grav}}} = F_{\text{grav}}h = mgh$ and $\Delta PE_{\text{grav}} = -mgh$. In summary, then, we have

Change in Gravitational Potential Energy

$$\Delta PE_{\text{grav}} = \begin{cases} +mgh, & \text{if the height of } m \text{ is increased by } h \\ -mgh, & \text{if the height of } m \text{ is decreased by } h \end{cases}$$

where it's assumed that we're close enough to the surface of the earth that g can be considered a constant.

The formulas above give the *change* in the gravitational potential energy of an object of mass *m*. If we designate the ground as our "$PE_{grav} = 0$" level, then we can say that the gravitational potential energy of an object at height *h* is equal to *mgh*.

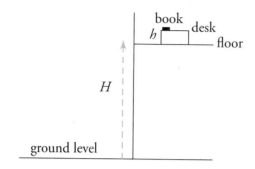

Potential energy is relative. Consider a book sitting on the desk in a second-floor office. Relative to the floor, the height of the book might be, say, half a meter. So, if the book has a mass of 1 kg, its gravitational potential energy is *mgh* = (1 kg)(10 N/kg)(0.5 m) = 5 J. But what if we were to measure the height of the book above the *ground*? Relative to the ground, the floor of the office might be at height *H* = 5 m, so the height of the book above the ground would be *H* + *h* = 5.5 m, and the book's gravitational potential energy is *mg*(*H* + *h*) = (1 kg)(10 N/kg)(5.5 m) = 55 J. Whenever we talk about "the" potential energy of an object, we must specify where we're choosing our "$PE = 0$" level.

The fact that potential energy is relative typically doesn't matter because it's only *changes* in potential energy that are important and physically meaningful. Let's go back to our book on the office desk example. If the book falls off the desk to the floor, what is the change in its potential energy? To the person who calls the floor of the office their "$PE = 0$" level, the change in the book's potential energy will be

$$\Delta PE_{grav} = PE_f - PE_i = 0 - mgh = -mgh = -(1\,kg)(10\,N/kg)(0.5\,m) = -5\,J$$

Now, to the person who calls the ground their "$PE = 0$" level, the change in the book's potential energy will be the same:

$$\Delta PE_{grav} = PE_f - PE_i = mgH - mg(H + h) = -mgh = -(1\,kg)(10\,N/kg)(0.5\,m) = -5\,J$$

Both people will always agree on the *change* in an object's potential energy, even if they disagree about what the potential energy *is* at a certain height (because they choose different "$PE = 0$" levels).

Example 6-15: A brick that weighs 25 N is lifted from the ground to a shelf that's 2 m high. What is its change in gravitational potential energy?

Solution: Because *mg* = 25 N, we have ΔPE_{grav} = *mgh* = (25 N)(2 m) = 50 J. Notice that since the brick was lifted *up*, its change in gravitational potential energy is *positive*.

Example 6-16: A 1 N apple in a tree is at height 4 m above the ground. The apple falls off its branch and lands on a branch that's only 1 m above the ground. What is the change in the apple's potential energy?

Solution: Because the apple *falls* through a distance of $h = 4 - 1 = 3$ m, the change in its gravitational potential energy is $-mgh = -(1 \text{ N})(3 \text{ m}) = -3$ J. We could also have answered the question like this: first, we choose, say, the ground to be our "$PE = 0$" level. Then the initial potential energy of the apple is $PE_i = mgh_i = (1 \text{ N})(4 \text{ m}) = 4$ J, and the final potential energy of the apple is $PE_f = mgh_f = (1 \text{ N})(1 \text{ m}) = 1$ J. The change in the potential energy is, therefore, $\Delta PE = PE_f - PE_i = (1 \text{ J}) - (4 \text{ J}) = -3$ J. Note that because the apple *falls*, the change in its gravitational potential energy must be *negative*.

Example 6-17: Which has more gravitational potential energy: an object of mass 2 kg at a height of 50 m, or an object of mass 50 kg at a height of 2 m? (Set $PE_{grav} = 0$ at the ground for both objects.)

Solution: Since the ground is the $PE_{grav} = 0$ level, then at height h an object's gravitational potential energy is $PE_{grav} = mgh$. The potential energy of the 2 kg object is

$$PE_1 = m_1 g h_1 = (2 \text{ kg})(10 \text{ N/kg})(50 \text{ m}) = 1000 \text{ J}$$

and the potential energy of the 50 kg object is

$$PE_2 = m_2 g h_2 = (50 \text{ kg})(10 \text{ N/kg})(2 \text{ m}) = 1000 \text{ J}$$

Therefore, these two objects have the *same* gravitational potential energy relative to the ground.

Gravity is a Conservative Force

Suppose we want to move a brick from the floor up to a shelf. One way we could do it would be to simply lift the brick straight up. Another way would be to set up a ramp and then push the brick up the ramp to the shelf. Let's figure out how much work gravity does in each of these cases. We'll assume that the brick has a mass of 3 kg and that the shelf is 2 m high.

The first case is easy. The gravitational force on the brick is $mg = (3 \text{ kg})(10 \text{ N/kg}) = 30$ N, directed straight downward. Since the displacement **h** of the brick is straight upward (that is, in the opposite direction from $\mathbf{F}_{grav}$), we know that the work done by gravity is negative F_{grav} times h:

$$W_{by \ F_{grav}} = -F_{grav} h = -(30 \text{ N})(2 \text{ m}) = -60 \text{ J}$$

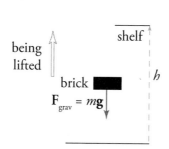
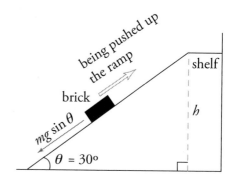

Now, let's look at the second case. Let's use a ramp whose incline angle θ is 30°. The gravitational force acting parallel to the ramp has magnitude $mg \sin \theta$, directed downward along the ramp. Because the displacement **d** is upward along the ramp (that is, in the opposite direction), we know the work done by gravity is negative, and equal to $-(mg \sin \theta)(d)$. Since the height of the shelf is $h = 2$ m, the length of the ramp (i.e., the hypotenuse of the right triangle) must be $d = h/(\sin \theta) = (2 \text{ m})/(\sin 30°) = 4$ m. Therefore, the work done by the gravitational force as the block is pushed up the ramp is

$$W_{\text{by F}_{\text{grav}}} = -(mg \sin \theta)(d) = -(30 \text{ N})(\sin 30°)(4 \text{ m}) = -(15 \text{ J})(4 \text{ m}) = -60 \text{ J}$$

This is the same answer as we found before! Since the change in the gravitational potential energy is defined to be the opposite of the work done by the gravitational force, $\Delta PE_{\text{grav}} = -W_{\text{by F}_{\text{grav}}}$, we can say that $\Delta PE_{\text{grav}} = -(-60 \text{ J}) = 60 \text{ J}$ in either case.

In the first case (lifting the brick straight upward), we exert a greater force over a smaller distance, while in the second case (moving the brick up a ramp), we exert a smaller force over a greater distance. However, the work done is the same in both cases.

These examples illustrate the following:

> *The work done by gravity*
>
> *depends only on the initial and final heights of the object,*
>
> *not on the path the object follows.*

Another way of saying this is to state that gravity is a **conservative** force. (In fact, it is the conservative nature of the gravitational force that allows us to define gravitational potential energy.)

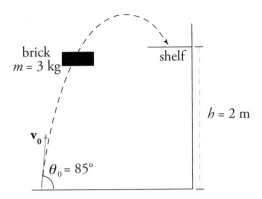

Example 6-18: In the situation pictured above, a brick is projected upward with an initial velocity $\mathbf{v}_0$ that makes an angle of 85° with the horizontal. The brick follows the path indicated and lands on the shelf. How much work did the gravitational force do on the brick?

Solution: The work done by gravity depends only on the initial and final positions of the object, not on the particular path the object takes. Since the initial height was $h_i = 0$ and the final height was $h_f = 2$ m, the change in the brick's gravitational potential energy is $\Delta PE_{grav} = mgh_f - mgh_i = mgh_f - 0 = mgh_f = (3\text{ kg})(10\text{ N/kg})(2\text{ m}) = 60$ J. Therefore, the work done by the gravitational force is

$$W_{by\ F_{grav}} = -\Delta PE_{grav} = -60\text{ J}$$

just as we found before.

Friction Is NOT a Conservative Force

Gravity is a conservative force because the work done by gravity depends only on the initial and final positions of the object, not on the path taken. We'll now show that friction is *not* a conservative force; the work done by kinetic friction *does* depend on the path taken.

Consider a flat tabletop and mark two points on it, A and B. We're going to slide a block from Point A to Point B along two different paths; the work done will be different for the two paths, which will show that friction is not a conservative force. The figure below shows the two points, A and B, separated by a distance of 5 m. Another way to get from A to B is to move from A to C and then from C to B; I've chosen a point C that's 3 m from A and 4 m from B.

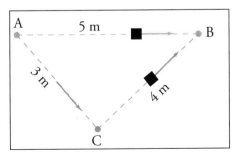

Assume the block has a mass of 1 kg; then its weight is $w = mg = (1 \text{ kg})(10 \text{ N/kg}) = 10 \text{ N}$, so the normal force on the block has magnitude 10 N also. If the coefficient of kinetic friction between the block and tabletop is 0.4, then, as the block slides, the magnitude of the force of kinetic friction is $F_f = \mu_k F_N = (0.4)(10 \text{ N}) = 4 \text{ N}$, always directed opposite to the direction in which the block is sliding.

Let's first figure out how much work friction does as we slide the block directly from A to B:

$$W_{\underset{A \to B}{\text{by } F_f}} = -F_f \cdot d_{A \to B} = -(4 \text{ N})(5 \text{ m}) = -20 \text{ J}$$

Now let's figure out how much work friction does as we slide the block from A to B by way of C:

$$W_{\underset{A \to C \to B}{\text{by } F_f}} = W_{\underset{A \to C}{\text{by } F_f}} + W_{\underset{C \to B}{\text{by } F_f}} = (-F_f \cdot d_{A \to C}) + (-F_f \cdot d_{C \to B}) = (-4 \text{ N})(3 \text{ m}) + (-4 \text{ N})(4 \text{ m}) = -28 \text{ J}$$

Even though we started at A and ended at B in both cases, we got a different amount of work done by friction for two different paths from A to B. Therefore, friction is *not* a conservative force. This means that there's no such thing as "frictional potential energy," because potential energy can be defined only for conservative forces.

6.5 TOTAL MECHANICAL ENERGY

Now that we've defined kinetic energy and potential energy, we can define an object's **total mechanical energy**, E. It's just the sum of the object's kinetic energy and potential energy:

> **Total Mechanical Energy**
> $$E = KE + PE$$

For example, consider an object of mass m sitting on a shelf that's at height h above the floor. Then, relative to the floor (where we'll set PE_{grav} equal to 0), the object's total mechanical energy is

$$E = KE + PE = 0 + mgh = mgh$$

Now, what if this same object falls off the shelf? What is its total mechanical energy when its height is, say, $h/2$? If v is the object's speed at this point, then the object's total mechanical energy is

$$E = KE + PE = \frac{1}{2}mv^2 + mg\frac{h}{2}$$

Example 6-19: An object of mass m is projected straight upward with an initial speed of v_0 at time $t = 0$.

a) What is the object's total mechanical energy at time $t = 0$?
b) At what time t will the object reach its maximum height?
c) What is the maximum height?
d) What is the object's total mechanical energy at this point?

Solution:

a) If we take the object's height at $t = 0$ to be $h = 0$, then its initial total mechanical energy is

$$E = KE + PE = \frac{1}{2}mv_0^2 + mg(0) = \frac{1}{2}mv_0^2$$

b) When the object reaches the highest point in its vertical path, its velocity is 0. Using Big Five #2 with $a = -g$, we find that

$$v = v_0 + at \;\rightarrow\; 0 = v_0 + (-g)t \;\rightarrow\; t = \frac{v_0}{g}$$

Applied Strategies

c) Using Big Five #5, we can find the object's maximum height:

$$v^2 = v_0^2 + 2ad \;\rightarrow\; (0)^2 = v_0^2 + 2(-g)d \;\rightarrow\; d = -\frac{v_0^2}{2(-g)} = \frac{v_0^2}{2g}$$

d) The object's total mechanical energy at this point is

$$E = KE + PE = \frac{1}{2}mv^2 + mgh = \frac{1}{2}m(0)^2 + mg\left(\frac{v_0^2}{2g}\right) = 0 + m\frac{v_0^2}{2} = \frac{1}{2}mv_0^2$$

Notice in this example that the answer to part (d) is the same as the answer to part (a): the object's total mechanical energy at its highest point is the same as it was at the object's initial point. This illustrates a very important concept: the **Conservation of Total Mechanical Energy**. If the only forces acting on an object during its motion are conservative (that means, for example, *no friction*), then the object's total mechanical energy will remain throughout the motion. Pick any two positions (or times) during the object's motion; for example, we could pick the initial position (initial time) and the final position (final time). Then

$$E_i = E_f$$

Writing E as $KE + PE$, we have

> ## Conservation of Total Mechanical Energy (no outside forces)
>
> $$KE_i + PE_i = KE_f + PE_f$$

Example 6-20: An object of mass m is projected straight upward with an initial speed of v_0 at time $t = 0$. Use Conservation of Total Mechanical Energy to find its maximum height.

Solution: If we take the object's height at $t = 0$ to be $h = 0$, then its initial total mechanical energy is

$$E = KE_i + PE_i = \tfrac{1}{2}mv_0^2 + mgh = \tfrac{1}{2}mv_0^2 + mg(0) = \tfrac{1}{2}mv_0^2$$

When the object reaches the highest point in its vertical path, its velocity is 0. Calling this height h, the object's total mechanical energy at this point is

$$E = KE_f + PE_f = \tfrac{1}{2}mv_0^2 + mgh = \tfrac{1}{2}m(0)^2 + mgh = mgh$$

Therefore, by Conservation of Total Mechanical Energy, we have

$$E_i = E_f$$

$$\frac{1}{2}mv_0^2 = mgh$$

$$\therefore h = \frac{v_0^2}{2g}$$

This is the same answer we found in Example 6-19(c) using the Big Five equations.

Another way to think about this problem is in terms of an energy *transfer*. At the moment the object was shot upward, it had only KE; at the top of its path, however, it has only PE. In other words, kinetic energy was transferred (or transformed) into gravitational potential energy:

$$KE \rightarrow PE \rightarrow \quad \frac{1}{2}mv_0^2 = mgh \quad \rightarrow \quad \therefore h = \frac{v_0^2}{2g}$$

It can be very helpful to think of Conservation of Total Mechanical Energy in terms of energy transfers between KE and PE. (The OAT likes to ask questions about such energy transfers.)

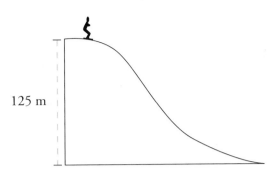

6.5

Example 6-21: A skier begins at rest at the top of a hill of height 125 m. If friction between her skis and the snow is negligible, what will be her speed at the bottom of the hill?

Solution: Let the bottom of the hill be $h = 0$, and call the top of the hill the skier's initial position and the bottom of the hill her final position. Then we have

$$KE_i + PE_i = KE_f + PE_f$$
$$0 + mgh = \tfrac{1}{2}mv^2 + 0$$
$$v = \sqrt{2gh}$$
$$= \sqrt{2(10 \text{ m/s}^2)(125 \text{ m})}$$
$$\therefore v = 50 \text{ m/s}$$

We could also think about this problem in terms of an energy transfer. At the top of the hill, the skier had only *PE*; at the bottom of the hill, she has only *KE*. In other words, gravitational potential energy was transferred (or transformed) into kinetic energy:

$$PE \rightarrow KE \rightarrow mgh = \tfrac{1}{2}mv_0^2 \rightarrow \therefore v = \sqrt{2gh}$$

Example 6-22: A roller-coaster car drops from rest down the track and enters a loop. If the radius of the loop is R, and the initial height of the car is $5R$ above the bottom of the loop, how fast is the car going at the top of the loop? Assume that $R = 15$ m and ignore friction.

Solution: Let's call the bottom of the loop our $h = 0$ level. At the car's initial position, we have $h_i = 5R$ and $v_i = 0$ (so $KE_i = 0$). At the top of the loop (the "final" position, for purposes of this question), we have $h_f = 2R$. The question is to find the car's speed, v, at this point. Using Conservation of Total Mechanical Energy, we get

$$KE_i + PE_i = KE_f + PE_f$$
$$0 + mgh_i = \tfrac{1}{2}mv^2 + mgh_f$$
$$gh_i = \tfrac{1}{2}v^2 + gh_f$$
$$v = \sqrt{2g(h_i - h_f)}$$
$$= \sqrt{2g(5R - 2R)}$$
$$= \sqrt{2g \cdot 3R}$$
$$= \sqrt{2(10 \text{ m/s}^2) \cdot 3(15 \text{ m})}$$

$$\therefore v = 30 \text{ m/s}$$

For extra practice, show that the car's speed when it's at the "9 o'clock" position within the loop is $\sqrt{1200}$ m/s ≈ 35 m/s, and that the car's speed when it's at the bottom of the loop is $\sqrt{1500}$ m/s ≈ 39 m/s.[1]

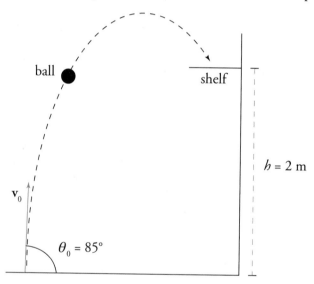

Example 6-23: In the situation pictured above, a ball is projected upward from the floor with an initial velocity v_0 of magnitude 12 m/s that makes an angle of 85° with the horizontal. The ball follows the path indicated and lands on the shelf. How fast is the ball traveling as it hits the shelf? (Ignore air resistance.)

---

[1] For even more practice, compute the centripetal acceleration at these points, and show that the amusement park operator is in danger of being sued. (As a benchmark, consider that fighter pilots with the benefit of pressurized suits risk blacking out at accelerations greater than about $9g \approx 88$ m/s^2.)

Solution: Let's call the floor our $h = 0$ level. At the object's initial position, we have $h_i = 0$ (so $PE_i = 0$). At the shelf (the final position), we have $h_f = 2$ m. The question is to find the speed of the ball, v, at this point. Using Conservation of Total Mechanical Energy, we get

$$KE_i + PE_i = KE_f + PE_f$$
$$\tfrac{1}{2}mv_0^2 + 0 = \tfrac{1}{2}mv^2 + mgh_f$$
$$\tfrac{1}{2}v_0^2 = \tfrac{1}{2}v^2 + gh_f$$
$$v = \sqrt{v_0^2 - 2gh_f}$$
$$= \sqrt{(12 \text{ m/s})^2 - 2(10 \text{ m/s}^2)(2\,\text{m})}$$
$$\therefore v \approx 10 \text{ m/s}$$

6.5

Notice that the direction of the initial velocity vector (given to be "at an angle of 85° with the horizontal") was irrelevant here. One of the most useful attributes of solving problems by Conservation of Total Mechanical Energy is that KE, PE, and E are all *scalars*. This makes it easier to solve questions because we don't have to worry about direction.

Using the Energy Method when There Is Friction

If friction acts during an object's motion, then total mechanical energy is no longer conserved. Consider this example. Let's say we give a block of mass 2 kg an initial speed of 6 m/s across a flat surface, where the coefficient of kinetic friction between the block and the surface is $\mu_k = 0.2$.

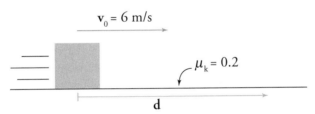

Kinetic friction will do work as the block slides. If d is the distance the block slides, then the work done by friction will be

$$W_{\text{by } F_f} = -F_f \cdot d = -\mu_k F_N d = -\mu_k mgd = -(0.2)(2 \text{ kg})(10 \text{ N/kg})d = -(4 \text{ N})d$$

In particular, when $d = 9$ m, the work done by friction will be

$$W_{\text{by } F_f} = -(4\,\text{N})d = -(4\,\text{N})(9\,\text{m}) = -36\,\text{J}$$

Since the initial kinetic energy of the block was

$$KE_i = \tfrac{1}{2}mv_0^2 = \tfrac{1}{2}(2\,\text{kg})(6 \text{ m/s})^2 = 36\,\text{J}$$

then the Work-Energy Theorem tells us that the final kinetic energy of the block will be 0:

$$W = \Delta KE = KE_f - KE_i \rightarrow KE_f = KE_i + W = \left(36\,J\right) + \left(-36\,J\right) = 0\,J$$

The block lost KE (and, therefore, E) as it moved because of friction. So, when friction acts, total mechanical energy is not a constant; in other words, it's not conserved.

Despite the fact that total mechanical energy is no longer conserved if friction acts, we can use a *modified* version of the Conservation of Total Mechanical Energy equation to handle questions with friction (or any force besides gravity). We can write this modified equation either in the form

$$\boxed{E_i + W_{by\,F} = E_f}$$

or as:

**Conservation of Total Mechanical Energy
(with outside forces)**

$$KE_i + PE_i + W_{by\,F} = KE_f + PE_f$$

Since $W_{by\,F_f}$ is negative, E_f will be less than E_i, just as we expect, since friction takes away mechanical energy.

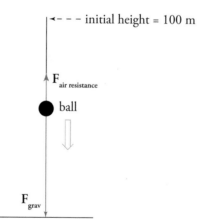

Example 6-24: A ball of mass 2 kg is dropped from a height of 100 m. As it falls, the ball feels an average force of air resistance of magnitude 4 N. What is the ball's speed as it strikes the ground?

Solution: Let's call the ground our $h = 0$ level. At the object's initial position, we have $h_i = 100$ m and $v_0 = 0$ (so $KE_i = 0$). As it hits the ground (the final position), we have $h_f = 0$ m (so $PE_f = 0$). The question is to find the speed of the ball, v, as it strikes the ground. Because the air resistance is given, and air resistance is friction exerted by the air on the moving object, we need to use the modified version of the energy equation, the one that includes the work done by friction.

Let's figure out the work done by the force of air resistance. Since the displacement of the ball is downward, the force of air resistance is upward; the opposite direction. This tells us that the work done by air resistance is negative, as we expect:

$$W_{\text{by } F_f} = -F_f \cdot h = -(4\,\text{N})(100\,\text{m}) = -400\,\text{J}$$

Therefore, using the modified equation for Conservation of Total Mechanical Energy, we find that

$$KE_i + PE_i + W_{\text{by } F_f} = KE_f + PE_f$$
$$0 + mgh + (-400\,\text{J}) = \tfrac{1}{2}mv^2 + 0$$
$$v = \sqrt{2gh - \frac{800\,\text{J}}{m}}$$
$$= \sqrt{2(10\ \text{m/s}^2)(100\,\text{m}) - \frac{800\,\text{J}}{2\,\text{kg}}}$$
$$= \sqrt{1600\ \text{m}^2/\text{s}^2}$$
$$v = 40\ \text{m/s}$$

Without air resistance, you can check that the ball's speed at impact would have been greater:

$$\sqrt{2000\ \text{m}^2/\text{s}^2} \approx 45\ \text{m/s}$$

6.6 MOMENTUM

For an object of mass m moving with velocity $\mathbf{v}$, we define the object's **momentum**, $\mathbf{p}$, as the product of m and $\mathbf{v}$. Notice that because $\mathbf{v}$ is a vector, momentum is a vector, too, pointing in the same direction as $\mathbf{v}$ (because m is always a *positive* scalar).

Momentum

$$\mathbf{p} = m\mathbf{v}$$

The SI unit of momentum is just the kg·m/s; there's no special name for it.

Example 6-25: A car whose mass is 2000 kg is traveling at a velocity of 15 m/s due east. What is its momentum? How does its momentum compare to that of a car whose mass is 2000 kg traveling at a velocity of 15 m/s due west?

Solution: Since $\mathbf{p} = m\mathbf{v}$, we have $\mathbf{p} = (2000\ \text{kg})(15\ \text{m/s, east}) = 30,000\ \text{kg·m/s, east}$. If we call *east* the positive direction, then we can write $\mathbf{p} = +30,000$ kg·m/s. For the car traveling west, the magnitude of its momentum will be the same, 30,000 kg·m/s, but the direction of its momentum will be to the west. So, if *east* is again the positive direction, then *west* is the negative direction, and we'd write $\mathbf{p} = -30,000$ kg·m/s. Remember, momentum is a vector, and its direction must be taken into account.

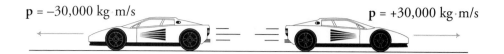

p = −30,000 kg·m/s   p = +30,000 kg·m/s

Example 6-26: An object of mass m is moving with velocity **v**. What will happen to its momentum if v doubles? What will happen to its kinetic energy?

Solution: Momentum has something in common with kinetic energy: namely, only moving objects have it. Also, the more massive an object, or the greater its velocity, the greater its momentum (and kinetic energy). However, there are two important differences. First, kinetic energy is a scalar, while momentum is a vector. Second, kinetic energy is proportional to v^2 whereas the magnitude of momentum is proportional only to v. So, if the object's speed doubles, then its momentum doubles while its kinetic energy increases by a factor of 4.

Now that we've defined momentum, let's see how it applies to the OAT.

Impulse

Let's say we exert a force **F** on an object of mass m over a time interval Δt. We can use Newton's Second Law, **F** = m**a**, to predict the effect of this force. Because **a** = Δ**v**/Δt, we can rewrite **F** = m**a** as

$$\mathbf{F} = m\frac{\Delta \mathbf{v}}{\Delta t}$$

Multiplying both sides by Δt gives

$$\mathbf{F}\Delta t = m\Delta \mathbf{v}$$

If the object's mass remains constant, then $m\Delta \mathbf{v}$ is the same as $\Delta(m\mathbf{v})$, so we get

$$\mathbf{F}\Delta t = \Delta(m\mathbf{v})$$

We now recognize the quantity on the right-hand side as Δ**p**, the change in momentum. The quantity on the left-hand side, force multiplied by time, is called **impulse**, denoted by **J**. (Don't confuse the variable for impulse, **J**, with the abbreviation for the joule, J.) So, this last equation can be written simply as **J** = Δ**p**. This alternative way of expressing Newton's Second Law is known as the

> ### Impulse-Momentum Theorem
> $$\mathbf{J} = \Delta\mathbf{p} = \Delta(m\mathbf{v}) = \mathbf{F}\Delta t$$

Example 6-27: A batter strikes a pitched baseball (mass = 0.15 kg) that was moving horizontally at 40 m/s, and it leaves his bat moving at speed of 50 m/s directly back toward the pitcher. The bat was in contact with the baseball for 15 ms.

6.6

a) What's the baseball's change in momentum?
b) What's the impulse of the force exerted by the batter?
c) What's the magnitude of the average force exerted by the bat on the ball?

Solution:

a) Since we're dealing with momentum, which is a vector, we need to define our positive direction. Let's choose *toward the pitcher* as the positive direction. This means that the initial momentum of the baseball (the momentum it had on its way from the pitcher to the batter) was negative, and the final momentum of the baseball (which is its momentum after the batter hits it) is positive. This gives

$$\mathbf{p}_i = m\mathbf{v}_i = \left(0.15\,\text{kg}\right)\left(-40\ \text{m/s}\right) = -6\ \text{kg}\cdot\text{m/s} \text{ and } \mathbf{p}_f = m\mathbf{v}_f = \left(0.15\,\text{kg}\right)\left(+50\ \text{m/s}\right) = 7.5\ \text{kg}\cdot\text{m/s}$$

So the change in the baseball's momentum is

$$\Delta\mathbf{p} = \mathbf{p}_f - \mathbf{p}_i = \left(+7.5\ \text{kg}\cdot\text{m/s}\right) - \left(-6\ \text{kg}\cdot\text{m/s}\right) = +13.5\ \text{kg}\cdot\text{m/s}$$

b) Impulse is equal to force multiplied by the time during which it acts. However, we are not told what the force is; in fact, we're asked that in part (c). So we need another way of figuring out the impulse. The Impulse-Momentum Theorem tells us that the impulse is equal to the change in momentum, which we just computed in part (a). Since $\Delta p = +13.5$ kg·m/s, this is also the impulse of the force. (We can also write the unit as a newton-second, N·s, which is the most natural unit for impulse: $J = F\Delta t$ implies that $[J] = [F][\Delta t] = $ N·s. However, the unit of momentum, kg·m/s, is the same as the unit of impulse, N·s, so we could say that $J = +13.5$ N·s.)

c) Now that we know J, we can use the definition $J = F\Delta t$ to find F:

$$J = F\Delta t \ \rightarrow \ F = \frac{J}{\Delta t} = \frac{13.5\,\text{N}\cdot\text{s}}{0.015\,\text{s}} = 900\,\text{N}$$

Because F usually varies while it acts, this is actually the *average* force exerted by the bat. To be more precise, we should place a bar over the F and write the definition of impulse as $J = \overline{F}\Delta t$.

Example 6-28: The graph at the right shows how a force **F** acting on an object of mass $m = 1$ kg varies as a function of time.

a) What is the magnitude of the impulse of this force?
b) If the object's initial velocity is +2 m/s, what will be the object's velocity after this force acts?

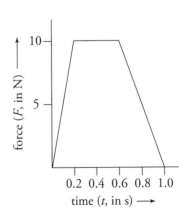

Solution:

a) Because impulse is equal to force × time, the area under a force vs. time graph gives the impulse. (Compare this to the statement from Chapter 1 that "The area under a velocity vs. time graph gives the displacement.") The area under the graph shown can be split into two right triangles and a rectangle, so the total area under the graph is

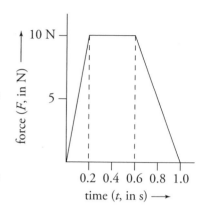

$$\text{area} = (\text{first triangle}) + (\text{rectangle}) + (\text{second triangle})$$
$$= \tfrac{1}{2}(0.2\,\text{s})(10\,\text{N}) + (0.6\,\text{s} - 0.2\,\text{s})(10\,\text{N}) + \tfrac{1}{2}(1\,\text{s} - 0.6\,\text{s})(10\,\text{N})$$
$$= (1\,\text{N}\cdot\text{s}) + (4\,\text{N}\cdot\text{s}) + (2\,\text{N}\cdot\text{s})$$
$$\therefore J = 7\,\text{N}\cdot\text{s}$$

b) The Impulse-Momentum Theorem says $\mathbf{J} = \Delta\mathbf{p} = \mathbf{p}_f - \mathbf{p}_i$, so

$$\mathbf{p}_f = \mathbf{p}_i + \mathbf{J} \rightarrow mv_f = mv_i + \mathbf{J}$$
$$\mathbf{v}_f = \mathbf{v}_i + \frac{\mathbf{J}}{m}$$
$$= (+2 \text{ m/s}) + \frac{7\,\text{N}\cdot\text{s}}{1 \text{ kg}}$$
$$= (+2 \text{ m/s}) + (7 \text{ m/s})$$

$$\therefore \mathbf{v}_f = +9 \text{ m/s}$$

Conservation of Momentum

Consider a pair of objects, 1 and 2, that exert forces (an action/reaction pair) on each other. Let $\mathbf{F}_{1\text{-on-}2}$ be the force exerted by Object 1 on Object 2, let $\mathbf{F}_{2\text{-on-}1}$ be the force exerted by Object 2 on Object 1, and let Δt be the time during which these forces act.

What's the impulse delivered by $\mathbf{F}_{1\text{-on-}2}$? It's $\mathbf{J}_{1\text{-on-}2} = \mathbf{F}_{1\text{-on-}2}\Delta t$.

What's the impulse delivered by $\mathbf{F}_{2\text{-on-}1}$? It's $\mathbf{J}_{2\text{-on-}1} = \mathbf{F}_{2\text{-on-}1}\Delta t$.

Now, since $\mathbf{F}_{1\text{-on-}2} = -\mathbf{F}_{2\text{-on-}1}$ by Newton's Third Law, we'll automatically have $\mathbf{J}_{1\text{-on-}2} = -\mathbf{J}_{2\text{-on-}1}$.

Okay, so the impulses are equal but opposite. What will that do? By the Impulse-Momentum Theorem, we know that $\mathbf{J}_{1\text{-on-}2} = \Delta\mathbf{p}_2$, where $\Delta\mathbf{p}_2$ is the change in momentum of Object 2, and that $\mathbf{J}_{2\text{-on-}1} = \Delta\mathbf{p}_1$, where $\Delta\mathbf{p}_1$ is the change in momentum of Object 1. So, because $\mathbf{J}_{1\text{-on-}2} = -\mathbf{J}_{2\text{-on-}1}$, we have

$$\Delta\mathbf{p}_2 = -\Delta\mathbf{p}_1$$

Therefore, the momentum changes if the two objects are equal but opposite too.

Now what if we ask, what's the change in momentum of both objects *together*? That is, what's $\Delta(\mathbf{p}_1 + \mathbf{p}_2)$? Well, if $\Delta\mathbf{p}_1$ and $\Delta\mathbf{p}_2$ are equal but opposite, then the total change in momentum is zero:

$$\Delta\mathbf{p}_2 + \Delta\mathbf{p}_1 \rightarrow \Delta\mathbf{p}_1 + \Delta\mathbf{p}_2 = 0 \rightarrow \Delta(\mathbf{p}_1 + \mathbf{p}_2) = 0$$

If the total momentum, $\mathbf{p}_1 + \mathbf{p}_2$, doesn't change, then it's a constant. We say that the total momentum is *conserved*.

In summary, what is shown above is simply that Newton's Third Law implies that when two objects interact only with each other, their total momentum doesn't change. That is, the total momentum *of the system* doesn't change. In fact, we could have any number of mutually interacting objects, not just two, and the result would be the same: the total momentum of the system will remain constant. This fact has the same stature as the Law of Conservation of Total Mechanical Energy, and it's called the Law of Conservation of Momentum:

6.6

Law of Conservation of Momentum

$$\Delta\mathbf{p}_{\text{system}} = 0$$

or

$$\text{total } \mathbf{p}_i = \text{total } \mathbf{p}_f$$

This law says that if a system of interacting objects feels no net external force (that is, if the forces the objects feel are only from other objects within the system) then the total momentum of the system will remain constant. The *individual* momenta of the objects in the system certainly can change, but always in such a way that their sum, the total momentum of all the objects, *doesn't* change. The second form of the law, total $\mathbf{p}_i$ = total $\mathbf{p}_f$, simply says that if we find the total momentum of an isolated system at one moment and then find the total momentum of the system at some later time, we'll get the same answer. We'll usually find it more convenient to use this second form when we solve problems, but of course, the two forms of the law say exactly the same thing.

Strictly speaking, the quantity $\mathbf{p} = m\mathbf{v}$ is known as **linear momentum**, so the law "$\Delta\mathbf{p}_{\text{system}} = 0$" or "total $\mathbf{p}_i$ = total $\mathbf{p}_f$" is known as the Law of Conservation of Linear Momentum. (There's another kind of momentum studied in physics: *angular momentum*. Since we rarely worry about this type of momentum for the OAT, we just use the word "momentum" for "linear momentum.")

Example 6-29: An astronaut (total mass, body + suit + equipment = 101 kg) is floating at rest in deep space near her ship, when she notices that the cord that's supposed to keep her connected to the ship has broken. She reaches into her pocket, finds a metal tool of mass 1 kg and throws it out into space with a velocity of 10 m/s, directly away from the ship. If she's 5 m away from the ship, how long will it take her to reach it?

Solution: Consider the astronaut and the metal tool as the system. Initially, both are at rest, so their total momentum is zero. Because of the Law of Conservation of Momentum, $\Delta\mathbf{p}_{system} = 0$, we know that after the astronaut throws the tool, the total momentum will still be zero:

$$m_{astronaut}\mathbf{v}'_{astronaut} + m_{tool}\mathbf{v}'_{tool} = 0$$

We can now solve for the astronaut's velocity after throwing the tool:

$$m_{astronaut}\mathbf{v}'_{astronaut} = -m_{tool}\mathbf{v}'_{tool}$$

$$\mathbf{v}'_{astronaut} = -\frac{m_{tool}\mathbf{v}'_{tool}}{m_{astronaut}}$$

$$= -\frac{(1\text{ kg})(-10\text{ m/s})}{100\text{ kg}}$$

$$\therefore \mathbf{v}'_{astronaut} = 0.1\text{ m/s}$$

The minus sign on $\mathbf{v}'_{tool}$ simply indicates that we're calling *away from the ship* the negative direction; as a result, the astronaut's velocity is in the opposite direction, toward the ship and positive. Now, the question is, traveling at a rate of 0.1 m/s, how long will it take her to move the 5 m to the ship? Using distance = rate × time, we find that

$$t = \frac{d}{v} = \frac{5\text{ m}}{0.1\text{ m/s}} = 50\text{ s}$$

Example 6-30: A radioactive atom of polonium-204, initially at rest, undergoes alpha decay. Show that, as a result of ejecting the alpha particle, the daughter nucleus recoils with a speed equal to 2% of the speed of the alpha particle.

Solution: Initially, the parent nucleus is at rest, so its total momentum is zero. Because of the Law of Conservation of Momentum, $\Delta\mathbf{p}_{system} = 0$, we know that after the decay, the total momentum of the daughter atom (actually, ion, but we'll ignore the electrons because they're such a small portion of the mass) and the alpha particle will still be zero; that is, $m_D\mathbf{v}_D + m_\alpha\mathbf{v}_\alpha = 0$, where D represents the daughter. This gives

$$m_D\mathbf{v}_D = -m_\alpha\mathbf{v}_\alpha \;\rightarrow\; \mathbf{v}_D = -\frac{m_\alpha}{m_D}\mathbf{v}_\alpha \;\rightarrow\; v_D = -\frac{m_\alpha}{m_D}v_\alpha$$

Now, since the daughter atom has a mass number that's 4 less than that of the parent, we'll have $m_D = 204 - 4 \approx 200$ u; and, since we know that $m_\alpha \approx 4$ u, we find that

$$v_D = -\frac{m_\alpha}{m_D}v_\alpha = -\frac{4\text{ u}}{200\text{ u}}v_\alpha = -\frac{1}{50}v_\alpha = -2\%\,v_\alpha$$

Collisions

Conservation of momentum is used to analyze collisions between objects. For example, consider this situation:

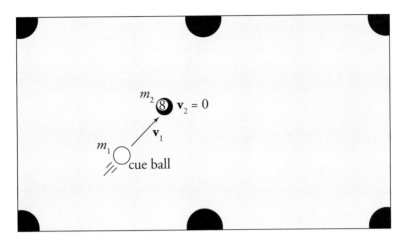

Let the cue ball and the 8-ball constitute our *system*, that is, the objects whose impending collision we're going to analyze. Before the collision, the cue ball is moving toward the 8-ball with a certain velocity, $\mathbf{v}_1$, and the 8-ball is at rest ($\mathbf{v}_2 = 0$). After the collision, the individual velocities of the objects change, to $\mathbf{v}_1'$ and $\mathbf{v}_2'$, respectively,

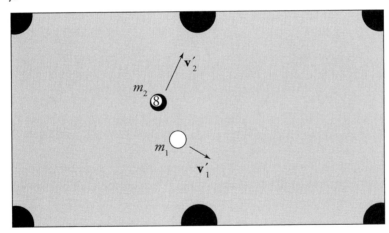

but in such a way that the *total* momentum *doesn't* change, because we must have $\Delta\mathbf{p}_{system} = 0$. Equivalently, we can say that $\mathbf{p}_{total}$ before the collision is equal to $\mathbf{p}_{total}$ after the collision:

$$\mathbf{p}_{total\ before} = \mathbf{p}_{total\ after}$$
$$m_1\mathbf{v}_1 + m_2\mathbf{v}_2 = m_1\mathbf{v}_1' + m_2\mathbf{v}_2'$$
$$m_1\mathbf{v}_1 = m_1\mathbf{v}_1' + m_2\mathbf{v}_2'$$

In this case, $\mathbf{v}_2 = 0$, which is why the term $m_2\mathbf{v}_2$ dropped out of the last equation.

Let's look at a simpler collision, one in which the motion of the objects is along a straight line.

Example 6-31: Ball 1 rolls with velocity $v_1 = 5$ m/s toward Ball 2, which is initially at rest. Ball 1 has a mass of $m_1 = 1$ kg, and Ball 2 has a mass of $m_2 = 4$ kg. After the collision, Ball 2 is observed to move with a velocity of $v_2' = 2$ m/s. What's the velocity of Ball 1 after the collision?

before the collision

$v_2 = 0$

$v_1 = 5$ m/s

① ⟶ ②

after the collision

$v_1' = ?$

$v_2' = 2$ m/s

① ② ⟶

Solution: Using Conservation of Momentum, we get

$$\mathbf{P}_{\text{total before}} = \mathbf{P}_{\text{total after}}$$
$$m_1 \mathbf{v}_1 + m_2 \mathbf{v}_2 = m_1 \mathbf{v}_1' + m_2 \mathbf{v}_2'$$
$$m_1 \mathbf{v}_1 = m_1 \mathbf{v}_1' + m_2 \mathbf{v}_2'$$
$$(1 \text{ kg})(5 \text{ m/s}) = (1 \text{ kg})\mathbf{v}_1' + (4 \text{ kg})(2 \text{ m/s})$$
$$\therefore \mathbf{v}_1' = -3 \text{ m/s}$$

Notice that the velocity of Ball 1 after the collision is negative; this means it points to the left (since we called velocities to the right positive). This isn't surprising. When an object collides with a heavier object, the lighter object often bounces backward.

after the collision

$v_1' = -3$ m/s $v_2' = 2$ m/s

⟵ ① ② ⟶

Example 6-32: Ball 1 and Ball 2 are rolling toward each other at the same speed, 5 m/s. Ball 1 has a mass of $m_1 = 8$ kg, and Ball 2 has a mass of $m_2 = 2$ kg. After the collision, Ball 1 is observed to move with a velocity of 2 m/s in the same direction as v_1. What's the velocity of Ball 2 after the collision?

before the collision

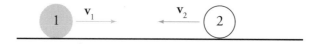

after the collision

$v'_2 = ?$

$v'_1 = 2$ m/s

1

2

Solution: Since v_1 and v_2 point in opposite directions, we need to choose which direction to call positive. Let's choose *to the right* as our positive direction; then $v_1 = +5$ m/s and $v_2 = -5$ m/s. Now, using Conservation of Momentum, we get

$$P_{\text{total before}} = P_{\text{total after}}$$
$$m_1 v_1 + m_2 v_2 = m_1 v'_1 + m_2 v'_2$$
$$(8 \text{ kg})(+5 \text{ m/s}) + (2 \text{ kg})(-5 \text{ m/s}) = (8 \text{ kg})(+2 \text{ m/s}) + (2 \text{ kg})v'_2$$
$$30 \text{ kg} \cdot \text{m/s} = 16 \text{ kg} \cdot \text{m/s} + (2 \text{ kg})v'_2$$
$$14 \text{ kg} \cdot \text{m/s} = (2 \text{ kg})v'_2$$
$$\therefore v'_2 = +7 \text{ m/s}$$

Notice that the velocity of Ball 2 after the collision is positive; this means it points to the right (since we called velocities to the right positive). This isn't surprising. When a heavy object collides with a lighter one, the lighter object often gets pushed forward.

after the collision

$v'_1 = 2$ m/s

1

$v'_2 = 7$ m/s

2

Now that we've looked at some collisions, it's time to classify them. Collisions can be grouped into two major types: elastic and inelastic. A collision is said to be **elastic** if the total *kinetic* energy is conserved also. (Notice I say "also," because total *momentum* is already conserved.) A collision is said to be **inelastic** if total kinetic energy is *not* conserved. Further, as a subcategory of inelastic collisions, we have **perfectly** (or **completely**) **inelastic** collisions; on the OAT, these are collisions in which the objects stick together afterwards.[2] *Perfectly inelastic collisions are the OAT's favorite type.*

> **Elastic Collision:** Total momentum *and* total kinetic energy are conserved.
> **Inelastic Collision:** Total momentum is conserved but total kinetic energy is not.
> **Perfectly Inelastic:** An inelastic collision in which the objects stick together afterwards.

---

[2] Technically, a perfectly inelastic collision is one in which the loss of kinetic energy is as great as possible (consistent with Conservation of Momentum). Luckily, we don't need to worry about this definition, because collisions in which the objects stick together are always perfectly inelastic.

Example 6-33: Ball 1 and Ball 2 are rolling toward each other at the same speed, 5 m/s. Ball 1 has a mass of $m_1 = 8$ kg, and Ball 2 has a mass of $m_2 = 2$ kg. After the collision, Ball 1 and Ball 2 stick together and slide frictionlessly across the table. What's their common velocity after the collision?

before the collision

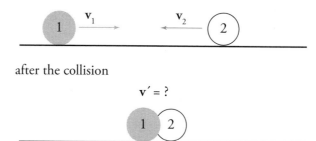

after the collision

$$\mathbf{v}' = ?$$

Solution: Choosing *to the right* as our positive direction, we have $\mathbf{v}_1 = +5$ m/s and $\mathbf{v}_2 = -5$ m/s. Now, using Conservation of Momentum, we get

$$\mathbf{P}_{\text{total before}} = \mathbf{P}_{\text{total after}}$$
$$m_1\mathbf{v}_1 + m_2\mathbf{v}_2 = (m_1 + m_2)\mathbf{v}'$$
$$(8 \text{ kg})(+5 \text{ m/s}) + (2 \text{ kg})(-5 \text{ m/s}) = (8 \text{ kg} + 2 \text{ kg})\mathbf{v}'$$
$$30 \text{ kg} \cdot \text{m/s} = (10 \text{ kg})\mathbf{v}'$$
$$\therefore \mathbf{v}' = +3 \text{ m/s}$$

The OAT likes these collisions because the math is easier; after the collision, we have just one object, with a combined mass of $m_1 + m_2$, moving with a *single* velocity, $\mathbf{v}'$.

after the collision

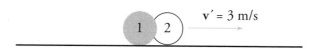

$$\mathbf{v}' = 3 \text{ m/s}$$

Example 6-34: Recall Example 6-31: Ball 1 rolled with velocity $\mathbf{v}_1 = 5$ m/s toward Ball 2, which was initially at rest. Ball 1's mass was $m_1 = 1$ kg, and Ball 2's mass was $m_2 = 4$ kg. After the collision, Ball 2 moved with a velocity of $\mathbf{v}_2' = 2$ m/s. We found that the velocity of Ball 1 after the collision was $\mathbf{v}_1' = -3$ m/s. Was this collision elastic or was it inelastic?

before the collision

$$\mathbf{v}_2 = 0$$
$$\mathbf{v}_1 = 5 \text{ m/s}$$

after the collision

$\mathbf{v}_1' = -3$ m/s   ① ② $\mathbf{v}_2' = 2$ m/s

Solution: We need to decide whether total kinetic energy was conserved. Consider the following:

$$KE_{\text{before collision}} = \tfrac{1}{2}m_1 v_1^2 + \tfrac{1}{2}m_2 v_2^2 = \tfrac{1}{2}(1 \text{ kg})(5 \text{ m/s})^2 + 0 = \tfrac{25}{2} \text{ J}$$

and

$$KE_{\text{after collision}} = \tfrac{1}{2}m_1 v_1'^2 + \tfrac{1}{2}m_2 v_2'^2 = \tfrac{1}{2}(1 \text{ kg})(3 \text{ m/s})^2 + \tfrac{1}{2}(4 \text{ kg})(2 \text{ m/s})^2 = \tfrac{25}{2} \text{ J}$$

Since the kinetic energy was conserved in this case, we can conclude that this collision was elastic.

Example 6-35: Recall Example 6-32: Ball 1 and Ball 2 were rolling toward each other at the same speed, 5 m/s. Ball 1's mass was $m_1 = 8$ kg, and Ball 2's mass was $m_2 = 2$ kg. After the collision, Ball 1 moved with a velocity of 2 m/s in the same direction as $\mathbf{v}_1$. We found that the velocity of Ball 2 after the collision was 7 m/s. Was this collision elastic or was it inelastic?

Solution: We need to check whether total kinetic energy was conserved. Consider the following:

$$KE_{\text{before collision}} = \tfrac{1}{2}m_1 v_1^2 + \tfrac{1}{2}m_2 v_2^2 = \tfrac{1}{2}(8 \text{ kg})(5 \text{ m/s})^2 + \tfrac{1}{2}(2 \text{ kg})(5 \text{ m/s})^2 = 125 \text{ J}$$

and

$$KE_{\text{after collision}} = \tfrac{1}{2}m_1 v_1'^2 + \tfrac{1}{2}m_2 v_2'^2 = \tfrac{1}{2}(8 \text{ kg})(2 \text{ m/s})^2 + \tfrac{1}{2}(2 \text{ kg})(7 \text{ m/s})^2 = 65 \text{ J}$$

Since the kinetic energy was not conserved in this case, we can conclude that this collision was inelastic. This is what happens with macroscopic objects that collide. Some of the initial kinetic energy is converted to other forms: heat (mostly) and sound. The objects may also suffer some permanent deformation, which can also use up some of the pre-collision kinetic energy.

Example 6-36: Recall Example 6-33: Ball 1 and Ball 2 were rolling toward each other at the same speed, 5 m/s. Ball 1's mass was $m_1 = 8$ kg, and Ball 2's mass was $m_2 = 2$ kg. After the collision, Ball 1 and Ball 2 stuck together. We found that the common velocity of the combined object after the collision was $\mathbf{v}' = 3$ m/s. Was this collision elastic or inelastic?

Solution: Actually, there's no need for a calculation. If the objects stick together after the collision, then the collision is perfectly inelastic. That's certainly an inelastic collision.

Here's the proof, just to be sure you're convinced!

$$KE_{\text{before collision}} = \tfrac{1}{2}m_1v_1^2 + \tfrac{1}{2}m_2v_2^2 = \tfrac{1}{2}(8 \text{ kg})(5 \text{ m/s})^2 + \tfrac{1}{2}(2 \text{ kg})(5 \text{ m/s})^2 = 1$$

and

$$KE_{\text{after collision}} = \tfrac{1}{2}(m_1 + m_2)v' = \tfrac{1}{2}(8 \text{ kg} + 2 \text{ kg})(3 \text{ m/s})^2 = 45 \text{ J}$$

Notice that in the previous example (which described a generic inelastic collision), only 125 − 65 = 60 J (which is less than 50%) of the initial kinetic energy was lost as a result of the collision. In this case, however (a completely inelastic collision), we lost 125 − 45 = 80 J (or over 60%) of the initial kinetic energy. Completely inelastic collisions always result in the maximum possible loss of kinetic energy.

After our work on the Conservation of Total Mechanical Energy, you might be tempted to solve collision problems by Conservation of Energy. *Don't.* Total kinetic energy is conserved only for elastic collisions, and these are very special. In the everyday world of macroscopic-sized objects, collisions result in a loss of energy due to heat, sound, and deformation, so all such collisions are, by definition, *not* elastic. (In the subatomic domain, when particles such as neutrons and protons run into each other, elastic collisions are common.) So, the moral is: Unless the question specifically says, "Assume the collision is elastic," or "Assume that energy losses are negligible," then you should never assume that a collision between macroscopic-sized objects is elastic. And even if a collision is (or can be treated as) elastic, you can still use Conservation of Momentum, because total momentum is conserved in both types of collisions, elastic *and* inelastic.

Example 6-37: A fast-moving neutron collides with another neutron initially at rest. Could such a collision be elastic? If so, describe what would happen.

Solution: Yes, a collision between subatomic particles could be elastic. Assume that before the collision, the moving neutron had velocity **v** and the target neutron was at rest. If the resulting collision is elastic, the moving neutron hits the target and stops, and the target neutron moves away with the same velocity, **v**, that the first one had coming in to the collision. In other words, the moving neutron gives up all its momentum and kinetic energy to the target neutron. This conserves both total momentum and kinetic energy, and describes an elastic collision.

before the collision   after the collision

Summary of Formulas

Work: $W = Fd\cos\theta$ (θ = angle between **F** and **d**)

Power: $P = \dfrac{W}{t}$

$P = Fv$ if F is parallel to **v** and constant.

Kinetic Energy: $KE = \dfrac{1}{2}mv^2$

Work-Energy Theorem: $W_{total} = \Delta KE$

Gravitational Potential Energy: $\Delta PE_{grav} = -W_{by\ F_{grav}} = -mg\Delta h$ (if g is constant)

Gravity is a conservative force (path independent).

Friction is NOT a conservative force (path dependent).

Total Mechanical Energy: $E = KE + PE$

Conservation of Total Mechanical Energy: $KE_i + PE_i = KE_f + PE_f$

If non-conservative forces (i.e., friction) act: $KE_i + PE_i + W_{other} = KE_f + PE_f$

Momentum: $\mathbf{p} = m\mathbf{v}$

Impulse-Momentum Theorem: $\mathbf{J} = \Delta\mathbf{p} = \mathbf{F}\Delta t$

Conservation of Total Momentum: total $\mathbf{p}_i$ = total $\mathbf{p}_f$

$m_1\mathbf{v}_1 + m_2\mathbf{v}_2... = m_1\mathbf{v}'_1 + m_2\mathbf{v}'_2...$

Collisions always conserve momentum

–Elastic collisions also conserve *KE*.

–Inelastic collisions do NOT conserve *KE* (lose *KE*).

–Perfectly inelastic collisions lose the most *KE* (objects stick together after collision).

Chapter 7
Fluid Statics

7.1 HYDROSTATICS: FLUIDS AT REST

In this section and the next, we'll discuss some of the fundamental concepts dealing with substances that can flow, which are known as **fluids**. *Both liquids and gases are fluids*, but there are distinctions between them. At the molecular level, a substance in the liquid phase is similar to one in the solid phase in that the molecules are close to, and interact with, one another. The molecules in a liquid are able to move around a little more freely than those in a solid, in which the molecules typically only vibrate around relatively fixed positions. By contrast, the molecules of a gas are not constrained and fly around in a chaotic swarm, with hardly any interaction. On a macroscopic level, there is another distinction between liquids and gases. If you pour a certain volume of a liquid into a container of a greater volume, the liquid will occupy its original volume, whatever the shape and size of the container. However, if you introduce a sample of gas into a container, the molecules will fly around and fill the *entire* container.

Density and Specific Gravity

The **density** of a substance is the amount of mass contained in a unit of volume. In SI units, density is usually expressed in kg/m^3 or g/cm^3.

$$density = \frac{mass}{volume}$$

$$\rho = \frac{m}{V}$$

There is one substance whose density you should memorize: the density of liquid water is taken to be 1000 kg/m^3 or 1 g/cm^3. (Another useful version of the same value: 1 kg/L, where L stands for a liter; a liter is 1000 cm^3.)

Sometimes the OAT mentions **specific gravity**. This (poorly named) unitless number tells us how dense something is compared to water:

$$specific\ gravity = \frac{density\ of\ substance}{density\ of\ water}$$

$$sp.\ gr. = \frac{\rho}{\rho_{H_2O}}$$

For solids, density doesn't change much with surrounding pressure or temperature. For example, the density of marble is pretty close to 2700 kg/m³ under most conditions. Liquids behave the same way: the density of water is pretty close to 1000 kg/m³ under all conditions at which it's a liquid. However, the density of a gas changes markedly with pressure and temperature. (The Ideal Gas Law tells us that $PV = nRT$, so the density of a sample of an ideal gas is given by the equation $\rho_{gas} = m/V = mP/nRT$, which depends on P and T.)

Example 7-1: Turpentine has a specific gravity of 0.9. What is the density of this liquid?

Solution: By definition, we have

$$\rho_{\text{turpentine}} = (\text{sp. gr.}_{\text{turpentine}})(\rho_{H_2O}) = (0.9)(1000 \text{ kg/m}^3) = 900 \text{ kg/m}^3$$

Example 7-2: A 2 cm³ sample of osmium, one of the densest substances on Earth, has a mass of 45 g. What's the specific gravity of this metal?

Solution: The density of osmium is

$$\rho = \frac{m}{V} = \frac{45\text{g}}{2\,\text{cm}^3} = 22.5 \text{ g/cm}^3$$

Since this is 22.5 times the density of water (which is 1 g/cm³), the specific gravity of osmium is 22.5.

Example 7-3: A cork has volume of 4 cm³ and weighs 0.01 N. What is its density? What is its specific gravity?

Solution: Because the cork weighs 10^{-2} N, its mass is

$$m = \frac{w}{g} = \frac{10^{-2} \text{ N}}{10 \text{ N/kg}} = 10^{-3} \text{ kg}$$

Therefore, its density is

$$\rho_{\text{cork}} = \frac{m}{V} = \frac{10^{-3} \text{ kg}}{4 \text{ cm}^3} \times \left(\frac{10^2 \text{ cm}}{1 \text{ m}}\right)^3 = \tfrac{1}{4} \times 10^3 \text{ kg/m}^3 = 2.5 \times 10^2 \text{ kg/m}^3$$

and its specific gravity is

$$\text{sp. gr.}_{\text{cork}} = \frac{\rho_{\text{cork}}}{\rho_{H_2O}} = \frac{\tfrac{1}{4} \times 10^3 \text{ kg/m}^3}{10^3 \text{ kg/m}^3} = \tfrac{1}{4} = 0.25$$

Force of Gravity for Fluids

When solving questions involving fluids, it is often handy to know how to find the force of gravity acting on the fluid itself or objects that are immersed in the fluid. In previous chapters, we have used $F_{grav} = mg$ without too much difficulty. However, with fluids, it is more difficult to remove a portion of fluid from a tank, place it on a scale, and find its mass. Using the relationship between mass, volume, and density, we can redefine the magnitude of F_{grav} for fluids questions:

$$\rho = \frac{m}{V} \rightarrow m = \rho V \rightarrow \therefore F_{grav} = mg = \rho V g$$

With this new formula $F_{grav} = \rho V g$, it is important to make sure that the density (ρ) and the volume (V) describe the properties of the correct object or fluid.

Pressure

If we place an object in a fluid, the fluid exerts a contact force on the object. If we look at how that force is *distributed* over any small area of the object's surface, we have the concept of **pressure**:

Pressure

$$P = \frac{\text{force}_\perp}{\text{area}} = \frac{F_\perp}{A}$$

The subscript $\perp$ (which means "perpendicular") indicates that pressure is defined as the magnitude of the force acting *perpendicular* to the surface, divided by the area. We don't need to worry very much about this, because (for OAT purposes) at any given point in a fluid the pressure is the same in all directions, which means that the force does not depend on the orientation of the force.

Although the formula for pressure involves "force," pressure is actually a *scalar* quantity, because the perpendicular force is the same for all orientations of surface. The unit of pressure is the N/m^2, which is called a **pascal** (abbreviated **Pa**). Because 1 N is a pretty small force and 1 m^2 is a pretty big area, 1 Pa is very small. Often, you'll see pressure expressed in kPa (or even in MPa). For example, at sea level, normal atmospheric pressure is about 100 kPa.

Let's imagine we have a tank of water with a lid on top. Suspended from the lid is a string attached to a thin metal sheet. The figures on the following page show you two views of this.

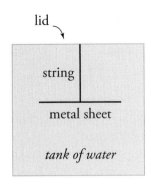

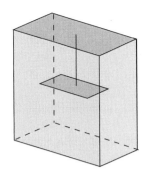

front view   side corner view

The weight of the water above the metal sheet produces a force that pushes down on the sheet. If we divide this force by the area of the sheet, w/A, we get the pressure, due to the water, on the sheet. The formula for calculating this pressure depends on the density of the fluid in the tank (ρ_{fluid}), the depth of the sheet (D), and the acceleration due to gravity (g).

$$P = \frac{w_{fluid}}{A} = \frac{m_{fluid}g}{A} = \frac{\rho_{fluid}V_{fluid}g}{A} = \frac{\rho_{fluid}ADg}{A} = \rho_{fluid}Dg$$

Hydrostatic Gauge Pressure

$$P_{gauge} = \rho_{fluid}gD$$

This formula gives the pressure due only to the fluid (in this case, the water) in the tank. This is called **hydrostatic gauge pressure**. It's called hydro*static*, because the fluid is at rest; and *gauge* pressure means that we don't take the pressure due to the atmosphere into account. If there were no lid on the water tank, then the water would be exposed to the atmosphere, and the *total* pressure at any point in the water would be equal to the atmospheric pressure pushing down on the surface *plus* the pressure due to the water (that is, the gauge pressure). So, below the surface, we'd have

$$P_{total} = P_{atm} + P_{gauge}$$

If the tank were closed to the atmosphere, but there were a layer of gas above the surface of the water, then the total pressure at a point below the surface would be the pressure of the gas pushing down at the surface plus the gauge pressure: $P_{total} = P_{gas} + P_{gauge}$. In general, we'll have

$$P_{total} = P_{at\,surface} + P_{gauge}$$

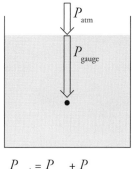
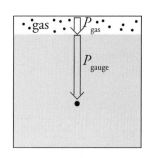

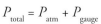

in either case:

$$P_{\text{total}} = P_{\text{at surface}} + P_{\text{gauge}}$$

Notice that hydrostatic gauge pressure, $P_{\text{gauge}} = \rho_{\text{fluid}} g D$, is proportional to both the depth and the density of the fluid. *Total* pressure, however, is *not* proportional to either of these quantities if $P_{\text{on surface}}$ isn't zero.

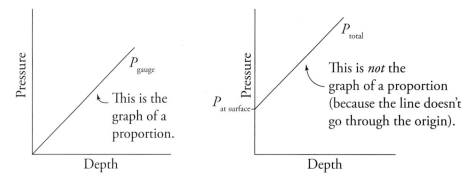

The lines in these graphs will be straight as long as the density of the liquid remains constant as the depth increases. Actually, ρ increases as the depth increases, but the effect is small enough that we generally consider liquids to be **incompressible**; that is, that the density of a liquid remains constant (so, in particular, the density doesn't increase with depth).

Example 7-4: The density of seawater is 1025 kg/m³. Consider a point X that's 10 m below the surface of the ocean.

a) What's the gauge pressure at X?
b) If the atmospheric pressure is 1.015×10^5 Pa, what is the total pressure at X?
c) Consider a point Y that's 50 m below the surface. How does the gauge pressure at Y compare to the gauge pressure at X? How does the total pressure at Y compare to the total pressure at X?

Solution:

a) The gauge pressure at X is

$$P_{gauge} = \rho_{fluid} gD = (1025 \text{ kg/m}^3)(10 \text{ N/kg})(10 \text{ m}) = 1.025 \times 10^5 \text{ Pa}$$

b) The total pressure at X is the atmosphere pressure plus the gauge pressure:

$$P_{total\,at\,X} = P_{atm} + P_{gauge} = (1.015 \times 10^5 \text{ Pa}) + (1.025 \times 10^5 \text{ Pa}) = 2.04 \times 10^5 \text{ Pa}$$

c) Since P_{gauge} is proportional to D, an increase in D by a factor of 5 will mean the gauge pressure will also increase by a factor of 5. Therefore, the gauge pressure at Y will be $5\left(P_{gauge\,at\,X}\right) = 5.125 \times 10^5 \text{ Pa}$. The total pressure at Y is equal to the atmospheric pressure plus the gauge pressure at Y, so

$$P_{total\,at\,Y} = P_{atm} + P_{gauge} = (1.015 \times 10^5 \text{ Pa}) + (5.125 \times 10^5 \text{ Pa}) = 6.14 \times 10^5 \text{ Pa}$$

Notice that $P_{total\,at\,Y}$ is not 5 times $P_{total\,at\,X}$. *Total* pressure is *not* proportional to depth.

Example 7-5: A large storage tank fitted with a tight lid holds a liquid. The space between the surface of the liquid and the lid of the tank is filled with molecules of the stored liquid in the gaseous phase. At a depth of 40 m, the total pressure is 520 kPa, while at a depth of 50 m, the total pressure is 600 kPa. What's the pressure of the gas above the surface of the liquid?

Solution: Let P_{gas} be the pressure that the gas exerts on the surface of the liquid. Then we have

$$P_{total\,at\,D_1 = 40\,m} = P_{gas} + \rho_{fluid} gD_1 = P_{gas} + \rho_{fluid} g(40 \text{ m}) = 520 \text{ kPa}$$
$$P_{total\,at\,D_2 = 50\,m} = P_{gas} + \rho_{fluid} gD_2 = P_{gas} + \rho_{fluid} g(50 \text{ m}) = 600 \text{ kPa}$$

We have two equations and two unknowns (P_{gas} and ρ_{fluid}). If we subtract the first equation from the second, we get $\rho_{fluid} g(10\,m) = 80\,kPa$, which tells us that $\rho_{fluid} g = 8$ kPa / m. Plugging this back into either one of the equations will give us P_{gas}. Choosing, say, the first one, we find that

$$P_{gas} + (8 \text{ kPa / m})(40\,m) = 520\,kPa \rightarrow P_{gas} = 200\,kPa$$

Example 7-6: The containers shown below are all filled with the same liquid. At which point (A, B, C, D, E, or F) is the gauge pressure the lowest?

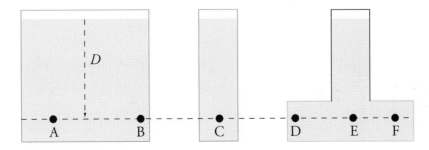

Solution: It's important to remember that the formula $P_{\text{gauge}} = \rho_{\text{fluid}} g D$ applies regardless of the shape of the container in which the fluid is held. If all the containers are filled with the same fluid, then the pressure is the *same* everywhere along the horizontal dashed line. This is because every point on this line (and within one of the containers) is at the same depth, D, below the surface of the fluid. The fact that the first container is wide, the second container is narrow, and the third container is wide at the base but has a narrow neck makes no difference. Even the fact that Points D and F (in the third container) aren't *directly* underneath a column of fluid of height D makes no difference either.

Pressure is the magnitude of the force per area, so pressure is a *scalar*. Pressure has no direction. The force *due to the pressure* is a vector, however, and the direction of this force on any small surface is always perpendicular to that surface. For example, in the figure below, the pressure at Point A is the same as the pressure at Point B, because they're at the same depth. But, as you can see, the direction of the force due to the pressure varies depending on the orientation of the surface (and even which side of the surface) the force is pushing on.

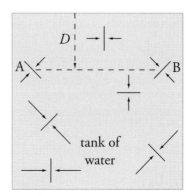

Buoyancy and Archimedes' Principle

Let's place a wooden block in our tank of water. Since the pressure on each side of the block depends on its average depth, we see that there's more pressure on the bottom of the block than there is on the top of it. Therefore, there's a greater force pushing up on the bottom of the block than there is pushing down on the top. The forces due to the pressure on the other four sides (left and right, front and back) cancel out, so the net fluid force on the block is upward. This net upward fluid force is called the **buoyant** force (or just **buoyancy** for short), which we'll denote by F_{Buoy} (or F_{B}).

We can calculate the magnitude of the buoyant force using Archimedes' principle:

Archimedes' Principle

The magnitude of the buoyant force
is equal to
the weight of the fluid displaced by the object.

When an object is partially or completely submerged in a fluid, the volume of the object that's submerged, which we call V_{sub}, is the volume of the fluid displaced.

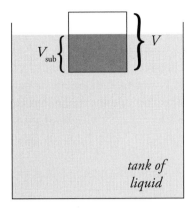

By multiplying V_{sub} by the density of the fluid, we get the *mass* of the fluid displaced; then, multiplying this mass by g gives us the weight of the fluid displaced. So, here's Archimedes' principle as a mathematical equation:

Archimedes' Principle

$$F_{Buoy} = \rho_{fluid} V_{sub} g$$

When an object floats, its submerged volume is just enough to make the buoyant force it feels balance its weight. That is, for a floating object, we always have $w_{object} = F_{Buoy}$. If an object's density is ρ_{object} and its volume is V, its weight will be $\rho_{object} V_{object} g$. The buoyant force it feels is $\rho_{fluid} V_{sub} g$. Setting these equal to each other, we find that

---

Floating Object in Equilibrium on Surface

$$w_{object} = F_{Buoy}$$

$$\frac{V_{sub}}{V} = \frac{\rho_{object}}{\rho_{fluid}}$$

So, if $\rho_{object} < \rho_{fluid}$, then the object will float; and the fraction of its volume that's submerged is the same as the ratio of its density to the fluid's density. *This is a very helpful fact to know for the OAT.* For example, if the object's density is 3/4 the density of the fluid, then 3/4 of the object will be submerged (and vice versa).

If an object is denser than the fluid, then the object will sink. In this case, even if the entire object is submerged (in an attempt to maximize the buoyant force), the object's weight is still greater than the buoyant force. This leaves a net force in the downwards direction, causing the object to sink by accelerating downwards. If an object just happens to have the same density as the fluid, it will be happy hovering (in static equilibrium) underneath the fluid.

For an object that is completely submerged in the surrounding fluid, the actual weight of the object ($w_{object} = \rho_{object} Vg$) remains unchanged. However, the object's "apparent" weight is less due to the buoyant force "buoying" the object upwards. This corresponds to the measurement of a scale placed at the bottom of a tank of liquid in order to measure the apparent weight of the submerged object, or the normal force acting on the object.

Since the volume of the object is equal to the submerged volume ($V = V_{sub}$), the buoyant force F_{Buoy} on the object is equal to $\rho_{fluid} Vg$. Therefore,

$$\frac{w_{object}}{F_{Buoy}} = \frac{\rho_{object} Vg}{\rho_{fluid} Vg} = \frac{\rho_{object}}{\rho_{fluid}}$$

If the fluid in which the object is submerged is water, the ratio of the object weight to the buoyant force is equal to the specific gravity of the object.

Example 7-7: Ethyl alcohol has a specific gravity of 0.8. If a cork of specific gravity 0.25 floats in a beaker of ethyl alcohol, what fraction of the cork's volume is submerged?

    A. 4/25
    B. 1/5
    C. 1/4
    D. 5/16

Solution: Because the cork has a lower density than the ethyl alcohol, we know that the cork will float. Furthermore, the fraction of the cork's volume that will be submerged is

$$\frac{V_{sub}}{V} = \frac{\rho_{object}}{\rho_{fluid}} = \frac{(0.25)\rho_{H_2O}}{(0.8)\rho_{H_2O}} = \frac{0.25}{0.8} = \frac{1/4}{4/5} = \frac{5}{16}$$

Therefore, the answer is (D).

Example 7-8: The density of ice is 920 kg/m³, and the density of seawater is 1025 kg/m³. Approximately what percent of an iceberg floats above the surface of the ocean (in other words, how much is "the tip of the iceberg")?

    A. 5%
    B. 10%
    C. 90%
    D. 95%

Solution: Because the ice has a lower density than the seawater, we know that the iceberg will float. Furthermore, the fraction of the iceberg's volume that will be submerged is

$$\frac{V_{sub}}{V} = \frac{\rho_{object}}{\rho_{fluid}} = \frac{920 \text{ kg/m}^3}{1025 \text{ kg/m}^3} = \frac{900}{1000} = 90\%$$

However, the answer is not (C). The question asked what percent of the iceberg floats *above* the surface. So, if 90% is submerged, then 10% is above the surface, and the answer is B. Watch for this kind of tricky wording; it is a common OAT tactic.

Example 7-9: A glass sphere of specific gravity 2.5 and volume 10^{-3} m³ is completely submerged in a large container of water. What is the apparent weight of the sphere while immersed?

Solution: Because the buoyant force pushes up on the object, the object's *apparent weight*, $w_{apparent} = w - F_{Buoy}$, is less than its true weight, w. Because the sphere is completely submerged, we have $V_{sub} = V$, so the buoyant force on the sphere is

$$\begin{aligned} F_{Buoy} &= \rho_{fluid} V_{sub} g \\ &= \rho_{H_2O} V g \\ &= (1000 \text{ kg/m}^3)(10^{-3} \text{ m}^3)(10 \text{ N/kg}) \\ &= 10 \text{ N} \end{aligned}$$

The true weight of the glass sphere is

$$\begin{aligned} w &= \rho_{glass} V g \\ &= (\text{sp. gr.}_{glass} \times \rho_{H_2O}) V g \\ &= (2.5 \times 1000 \text{ kg/m}^3)(10^{-3} \text{ m}^3)(10 \text{ N/kg}) \\ &= 25 \text{ N} \end{aligned}$$

Therefore, the apparent weight of the sphere while immersed is

$$w_{apparent} = w - F_{Buoy} = 25 \text{ N} - 10 \text{ N} = 15 \text{ N}$$

Example 7-10: An object weighs 50 N, but weighs only 30 N when it's completely immersed in a liquid of specific gravity 0.8. What's the specific gravity of this object?

Solution: The weight of the object is $w_{object} = \rho_{object} V g$, and the buoyant force it feels when completely immersed (that is, when $V_{sub} = V$) is $F_{Buoy} = \rho_{fluid} V g$. Therefore,

$$\frac{w_{object}}{F_{Buoy}} = \frac{\rho_{object} V g}{\rho_{fluid} V g} = \frac{\rho_{object}}{\rho_{fluid}}$$

Now, since this 50 N object weighs only 30 N when immersed, the buoyant force must be 20 N. So, we can write

$$\frac{w_{object}}{F_{Buoy}} = \frac{50\,N}{20\,N} = \frac{5}{2}$$

We now have two expressions for the ratio w_{object} / F_{Buoy}. Therefore,

$$\frac{\rho_{object}}{\rho_{fluid}} = \frac{5}{2}$$

If the object's density is 5/2 times the fluid's density, then the object's specific gravity is 5/2 times the fluid's specific gravity; that is,

$$sp.\,gr._{object} = \tfrac{5}{2}(sp.\,gr._{fluid}) = \tfrac{5}{2}(0.8) = 2$$

Example 7-11: A balloon that weighs 0.18 N is then filled with helium so that its volume becomes 0.03 m³. (Note: The density of helium is 0.2 kg/m³.)

a)   What is the net force on the balloon if it's surrounded by air? (Note: The density of air is 1.2 kg/m³.)
b)   What will be the initial upward acceleration of the balloon if it's released from rest?

Solution:

a)   Remember that gases are fluids, so they also exert buoyant forces. If an object is immersed in a gas, the object experiences a buoyant force equal to the weight of the gas it displaces. In this case, the balloon is completely immersed in a "sea" of air (so $V_{sub} = V$), and Archimedes' principle tells us that the buoyant force on the balloon due to the surrounding air is

$$\begin{aligned}
F_{Buoy} &= \rho_{fluid} V_{sub} g \\
&= \rho_{air} V g \\
&= (1.2\ \text{kg/m}^3)(0.03\,\text{m}^3)(10\ \text{N/kg}) \\
&= 0.36\,\text{N}
\end{aligned}$$

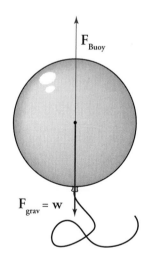

F_{Buoy}

$F_{grav} = w$

The weight of the inflated balloon is equal to the weight of the balloon material (0.18 N) plus the weight of the helium:

$$w_{total} = w_{material} + w_{helium}$$
$$= w_{material} + \rho_{helium}Vg$$
$$= 0.18\,N + (0.2\ kg/m^3)(0.03\ m^3)(10\ N/kg)$$
$$= 0.18\,N + 0.06\,N$$
$$= 0.24\,N$$

Because $F_{Buoy} > w_{total}$, the net force on the balloon is upward and has magnitude

$$F_{net} = F_{Buoy} - w_{total} = (0.36\,N) - (0.24\,N) = 0.12\,N$$

b)   Using Newton's Second Law, $a = F_{net}/m$, we find that

$$a = \frac{F_{net}}{m} = \frac{F_{net}}{\frac{w}{g}} = \frac{0.12\ N}{\left(\frac{0.24\ N}{10\ m/s^2}\right)} = \frac{(0.12\ N)(10\ m/s^2)}{0.24\ N} = \frac{10\ m/s^2}{2} = 5\ m/s^2$$

Pascal's Law

Pascal's Law is a statement about fluid pressure. It says that a confined fluid will transmit an externally applied pressure change to all parts of the fluid and the walls of the container without loss of magnitude. In less formal language, if you squeeze a container of fluid, the fluid will transmit your squeeze perfectly throughout the container. The most important application of Pascal's Law is to hydraulics.

Consider a simple hydraulic jack consisting of two pistons resting above two cylindrical vessels of fluid that are connected by a pipe. If you push down on one piston, the other one will rise. Let's make this more precise. Let F_1 be the magnitude of the force you exert down on one piston (whose cross-sectional area is A_1), and let F_2 be the magnitude of the force that the other piston (cross-sectional area A_2) exerts upward as a result.

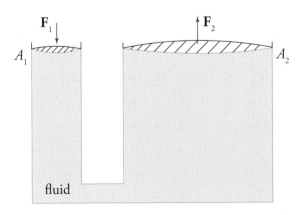

Pushing down on the left-hand piston with a force F_1 introduces a pressure increase of F_1/A_1. Pascal's Law tells us that this pressure change is transmitted, without loss of magnitude, by the fluid to the other end. Since the pressure change at the other piston is F_1/A_1, we have, by Pascal's Law,

$$\frac{F_1}{A_1} = \frac{F_2}{A_2}$$

Solving this equation for F_2, we get

$$F_2 = \frac{A_2}{A_1} F_1$$

So, if A_2 is greater than A_1 (as it is in the figure), then the ratio of the areas, A_2/A_1, will be greater than 1, so F_2 will be greater than F_1; that is, *the output force, F_2, is greater than your input force, F_1.* This is why hydraulic jacks are useful; we end up lifting something very heavy (a car, for example) by exerting a much smaller force (one that would be insufficient to lift the car if it were just applied directly to the car).

This seems too good to be true; doesn't this violate some conservation law? No, since there's no such thing as a "Conservation of Force" law. However, there *is* a price to be paid for the magnification of the force. Let's say you push the left-hand piston down by a distance d_1, and that the distance the right-hand piston moves upward is d_2. Assuming the fluid is incompressible, whatever fluid you push out of the left-hand cylinder must appear in the right-hand cylinder. Since volume is equal to cross-sectional area times distance, the volume of the fluid you push out of the left-hand cylinder is $A_1 d_1$, and the extra volume of fluid that appears in the right-hand cylinder is $A_2 d_2$.

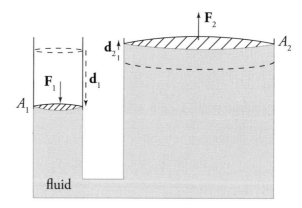

But these volumes have to be the same, so $A_1 d_1 = A_2 d_2$. Solving this equation for d_2, we get

$$d_2 = \frac{A_1}{A_2} d_1$$

If the area of the right-hand piston (A_2) is greater than the area of the left-hand piston (A_1), the ratio A_1/A_2 will be *less* than 1, so d_2 will be less than d_1. In fact, the decrease in d is the same as the increase in F. For example, if A_2 is five times larger than A_1, then F_2 will be five times greater than F_1, but d_2 will only be *one-fifth* of d_1. We can now see that the product of F and d will be the same for both pistons:

$$F_2 d_2 = \left(\frac{A_2}{A_1} F_1 \right) \cdot \left(\frac{A_1}{A_2} d_1 \right) = F_1 d_1$$

Recall that the product of F and d is the amount of work done. What we have shown is that the work you do pushing the left-hand piston down is equal to the work done by the right-hand piston as it pushes upward. Remember that we can't cheat when it comes to work. True, we can do the same job with less force, but we will always pay for that by having to exert that smaller force through a greater distance. This is the whole idea behind all simple machines, not just a hydraulic jack.

Surface Tension

To complete our section on fluids at rest, we introduce the phenomenon of **surface tension**. We have all seen long-legged bugs that can walk on the surface of a pond or have watched a slowly-leaking faucet form a drop of water that grows until it finally drops into the sink. Both of these are illustrations of surface tension. The surface of a fluid can behave like an elastic membrane or thin sheet of rubber. A liquid will form a drop because the surface tends to contract into a sphere (to minimize surface area); however, when you see a drop hanging precariously from a faucet, its spherical shape is distorted by the pull of gravity. In fact, the reason it eventually falls into the sink is that the force due to surface tension causing the drop to cling to the head of the faucet is overwhelmed by the increasing weight of the drop. It can't hang on, and away it goes.

A standard way to define the surface tension is as follows. Imagine a rectangular loop of thin wire with one side able to slide up and down freely, thereby changing the enclosed area. If this apparatus is dipped into a fluid, a thin film will form in the enclosed area. Both the front face and the back face of the film are pulling upward on the free horizontal wire with a total upward force **F** against the wire's weight.

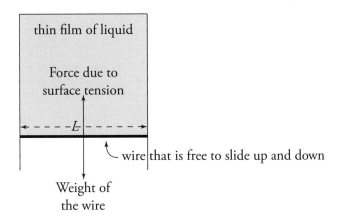

The strength of the surface tension force depends on the particular liquid and is determined by the *coefficient of surface tension*, γ, which is the force per unit length. Since there are *two* surfaces here (the front and the back), each of which acts along a length L, the force F due to surface tension acts along a total length of $2L$. The coefficient of surface tension is defined to be $\gamma = F / 2L$, so $F_{\text{surf tension}} = 2\gamma L$. To give you an idea of the values of γ, the surface tension coefficient of water is 0.07 N/m at room temperature (and decreases as the temperature increases). A fluid with one of the highest surface tension coefficients is mercury. Its surface tension coefficient is nearly seven times greater than that of water: $\gamma_{\text{Hg}} = 0.46\,\text{N/m}$ at room temperature. Note that these values are really quite small. The surface of a pond of water can support the weight of a bug, but a frog isn't about to walk across the pond supported by surface tension.

Summary of Formulas

HYDROSTATICS

Assume liquids are incompressible unless otherwise stated.

Standard atmospheric pressure = 1 atm = 760 mmHg = 760 torr ≈ 100 kPa

Density: $\rho = \dfrac{m}{V}$

Specific gravity: $\text{sp.gr.} = \dfrac{\rho}{\rho_{H_2O}}$

$$\left(\rho_{H_2O} = 1000 \text{ kg/m}^3 \text{ or } 1 \text{ g} / \text{cm}^3 \text{ or } 1 \text{ kg} / \text{L} \right)$$

Force of gravity: $mg = \rho V g$

Pressure: $P = \dfrac{F_\perp}{A}$

Hydrostatic gauge pressure: $P_{gauge} = \rho_{fluid} g D$

>   Hydrostatic gauge pressure is proportional to depth. Total hydrostatic pressure increases with increasing depth but is NOT proportional to depth.

>   Total hydrostatic pressure: $P_{total} = P_{at\ surface} + P_{gauge}$

Archimedes' principle: $F_{Buoy} = \rho_{fluid} V_{sub} g$

>   Buoyant force is equal to the weight of the displaced fluid.

Floating object: $\rho_{object} < \rho_{fluid} \rightarrow w_{object} = F_{Buoy}$

$$\frac{V_{sub}}{V} = \frac{\rho_{object}}{\rho_{fluid}}$$

Apparent weight of submerged object: $w_{apparent} = w_{object} - F_{Buoy}$

Pascal's Law: $\dfrac{F_1}{A_1} = \dfrac{F_2}{A_2}$

Chapter 8
Electrostatics

8.1 ELECTRIC CHARGE

An atom is composed of a central nucleus (which is itself composed of protons and neutrons) surrounded by a cloud of one or more electrons. The fact that an atom is held together as a single unit is due to the fact that protons and electrons have a special property: they carry **electric charge**, which gives rise to an attractive force between them.

Electric charge exists in two varieties, which are called **positive** and **negative**. By convention, we say that protons carry positive charge and electrons carry negative charge. (Neutrons are well-named: they're neutral, because they have no electric charge.) The charge of a proton is +e, where e is called the **elementary charge**, and the charge of an electron is −e. Notice that the proton and the electron carry exactly the same amount of charge; the only difference in their charges is that one is positive and the other is negative.

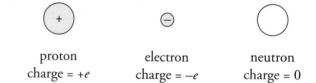

| proton | electron | neutron |
| charge = +e | charge = −e | charge = 0 |

In SI units, electric charge is measured in **coulombs** (abbreviated **C**), and the value of the elementary charge, e, is 1.6×10^{-19} C.

Elementary Charge

$$e = 1.6 \times 10^{-19} \text{ C}$$

When an atom (or any other object) contains the same number of electrons as protons, its total charge is zero because the individual positive and negative charges add up and cancel. So, when the number of electrons (#e) equals the number of protons (#p), the object is *electrically neutral*. We say that an object is **charged** when there's an imbalance between the number of electrons and the number of protons. When an object has one or more extra electrons (#e > #p), the object is *negatively charged*, and when an object has a deficit of electrons (#e < #p), the object is *positively charged*. If a neutral atom has electrons removed or added, we say that it has been **ionized**, and the resulting electrically charged atom is called an **ion**. A positively charged ion is called a **cation**, and a negatively charged ion is called an **anion**. (An object can also become charged by gaining or losing protons, but these are usually locked up tight within the nuclei of the atoms. In virtually all cases, objects become charged by the transfer of *electrons*.)

Because an object can become charged only by losing or gaining electrons or protons, which can't be "sliced" into smaller pieces with fractional amounts of charge, the charge on an object can only be a whole number of ±e's; that is, charge is **quantized**. So, for any object, its charge is always equal to n(±e), where n is a whole number. To remind us that charge is *quantized*, electric charge is usually denoted by the letter q (or Q).

Charge is Quantized

$$q = n(\pm e)$$

where $n = 0, 1, 2...$

In chemistry, it's common to talk about the charge of an atom in terms of whole numbers like +1 or –2, etc. For example, we say that the charge of the fluoride ion, F^-, is –1, and the charge of the calcium ion, Ca^{+2}, is +2. This is just a convenient way of saying that the charge of the fluoride ion is –1 elementary unit (in other words, $-1e$), and the charge of the calcium ion is +2 elementary units, $+2e$. When we want to find the electric force between ions, we will express their charges in the proper unit (coulombs), and say, for example, that the charge of the fluoride ion is $-1e = -1.6 \times 10^{-19}$ C and the charge of the calcium ion is $+2e = +3.2 \times 10^{-19}$ C.

Finally, total electric charge is always conserved; that is, the total amount of charge before any process must always be equal to the total amount of charge afterward.[1]

Example 8-1: When you pet a cat, you rub electrons off the cat's fur, which are transferred to your hand. Assuming that you transfer 5×10^{10} electrons to your hand, what is the electric charge on your hand? What's the charge on the cat?

Solution: Because each electron carries a charge of $-e = -1.6 \times 10^{-19}$ C, and you've gained 5×10^{10} of them, the charge on your hand will be

$$(5 \times 10^{10})(-e) = (5 \times 10^{10})(-1.6 \times 10^{-19}) = -8 \times 10^{-9} \text{ C}$$

Since the cat has lost 5×10^{10} electrons, the charge on the cat will be

$$(5 \times 10^{10})(+e) = (5 \times 10^{10})(1.6 \times 10^{-19}) = +8 \times 10^{-9} \text{ C}$$

Notice that the *net* charge before and after petting the cat was zero; all you've done is transferred charge.

---

[1] This does not mean that electric charge cannot be created or destroyed, which happens all the time. For example, in the reaction $e^- + e^+ \rightarrow \gamma + \gamma$, an electron ($e^-$) and its antiparticle (the positron, e^+, which is, in effect, a positively charged electron) meet and annihilate each other, producing energy in the form of two gamma-ray photons (γ), which carry no charge. Charge has been destroyed, but the total charge (zero, in this case) has been conserved. Conversely, charge can be created in the opposite process, when energy is converted to mass and charge (but always with zero total charge).

Example 8-2: How much positive charge is contained in 1 mole of carbon atoms? How much negative charge? What is the total charge?

Solution: Every atom of carbon contains 6 protons, so the amount of positive charge in one carbon atom is $q_+ = +6e$. Therefore, if N_A denotes Avogadro's number, the total amount of positive charge in 1 mole of carbon atoms is

$$Q_+ = N_A \times q_+ = N_A \times (+6e) = (6.02 \times 10^{23}) \times (6)(+1.6 \times 10^{-19} \text{ C}) \approx +6 \times 10^5 \text{ C}$$

Because every neutral carbon atom also contains 6 electrons, the amount of negative charge in a carbon atom is $q_- = 6(-e) = -6e = -q_+$, so the total amount of negative charge in 1 mole of carbon atoms is $Q_- = N_A \times q_- = -Q_+ \approx -6 \times 10^5 \text{ C}$. The total charge on the carbon atoms, $Q_+ + Q_-$, is zero.

8.2 ELECTRIC FORCE AND COULOMB'S LAW

If two charged particles are a distance r apart,

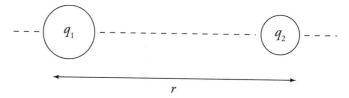

then the electric force between them, $\mathbf{F_E}$, is directed along the line joining them. The magnitude of this force is proportional to the charges (q_1 and q_2) and inversely proportional to r^2, as given by

---

Coulomb's Law

$$F_E = k \frac{q_1 q_2}{r^2}$$

The proportionality constant is k, and in general, its value depends on the material between the particles. However, in the usual case where the particles are separated by empty space (or by air, for all practical purposes), the proportionality constant is denoted by k_0 and called **Coulomb's constant**. This is a fundamental constant of nature (equal in magnitude, by definition, to 10^{-7} times the speed of light squared), and its value is $k_0 = 9 \times 10^9 \text{ N} \cdot \text{m}^2 / \text{C}^2 / \text{C}^2$:

Coulomb's Constant

$$k_0 = 9 \times 10^9 \ \text{N} \cdot \text{m}^2 / \text{C}^2$$

This is the value of k you should use unless you're specifically given another value (which would happen only if the charges were embedded in some insulating material that weakens the electric force).

If we retain the signs of the charges q_1 and q_2 when we use the formula $F_E = kq_1q_2 / r^2$, then a positive F_E means that the particles repel each other; a negative F_E means they attract each other. This is consistent with the fact that like charges (two positives or two negatives) repel each other, and opposite charges (one positive and one negative) attract. Note that the two electric forces in each of the following diagrams form an action–reaction pair.

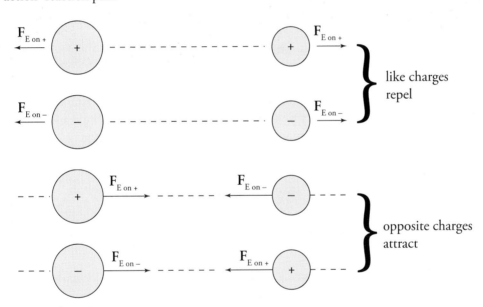

Example 8-3: Two charges, $q_1 = -2 \times 10^{-6} \ \text{C}$ and $q_2 = +5 \times 10^{-6} \ \text{C}$, are separated by a distance of 10 cm. Describe the electric force between these particles.

Solution: Using Coulomb's Law, we find that

$$F_E = k_0 \frac{q_1 q_2}{r^2} = (9 \times 10^9 \ \text{N} \cdot \text{m}^2 / \text{C}^2) \frac{(-2 \times 10^{-6} \ \text{C})(+5 \times 10^{-6} \ \text{C})}{(10^{-1} \ \text{m})^2} = -9 \ \text{N}$$

The minus sign on F_E tells us that the electric force between the charges is attractive, which we expected since q_1 is negative and q_2 is positive. Therefore, the electric force on q_1 is directed toward q_2, the electric force on q_2 is directed toward q_1, and the magnitude of the electric force that each charge feels due to the other is 9 N.

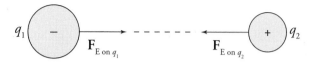

Example 8-4: A coulomb is a *lot* of charge. To get some idea just how much, imagine that we had two objects, each with a charge of 1 C, separated by a distance of 1 m. What would be the electric force between them?

Solution: Using Coulomb's Law, we'd find that

$$F_E = k_0 \frac{q_1 q_2}{r^2} = (9 \times 10^9 \ \text{N} \cdot \text{m}^2 \, / \, \text{C}^2) \frac{(1 \ \text{C})(1 \ \text{C})}{(1 \ \text{m})^2} = 9 \times 10^9 \ \text{N}$$

To write this answer in terms of a more familiar unit, let's use the fact that 1 pound (1 lb) is about 4.5 N, and 1 ton is 2000 lb:

$$F_E = (9 \times 10^9 \ \text{N}) \cdot \frac{1 \ \text{lb}}{4.5 \ \text{N}} \cdot \frac{1 \ \text{ton}}{2000 \ \text{lb}} = \text{one million tons}$$

That's equivalent to the weight of about 2500 Boeing 747s! It's now easy to understand why most real-life situations deal with charges that are very tiny fractions of a coulomb; the *microcoulomb* (1 μC $= 10^{-6}$ C) and the *nanocoulomb* (1 nC $= 10^{-9}$ C) are more common "practical" units of charge.

Example 8-5: Consider a charge, $+q$, initially at rest near another charge, $-Q$. How would the magnitude of the electric force on $+q$ change if $-Q$ were moved away, doubling its distance from $+q$?

Solution: Coulomb's Law is an inverse-square law, $F_E \propto 1 \, / \, r^2$, so if r increases by a factor of 2, then F_E will *decrease* by a factor of 4 (because $2^2 = 4$).

Example 8-6: Consider two plastic spheres, 1 meter apart: a little sphere with a mass of 1 kg and an electric charge of $+1$ nC, and a big sphere with a mass of 11 kg and an electric charge of $+11$ μC.

a) Find the electric force and the gravitational force between these spheres. Which force is stronger?
b) If the big sphere is fixed in position, and the little sphere is free to move, describe the resulting motion of the little sphere if it's released from rest.

Solution:

a) Using Coulomb's Law, we find that the electric force between the spheres is

$$F_E = k_0 \frac{Qq}{r^2} = (9 \times 10^9 \text{ N} \cdot \text{m}^2 / \text{C}^2) \frac{(11 \times 10^{-6} \text{ C})(1 \times 10^{-9} \text{ C})}{1 \text{m}^2} = 9.9 \times 10^{-5} \text{ N} \approx 10^{-4} \text{ N}$$

Using Newton's Law of Gravitation, the gravitational force between them is

$$F_G = G \frac{Mm}{r^2} = (6.7 \times 10^{-11} \text{ N} \cdot \text{m}^2 / \text{kg}^2) \frac{(1 \text{ kg})(11 \text{ kg})}{1 \text{ m}^2} \approx 7.4 \times 10^{-10} \text{ N}$$

Which force is stronger? It's no contest: The electric force is *much* stronger than the gravitational force. So, even though the spheres experience an attraction due to gravity, it is many orders of magnitude weaker than their electrical repulsion and can therefore be ignored.

b) The net force on the little sphere is essentially equal to the electrical repulsion it feels from the big sphere (since the gravitational force is *so* much smaller, it can be ignored). Therefore, the initial acceleration of the little sphere is

$$a = \frac{F_E}{m} = \frac{10^{-4} \text{ N}}{1 \text{ kg}} = 10^{-4} \text{ m/s}^2$$

directed away from the big sphere. Notice that as the little sphere moves away, its acceleration does not remain constant. Because the electric force is inversely proportional to the square of the distance between the charges, as the little sphere moves away, the repulsive force it feels weakens, so its acceleration decreases. Therefore, the little sphere moves directly away from the big sphere with decreasing acceleration.

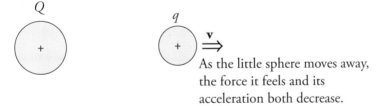

As the little sphere moves away, the force it feels and its acceleration both decrease.

Nevertheless, because the acceleration of the little sphere always points in the same direction (namely, away from the big sphere), the speed of the little sphere is always increasing, although the rate of increase of speed gets smaller as the little sphere gets farther away.

The Principle of Superposition for Electric Forces

Coulomb's Law tells us how to calculate the force that one charge exerts on another one. What if two (or more) charges affect a third one? For example, what is the electric force on q_3 in the following figure?

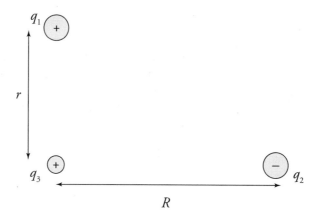

Here's the answer: If $\mathbf{F}_{\text{1-on-3}}$ is the force that q_1 *alone* exerts on q_3 (ignoring the presence of q_2) and if $\mathbf{F}_{\text{2-on-3}}$ is the force that q_2 *alone* exerts on q_3 (ignoring the presence of q_1), then the total force that q_3 feels is simply the vector sum $\mathbf{F}_{\text{1-on-3}} + \mathbf{F}_{\text{2-on-3}}$. The fact that we can calculate the effect of several charges by considering them individually and then just adding the resulting forces is known as the **principle of superposition**. (This important property will also be used when we study electric field vectors, electric potential, magnetic fields, and magnetic forces.)

The Principle of Superposition

The net electric force on a charge (q) due to a collection of other charges (Q's)

is equal to

the sum of the individual forces that each of the Q's alone exerts on q.

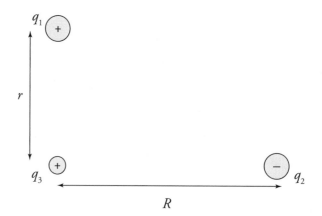

Example 8-7: In the figure above, assume that $q_1 = 2$ C, $q_2 = -8$ C, and $q_3 = 1$ nC. If $r = 1$ m and $R = 2$ m, which one of the following vectors best illustrates the direction of the net electric force on q_3?

A.   C.

B.   D.

Solution: The individual forces $\mathbf{F}_{1\text{-on-3}}$ and $\mathbf{F}_{2\text{-on-3}}$ are shown in the figure below. Adding these vectors gives $\mathbf{F}_{\text{on }3}$, which points down to the right, so the answer is (C).

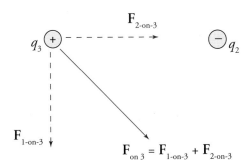

$$F_{1-\text{on}-3} = k_0 \frac{q_1 q_3}{r^2} = \left(9 \times 10^9 \text{ N} \cdot \text{m}^2 / \text{C}^2\right)\frac{(2\,\text{C})(1 \times 10^{-9}\,\text{C})}{(1\,\text{m})^2} = 18\,\text{N}$$

(repulsive; away from q_1)

$$F_{2-\text{on}-3} = k_0 \frac{q_2 q_3}{R^2} = \left(9 \times 10^9 \text{ N} \cdot \text{m}^2 / \text{C}^2\right)\frac{(-8\,\text{C})(1 \times 10^{-9}\,\text{C})}{(2\,\text{m})^2} = -18\,\text{N}$$

(attractive; toward q_2)

If the question had asked for the magnitude of the net electric force on q_3, then we'd use the Pythagorean Theorem to find the length of the vector $\mathbf{F}_{\text{on }3}$. The vector $\mathbf{F}_{\text{on }3}$ is the hypotenuse of the right triangle whose legs are $\mathbf{F}_{1\text{-on-3}}$ and $\mathbf{F}_{2\text{-on-3}}$, so the magnitude of $\mathbf{F}_{\text{on }3}$ is found like this:

$$\left(F_{\text{on }3}\right)^2 = \left(F_{1-\text{on}-3}\right)^2 + \left(F_{2-\text{on}-3}\right)^2$$
$$= 18^2 + 18^2$$
$$= (18^2)(2)$$
$$\therefore F_{\text{on }3} = 18\sqrt{2} \approx 25\,\text{N}$$

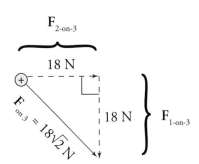

Example 8-8: In the figure below, assume that q_1 = 1 C, q_2 = −1 nC, and q_3 = 8 C. If q_4 is a negative charge, what must its value be in order for the net electric force on q_2 to be zero?

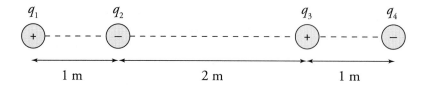

Solution: The individual forces $\mathbf{F}_{1\text{-on-}2}$, $\mathbf{F}_{3\text{-on-}2}$, and $\mathbf{F}_{4\text{-on-}2}$ are shown in the figure below. Notice that $\mathbf{F}_{1\text{-on-}2}$ and $\mathbf{F}_{4\text{-on-}2}$ point to the left, while $\mathbf{F}_{3\text{-on-}2}$ points to the right.

If we let $q_4 = -x$ C, then the magnitudes of the individual forces on q_2 are

$$\left|F_{1\text{-on-}2}\right| = k_0 \frac{q_1 |q_2|}{(r_{1-2})^2} = (9 \times 10^9 \ \text{N} \cdot \text{m}^2 / \text{C}^2) \frac{(1\text{C})(1\text{nC})}{(1\text{m})^2} = 9 \ \text{N}$$

$$\left|F_{3\text{-on-}2}\right| = k_0 \frac{q_2 |q_3|}{(r_{2-3})^2} = (9 \times 10^9 \ \text{N} \cdot \text{m}^2 / \text{C}^2) \frac{(1\text{nC})(8\text{C})}{(2\text{m})^2} = 18 \ \text{N}$$

$$\left|F_{4\text{-on-}2}\right| = k_0 \frac{q_2 |q_4|}{(r_{2-4})^2} = (9 \times 10^9 \ \text{N} \cdot \text{m}^2 / \text{C}^2) \frac{(1\text{nC})(x\text{C})}{(3\text{m})^2} = x \ \text{N}$$

In order for the net electric force on q_2 to be zero, the sum of the magnitudes of $\mathbf{F}_{1\text{-on-}2}$ and $\mathbf{F}_{4\text{-on-}2}$ must be equal to the magnitude of $\mathbf{F}_{3\text{-on-}2}$. That is, 9 N + x N = 18 N so x = 9. Therefore, $q_4 = -x$ C = −9 C.

8.3 ELECTRIC FIELDS

There are several advantages to regarding electrical interactions in a slightly different way from the simple "charge Q exerts a force on charge q" mode of thinking. In this more sophisticated interpretation, the very existence of a charge (or a more general distribution of charge) alters the space around it, creating what we call an **electric field** in its vicinity. If a second charge happens to be there or to roam by, it will feel the effect of the field created by the original charge. That is, we think of the electric force on a second charge q as exerted *by the field*, rather than directly by the original charge(s). Qualitatively, we can represent electrical interactions as follows:

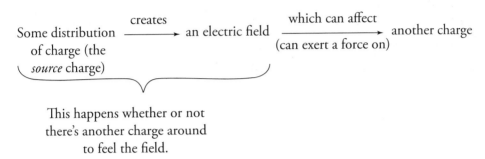

The charge(s) creating the electric field is/are called the **source charge(s)**; they're the source of the electric field. You may like to think of a source charge as a spider and its electric field as the spider's web. After a spider creates a web, when a small insect roams by, it is the web that ensnares the unfortunate bug, not the spider directly.

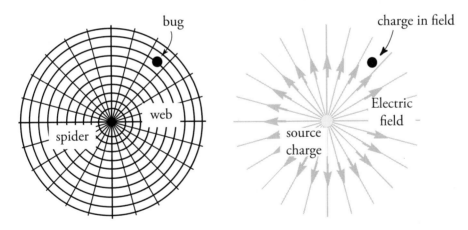

The figure on the right above illustrates one way to picture an electric field, but a few words of explanation are needed. First, an electric field is a **vector field**, which means that at each point in space surrounding the source charge, we associate a specific vector. The length of this vector will tell us the magnitude, or strength, of the field at that point, and the direction of the vector will tell us the direction of the resulting electric force that a *positive* test charge would feel if it were placed at that point. That's the convention: although the charge that finds itself in an electric field can of course be positive or negative, for purposes of *illustrating* the field, we always think of a *positive* test charge. Because of this convention, *electric field vectors always point away from positive source charges and toward negative ones*. Also, the closer we are to the source charge, the stronger the resulting electric force a test charge would feel (because Coulomb's Law is an *inverse*-square law). So, we expect the electric field vectors to be long at points close to the source charge and shorter at points farther away. The following figures illustrate the electric field due to a positive source charge and the electric field due to a negative source charge.

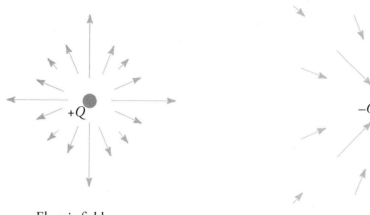

Electric field vectors
point away from
a positive source charge.

Electric field vectors
point toward
a negative source charge.

We can use Coulomb's Law to find a formula for the strength of the electric field. Remember that a source charge creates an electric field whether or not there's another charge in the field to feel it. It takes *two* charges to create an electric *force*, but it takes only *one* (the source charge) to create an electric *field*. So, let's imagine we have a single source charge, Q, and another charge, q, at a distance r from Q.

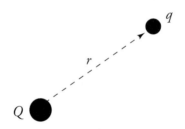

The force by Q, on the charge q, is, by Coulomb's Law,

$$F_{\text{by } Q} = k\frac{Qq}{r^2}$$

Now we ask, "What if q weren't there? Do we still have something?" The answer is *yes*, we have the electric field created by the source charge, Q. "So, if q weren't there, what if we removed q from the formula for the force exerted on it by Q? Would we still have something?" The answer is *yes*, we'd have the formula for the electric field, **E**, created by the single source charge Q.

Electric Field

$$E_{\text{by } Q} = k\frac{Q}{r^2}$$

In the formula for the force by Q on q, the variable r represents the distance from Q to q. However, if q is not there, what does r mean now? Answer: It's simply the distance from Q to the point in space where we want to know the electric field vector.

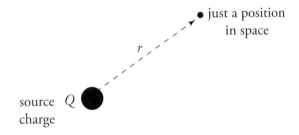

A final note: If we retain the sign of the source charge Q when we use the formula $E = kQ / r^2$, then a positive value for E means that the source charge Q is positive and the electric field vector at that point in space points away from Q; a negative value for E means that the source charge Q is negative and the electric field vector at that point in space points toward Q. (This makes the formula conform to the convention that electric field vectors are always pictured from the point of view of the force that a *positive* test charge would feel.)

Example 8-9: Let Q = +4 nC be a charge that is fixed in position at the origin of an *x-y* coordinate system. What is the magnitude and direction of the electric field at the point (10 cm, 0)? At the point (–20 cm, 0)?

Solution: In the figure below, the point A is (10 cm, 0), which is 10 cm directly to the right of Q, and B is the point (–20 cm, 0), which is 20 cm directly to the left of Q.

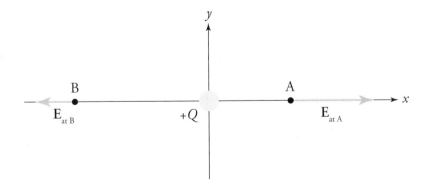

The electric field at point A is

$$E_{\text{at A}} = k_0 \frac{Q}{(r_{\text{to A}})^2} = (9 \times 10^9 \text{ N} \cdot \text{m}^2 / \text{C}^2) \frac{(4 \times 10^{-9} \text{ C})}{(10^{-1} \text{ m})^2} = 3600 \text{ N/C}$$

Since $E_{\text{at A}}$ is positive, this means the electric field vector, $\mathbf{E}_{\text{at A}}$, points away from the source charge. Therefore, $\mathbf{E}_{\text{at A}}$ points in the positive x direction, which is usually written as the direction $\mathbf{i}$. So, if we wanted to write the complete electric field vector at point A, we'd write $\mathbf{E}_{\text{at A}} = (3600 \text{ N/C})\mathbf{i}$.

The electric field at point B is

$$E_{\text{at B}} = k_0 \frac{Q}{(r_{\text{to B}})^2} = (9 \times 10^9 \text{ N} \cdot \text{m}^2 / \text{C}^2) \frac{(4 \times 10^{-9} \text{ C})}{(2 \times 10^{-1} \text{ m})^2} = 900 \text{ N/C}$$

Since $E_{\text{at B}}$ is negative, this means the electric field vector, $\mathbf{E}_{\text{at B}}$, points away from the source charge. Therefore, $\mathbf{E}_{\text{at B}}$ points in the negative x direction, which is usually written as the direction $-\mathbf{i}$. So, if we wanted to write the complete electric field vector at point B, we'd write $\mathbf{E}_{\text{at B}} = (900 \text{ N/C})(-\mathbf{i})$ or $-(900 \text{ N/C})\mathbf{i}$.

Notice from the formula $E = kQ / r^2$ that the electric field obeys an inverse-square law, like the electric force. So the strength of an electric field from a single source charge decreases as we get farther from the source; in particular, $E \propto 1 / r^2$. Also, for a given source charge Q, the electric field strength depends only on r, the distance from Q. So at every point on a circle (or more generally a sphere) of radius r centered on the source charge, the electric field strength is the same. In the electric field vector diagram below on the left, all the field vectors at the points on the smaller dashed circle have the same length, indicating that the electric field magnitude is the same at all points on this circle. Similarly, all the field vectors at the points on the larger dashed circle have the same length, indicating that the electric field magnitude is the same at all points on *this* circle. (Note that the field vectors at the points on the larger circle are shorter than those at the points on the smaller circle.) However, notice that the magnitude may be the same at every point on each circle (because they're all the same distance r from the source charge) but the directions of the electric field vectors are all different on each circle. Therefore, we're forced to say that the electric field isn't the same at every point a distance r from Q because the directions are all different.

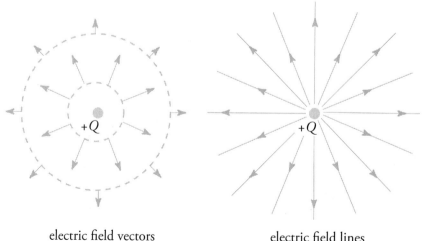

electric field vectors   electric field lines

The diagram on the left above and the two given earlier for the electric field produced by a positive source charge and by a negative source charge show the field represented by individual vectors. However, this is not the easiest way to draw an electric field.

Instead of drawing a bunch of separate vectors, we instead draw *lines* through them, like in the diagram on the right above. This drawing depicts the electric field using **field lines**. The direction of the field is indicated as usual; remember that, by convention, the electric field points away from positive source charges and toward negative ones and indicates the direction of the electric force that a positive test charge would feel if it were placed in the field.

Now that we've eliminated the separate vectors, it seems as though we've lost some information, namely, where the field is strong and where it's weak because we got this information from the lengths of the individual vectors. (Where the vectors were long, the field was strong, and where the vectors were shorter, the field was weaker.) However, we can still get a general idea of where the field is strong and where it's weak by looking at the *density* of the field lines: Where the field lines are cramped close together, the field is stronger; where the field lines are more spread out, the field is weaker.

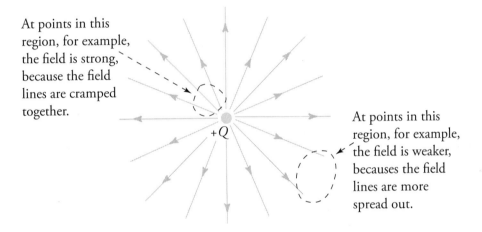

At points in this region, for example, the field is strong, because the field lines are cramped together.

$+Q$

At points in this region, for example, the field is weaker, becauses the field lines are more spread out.

Now, let's imagine that we have a source charge Q creating an electric field, and another charge, q, roams in to the field. What force will q feel? We want to find an equation for the force on q due to the electric field. Recall the formulas above: $F_{on\ q} = kQq\ /\ r^2$ and $E_{by\ Q} = kQ\ /\ r^2$. What would we need to do to E to get F? Just multiply it by q! That is, $F_{on\ q} = qE_{by\ Q}$. It turns out that this very important formula works not just for the electric field created by a single source charge; it works for *any* electric field:

Electric Force and Field

$$\mathbf{F}_{on\ q} = q\mathbf{E}$$

Notice also from this formula that $E = F\ /\ q$, so the units of E are N/C, which you saw in Example 8-9. The equation $\mathbf{E} = \mathbf{F}\ /\ q$ also gives us the definition of the electric field: it's the force per unit charge.

Finally, before we get to some more examples, realize that we've had two important (boxed) formulas in this section on the electric field: $E = kQ / r^2$ and $\mathbf{F} = q\mathbf{E}$. In the first formula, Q is the charge that *makes* the field, while in the second formula, q is the charge that *feels* the field.

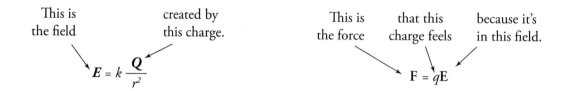

Example 8-10: A particle with charge $q = 2\ \mu C$ is placed at a point where the electric field has magnitude 4×10^4 N/C. What will be the strength of the electric force on the particle?

Solution: From the equation $F_{on\ q} = qE$, we find that

$$F = (2 \times 10^{-6}\ C)(4 \times 10^4\ N/C) = 8 \times 10^{-2}\ N$$

Notice that we didn't need to know what created the field. If E is given, and the question asks for the force that some charge q feels in this field, all we have to do is multiply, $F = qE$, and we're done.

Example 8-11: In the diagram on the left below, the electric field at Point A points in the positive y direction and has magnitude 5×10^6 N/C. (The source charge is not shown.) If a particle with charge $q = -3\ nC$ is placed at point A, what will be the electric force on the particle?

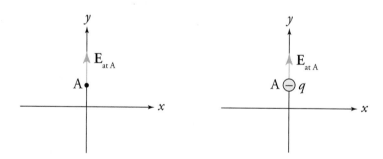

Solution: $\mathbf{E}_{at\ A}$ points in the positive y direction, which is usually written as the direction $\mathbf{j}$, so $\mathbf{E}_{at\ A} = (5 \times 10^6\ N/C)\mathbf{j}$. The equation $\mathbf{F}_{on\ g} = q\mathbf{E}$ then gives us

$$\mathbf{F} = (-3 \times 10^{-9}\ C)(5 \times 10^6\ \tfrac{N}{C})\mathbf{j} = (1.5 \times 10^{-2}\ N)(-\mathbf{j})$$

That is, the force will have magnitude 1.5×10^{-2} N and point in the negative y direction $(-\mathbf{j})$. Notice that whenever q is negative, the force $F_{on\ q}$ will always point in the direction *opposite* to the electric field.

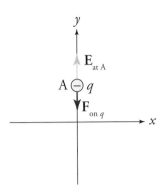

Example 8-12: A particle of mass m and charge q is placed at a point where the electric field is E. If the particle is released from rest, find its initial acceleration, **a**.

Solution: The acceleration of the particle is the force it feels divided by its mass: **a** = F/m. Because **F** = q**E**, we get

$$\mathbf{a} = \frac{\mathbf{F}}{m} = \frac{q\mathbf{E}}{m}$$

Notice that if q is negative, then **F** (and, consequently, **a**) will be directed *opposite* to the electric field **E**. Also, the question asked only for the *initial* acceleration, because once the particle starts moving, it will most likely move through locations where the electric field is different (in magnitude or direction or both), so the force on the particle will change; and if the force on the particle changes, so will the acceleration.

Example 8-13: The magnitude of the electric field at a distance r from a source charge $+Q$ is equal to E. What will be the magnitude of the electric field at a distance $4r$ from a source charge $+2Q$?

Solution: The first sentence tells us that $kQ/r^2 = E$. Now, if we change Q to $2Q$ and r to $4r$, we find that E decreases by a factor of 8, because

$$E' = k\frac{Q'}{(r')^2} = k\frac{2Q}{(4r)^2} = \frac{2}{16} \cdot k\frac{Q}{r^2} = \frac{1}{8}E$$

Example 8-14: The electric field at a distance y above the center of a ring of charge is given by the formula $E = k_0 Qy / \left(y^2 + R^2 \right)^{\frac{3}{2}}$, where Q is the charge on the ring and R is its radius.

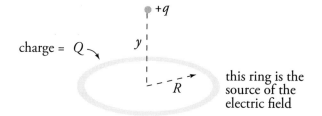

If $Q = +25$ mC and $R = 3$ m, find the force that a charge $q = +25/9$ nC would feel if it were placed at $y = 4$ m.

Solution: Even though the source of the electric field is not a point charge, we can still use the formula $F = qE$:

$$F = q \cdot E$$

$$= q \cdot k_0 \frac{Qy}{(y^2 + R^2)^{\frac{3}{2}}}$$

$$= (\tfrac{25}{9} \times 10^{-9} \text{ C}) \cdot (9 \times 10^9 \text{ N} \cdot \text{m}^2 / \text{C}^2) \frac{(25 \times 10^{-3} \text{ C})(4 \text{ m})}{[(4 \text{ m})^2 + (3 \text{ m})^2]^{\frac{3}{2}}}$$

$$= (25 \text{ N} \cdot \text{m}^2 / \text{C}) \frac{(10^{-1}) \text{ C} \cdot \text{m}}{(5^3) \text{ m}^3}$$

$$= 2 \times 10^{-2} \text{ N}$$

The Principle of Superposition for Electric Fields

The pictures we've drawn so far have been of electric fields created by a single source charge. However, we can also have two or more charges whose electric fields overlap, creating one combined field. For example, let's consider an **electric dipole**, which, by definition, is a pair of equal but opposite charges:

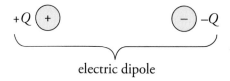

electric dipole

What if we regarded *both* of them as source charges; how would we find the electric field that they create together? By using the principle of superposition. If we wanted to find the electric field vector at, say, the point P in the diagram below,

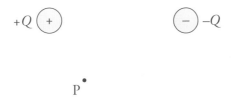

we'd first find the electric field vector, E_+, at P due to the +Q charge alone (ignoring the presence of the −Q charge) and then we'd find the electric field vector, E_-, at P due to the −Q charge alone (ignoring the presence of the +Q charge). The net electric field vector at P will then be the vector sum, $E_+ + E_-$.

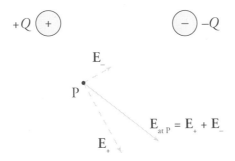

We can do this for as many points as we like and obtain a diagram of the electric field as a collection of vectors. The diagram in terms of electric field lines would look like this:

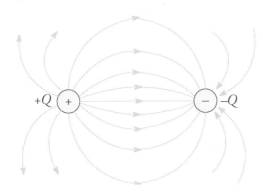

Notice that between the charges, where the field lines are dense, the field is strong; and as we move away from the charges, the field lines get more spread out, indicating that the field gets weaker.

Example 8-15: An electric dipole consists of two charges, $+Q$ and $-Q$, where $Q = 4\ \mu C$, separated by a distance of $d = 20$ cm. Find the electric field at the point midway between the charges.

Solution: The electric field at P due to the positive charge is $E_+ = k_0 Q / \left(\frac{1}{2}d\right)^2$, pointing away from $+Q$, and the electric field at P due to the negative charge is $E_- = k_0 Q / \left(\frac{1}{2}d\right)^2$, pointing toward $-Q$ (which is in the same direction as $\mathbf{E}_+$).

$$+Q\ \textcircled{+} \qquad\qquad \text{P}\cdot \overset{\mathbf{E}_+}{\underset{\mathbf{E}_-}{\longrightarrow}} \qquad \textcircled{-}\,-Q$$

$$\longleftarrow \tfrac{1}{2}d \longrightarrow \longleftarrow \tfrac{1}{2}d \longrightarrow$$

By the principle of superposition, the net electric field at P is the sum: $\mathbf{E} = \mathbf{E}_+ + \mathbf{E}_-$. The magnitude of $E_{\text{at P}}$ is $E_+ + E_- = k_0 Q / \left(\frac{1}{2}d\right)^2 + k_0 Q / \left(\frac{1}{2}d\right)^2 = 2k_0 Q / \left(\frac{1}{2}d\right)^2$:

$$E = 2k_0 \frac{Q}{\left(\frac{1}{2}d\right)^2}$$

$$= 2(9 \times 10^9\ \text{N} \cdot \text{m}^2 / \text{C}^2) \frac{4 \times 10^{-6}\ \text{C}}{(1 \times 10^{-1}\ \text{m})^2}$$

$$= 7.2 \times 10^6\ \text{N/C}$$

The direction of $\mathbf{E}_{\text{at P}}$ is away from $+Q$ and toward $-Q$:

$$+Q\ \textcircled{+} \qquad\qquad \underset{\text{P}}{\cdot}\ \overset{\mathbf{E}}{\dashrightarrow} \qquad \textcircled{-}\,-Q$$

Example 8-16: A positive charge, $+q$, is placed at the point labeled P in the field of the dipole shown below. Describe the direction of the resulting electric force on the charge. Do the same for a negative charge, $-q$, placed at the point labeled N.

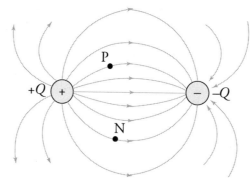

Solution: The electric field vector at any point is always *tangent* to the field line passing through that point and its direction is the same as that of the field line. Since $\mathbf{F} = q\mathbf{E}$, the force on a positive charge is in the same direction as $\mathbf{E}$ and the force on a negative charge is in the opposite direction from $\mathbf{E}$. The directions of $\mathbf{F}_{\text{on }+q}$ and $\mathbf{F}_{\text{on }-q}$ are shown in the figure below.

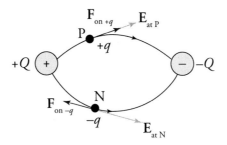

Conductors, Insulators, and Polarization

Most everyday materials can be classified into one of two major categories: *conductors* or *insulators* (also known as *dielectrics*). A material is a **conductor** if it contains charges that are free to roam throughout the material. Metals are the classic and most important conductors. In a metal, one or more valence electrons per atom are not strongly bound to any particular atom and are thus free to roam. If a metal is placed in an electric field, these free charges (called **conduction electrons**) will move in response to the field. Another example of a conductor would be a solution that contains lots of dissolved ions (such as saltwater).

Here's an interesting property of conductors: imagine that we place a whole bunch of electrons on a piece of metal. It's now negatively charged. Since electrons repel each other, they'll want to get as far away from each other as possible. As a result, all this excess charge moves (rapidly) to the surface. Any net charge on a conductor resides on its surface. Since there's no excess charge within the body of the conductor, there cannot be an electrostatic field inside a conductor. You can block out external electric fields simply by surrounding yourself with metal; the free charges in the metal will move to the surface to shield the interior and keep **E** = 0 inside.

By contrast, an **insulator** (**dielectric**) is a material that doesn't have free charges. Electrons are tightly bound to their atoms and thus are not free to roam throughout the material. Common insulators include rubber, glass, wood, paper, and plastic.

Now, let's study this situation: start with a neutral metal sphere and bring a charge (a positive charge) Q nearby without touching the original metal sphere. What will happen? The positive charge will attract free electrons in the metal, leaving the far side of the sphere positively charged. Since the negative charge is closer to Q than the positive charge, there'll be a net attraction between Q and the sphere. So, even though the sphere as a whole is electrically neutral, the separation of charge induced by the presence of Q will create a force of electrical attraction between them.

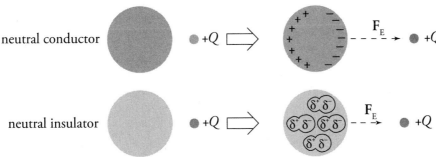

Now what if the sphere was made of glass (an insulator)? Although there aren't free electrons that can move to the near side of the sphere, the atoms that make up the sphere will become **polarized**. That is, their electrons will feel a tug toward Q, causing the atoms to develop a partial negative charge pointing toward Q (and a partial positive charge pointing away from Q). The effect isn't as dramatic as the mass movement of free electrons in the case of a metal sphere, but the polarization is still enough to cause an electrical attraction between the sphere and Q. For example, if you comb your hair, the comb will pick up extra electrons, making it negatively charged. If you place this electric field source near little bits of paper, the paper will become polarized and will then be attracted to the comb.[2]

8.4 ELECTRIC POTENTIAL

So far, we have viewed the electric field due to a source charge (or a more general charge distribution, such as a pair of charges, a ring, or a plate) as a collection of vectors. This point of view allowed us to answer questions about other *vector* quantities, like force and acceleration. The basic equations for finding these quantities were $\mathbf{F} = q\mathbf{E}$ and $\mathbf{a} = \mathbf{F}/m = q\mathbf{E}/m$.

What if we wanted to answer questions about *scalar* quantities, like energy, work, or speed? It turns out that the easiest way to answer these questions is to view the electric field in a different way, in terms of a scalar field. That is, instead of thinking of a vector at each point in the space around a source charge, we'll think of a scalar (just a *number*) at each point in space around a source charge. This scalar has a name: it's called **electric potential** (or just **potential** for short).

Let Q be a point source charge. At any point P that's a distance r from Q, we say that the electric potential at P is the scalar given by this formula:

Electric Potential

$$\phi = k\frac{Q}{r}$$

---

[2] The same phenomenon, in which the presence of a charge tends to cause polarization in a nearby collection of charges, is responsible for a kind of intermolecular force: Dipole-induced dipole forces are caused by a shifting of the electron cloud of a neutral molecule toward positively charged ions or away from a negatively charged ion; in each case, the resulting force between the ion and the atom is attractive.

The **London dispersion force**, in which electrically neutral molecules temporarily induce polarization in each other, is a much weaker version of the same phenomenon—again, electron clouds shift a little bit to create dipoles.

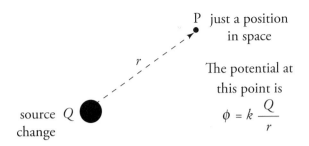

source Q change

P just a position in space

The potential at this point is

$$\phi = k\frac{Q}{r}$$

Notice the differences between this formula and the one for the electric field. First, the potential is kQ divided by r, while the electric field is kQ divided by r^2. Second, the electric field has a specific direction at each point (because it's a vector quantity); the potential, on the other hand, is not a vector, so it has no direction. While the electric field has the same magnitude at every point a distance r from Q, the field has a different direction at every point on the circle (or, more generally, the sphere) of radius r centered on Q. Therefore, we're forced to say that the electric field isn't the same at every point a distance r from Q because the directions are all different. The potential, however, is easier because it has no direction: the potential *is* the same at every point that's a distance r from Q.

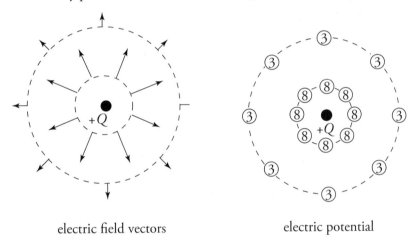

electric field vectors   electric potential

The dashed circles shown in the figure on the right above are called **equipotentials** ("equal potentials"), because the potential is the same at every point on them. For example, the potential is equal to 8 units everywhere on the inner dashed circle, and equal to 3 units everywhere on the outer dashed circle. As we move around on either dashed circle, the electric field changes (because the direction of **E** changes), but the potential doesn't change.

The formula given above for the potential, $\phi = kQ/r$, assumes that the potential decreases to 0 as we move far away from the source charges (that is, as $r \to \infty$); this is the standard, conventional assumption. With this formula, you can see that if Q is a positive charge, then the values of the potential due to this source charge are also positive (if Q is positive, then kQ/r is positive); on the other hand, the values of the potential due to a negative source charge are negative (if Q is negative, then kQ/r is negative). The sign of the potential (that is, whether it's positive or negative) is not an indication of a direction; remember, potential is a scalar, so it has no direction.

Before we get to some examples, it's important to mention that while there's no special name for the unit of electric field, there *is* a special name for the unit of electric potential:

$$[\phi]=[k]\frac{[Q]}{[r]}=(N\cdot m^{2}/C^{2})\frac{C}{m}=\frac{N\cdot m}{C}=\frac{J}{C}$$

A joule per coulomb (J/C) is called a **volt**, abbreviated V.

Example 8-17: What is the electric potential at a distance of r = 30 cm from a source charge Q = –20 nC ?

Solution: Using the formula $\phi = k_0 Q / r$, we find that

$$\phi = k_0 \frac{Q}{r}=(9\times 10^{9}\ N\cdot m^{2}/C^{2})\frac{-20\times 10^{-9}\ C}{30\times 10^{-2}\ m}=-600\ V$$

Example 8-18: In the figure below, the potential at Point A is 1,000 V. What's the potential at Point B ?

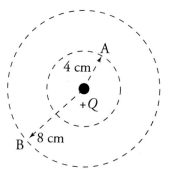

Solution: From the formula $\phi = k_0 Q / r$, we see that the potential is inversely proportional to r: Thus, $\phi \propto 1/r$. Because the distance from Q to B is twice the distance from Q to A, the potential at B should be half the potential at A. Therefore, $\phi_{at\,B} = 500\,V$. (Notice that because the potential at A is 1,000 V, the potential at *every* point on the inner circle is 1,000 V; and since the potential at B is 500 V, the potential at *every* point on the outer circle is 500 V.)

Now that we know how to calculate electric potential, how do we use it to answer questions about the scalar quantities energy, work, and speed? The applications of electric potential all follow from this one fundamental equation:

Change in Electrical Potential Energy

$$\Delta PE = q\Delta\phi = qV$$

That is, the change in potential energy of a charge q that moves between two points whose potential difference is $\Delta\phi$ is just given by the product, $q\Delta\phi$; it also can be expressed as qV, where V is defined in the change in potential and is known as the *voltage*. For example, let's say a charge $q = +0.03\,\text{C}$ moves from a point on the inner circle to a point on the outer circle in the figure accompanying the preceding example:

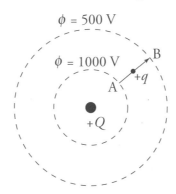

$\phi = 500\text{ V}$

$\phi = 1000\text{ V}$

B

$+q$

A

$+Q$

Then the change in the electrical potential energy of the charge q is

$$\Delta PE_{A \to B} = q\Delta\phi_{A \to B} = q(\phi_B - \phi_A) = (+0.03\,\text{C})(500\,\text{V} - 1000\,\text{V}) = -15\,\text{J}$$

We expected that the change in potential energy would be negative (that is, the potential energy would decrease), because the positive charge is moving farther from the positive source charge; because q moves in a way it naturally "wants" to move (since the positive charge q is naturally repelled by the positive charge Q), its potential energy should decrease.

If the charge q were instead pushed (by some outside force) from Point B to Point A, then its potential energy would increase:

$$\Delta PE_{B \to A} = q\Delta\phi_{B \to A} = q(\phi_A - \phi_B) = (+0.03\,\text{C})(1000\,\text{V} - 500\,\text{V}) = +15\,\text{J}$$

What if the charge q were moved from one point on the outer circle (Point B, say) to another point on the outer circle, B′?

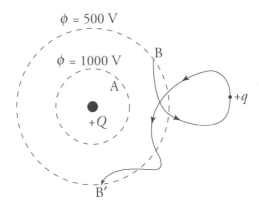

$\phi = 500\text{ V}$

$\phi = 1000\text{ V}$

B

A

$+Q$

$+q$

B′

Its potential energy would not change. Because the potential is the same everywhere on the outer circle, the potential at B is the same as the potential at B′, so the potential *difference* between Points B and B′ is zero; and if $\Delta\phi = 0$, then $\Delta PE = 0$ as well. *A charge experiences no change in potential energy when its initial and final positions are at the same potential.*

The figure above also illustrates that the path taken by the charge is irrelevant. Like the gravitational force, the electric force is conservative; all that matters is where the charge began and where it ended; the specific path it takes doesn't matter.

Example 8-19: A charge $q = -8$ nC is moved from a position that's 10 cm from a charge $Q = +2$ μC to a position that's 20 cm away. What is the change in its electrical potential energy?

Solution: Let A be the initial point and B the final point; then the change in potential from Point A to Point B is

$$\Delta\phi = \phi_B - \phi_A = \frac{k_0 Q}{r_B} - \frac{k_0 Q}{r_A} = k_0 Q\left(\frac{1}{r_B} - \frac{1}{r_A}\right)$$
$$= (9\times10^9 \text{ N}\cdot\text{m}^2/\text{C}^2)(2\times10^{-6}\text{ C})\left(\tfrac{1}{0.2\text{ m}} - \tfrac{1}{0.1\text{ m}}\right)$$
$$= -9\times10^4 \text{ V}$$

Therefore, the change in potential energy of the charge q is

$$\Delta PE = q\Delta\phi = (-8\times10^{-9}\text{ C})(-9\times10^4\text{ V}) = 7.2\times10^{-4} \text{ J}$$

Now that we've seen examples of how to calculate changes in potential energy in an electric field by using the concept of electric potential, how do we answer questions about work or kinetic energy? By using equations we already know from mechanics.

What if we want to find the work done by the electric field as a charge moves? If we move objects around in a *gravitational* field, we remember that the change in gravitational potential energy is equal to the opposite of the work done by the gravitational field. That is, $\Delta PE_{grav} = -W_{by\,gravity}$, which is the same as $W_{by\,gravity} = -\Delta PE_{grav}$. Applying this same idea to an electric field, we can say that the work done by the electric field is equal to $-\Delta PE_{elec}$:

Work Done by Electric Field

$$W_{by\,electric\,field} = -\Delta PE_{elec}$$

Now what about kinetic energy? Well, if there's no friction (which will be the case for charges moving around in empty space) or other forces doing work as a charge moves, then mechanical energy is conserved; that is, $KE + PE$ will remain constant. And if $KE + PE$ is constant, then $\Delta(KE + PE)$ will be zero.

That is, ΔKE will be equal to $-\Delta PE$. Since we know how to calculate ΔPE, we can calculate ΔKE by just changing the sign of ΔPE:

$$\Delta KE = -\Delta PE$$

So, as long as you remember the fundamental formula for potential energy changes in an electric field, $\Delta PE = q\Delta\phi$, you can answer questions about work or kinetic energy in an electric field by just using the formulas above.

Example 8-20: In the figure below, a particle whose charge q is +4 nC moves in the electric field created by a negative source charge, $-Q$.

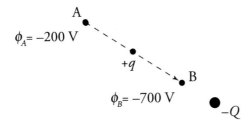

Find:

a) the change in potential energy,
b) the work done by the electric field, and
c) the change in kinetic energy of the particle as it moves from position A to position B.
d) If the mass of the particle is 10^{-8} kg and it started from rest at Point A, what will be its speed as it passes through Point B?

Solution:

a) $\Delta PE = q\Delta\phi = q(\phi_B - \phi_A) = (4\times10^{-9}\,\text{C})\left[(-700\,\text{V})-(-200\,\text{V})\right]$
   $= -2\times10^{-6}\,\text{J}$

b) $W_{\text{by electric field}} = -\Delta PE_{\text{elec}} = -(-2\times10^{-6}\,\text{J}) = 2\times10^{-6}\,\text{J}$

c) $\Delta KE = -\Delta PE_{\text{elec}} = -(-2\times10^{-6}\,\text{J}) = +2\times10^{-6}\,\text{J}$

d) If the particle started from rest at Point A, then $KE_{\text{at B}} = \Delta KE = +2\times10^{-6}\,\text{J}$, so

$$\frac{1}{2}mv_B^2 = 2\times10^{-6}\,\text{J} \;\rightarrow\; v_B^2 = \frac{2(2\times10^{-6}\,\text{J})}{m} \;\rightarrow\; v_B = \sqrt{\frac{4\times10^{-6}\,\text{J}}{10^{-8}\,\text{kg}}} = \sqrt{400\,\text{m}^2/\text{s}^2} = 20\;\text{m/s}$$

Example 8-21: Verify these statements:

a) Positive charges spontaneously accelerate (increase in kinetic energy) when they move toward a point of lower potential.
b) Negative charges spontaneously accelerate (increase in kinetic energy) when they move toward a point of higher potential.

Solution:

a) A charge will acquire more kinetic energy if it loses potential energy; that is, ΔKE will be positive if ΔPE is negative. So statement (a) is equivalent to this one: "A positive charge loses potential energy when it moves to a point of lower potential." To see that this is correct, notice first that if the charge moves to a point of lower potential, then the potential decreases, so $\Delta\phi$ is negative. It's now easy to see that if q is positive, then ΔPE will indeed be negative here, since $\Delta PE = q\Delta\phi = (+)(-) = (-)$.

b) Here, we want to show that if q is negative, then ΔPE will be negative if $\Delta\phi$ is positive. Thus, $\Delta PE = q\Delta\phi = (-)(+) = (-)$.

Here's a mnemonic for the statements in this example: the basic unit of positive charge is that of the proton, and the basic unit of negative charge is that of the electron. Protons are much heavier than electrons, so think of the heavy proton (or anything with a positive charge) like a rock and the light electron (or anything with a negative charge) like a helium balloon. Rocks naturally fall and helium balloons naturally rise; that is, positive charges naturally fall (to points at lower potential), while negative charges naturally rise (to points at higher potential).

Example 8-22: An electric field pulls an electron from one position to another such that the change in potential is +1 V. By how much does the electron's kinetic energy change?

Solution: The change in potential energy is

$$\Delta PE = q\Delta\phi = (-1.6\times10^{-19}\ \text{C})(+1\ \text{V}) = -1.6\times10^{-19}\ \text{J}$$

so the change in kinetic energy is the opposite of this, $+1.6\times10^{-19}$ J. This amount of energy is known as 1 **electron volt** (**eV**). In fact, the abbreviation for this unit makes the definition easy to remember: an electron (e^-) moving through a potential difference of 1 V experiences a kinetic energy change of $-q\Delta\phi = (e)(1\ \text{V}) = 1.6\times10^{-19}$ J $= 1$ eV. While the joule is the SI unit for energy, it's too big to be convenient when discussing atomic-sized systems. The electron volt is commonly used instead.

Example 8-23: An electric field pushes a proton from one position to another such that the change in potential is -500 V. By how much does the kinetic energy of the proton increase, in electron volts?

Solution: The change in potential energy is

$$\Delta PE = q\Delta\phi = (+e)(-500\ \text{V}) = -500\,\text{eV}$$

so the change in kinetic energy, ΔKE, is $-\Delta PE = -(-500\ \text{eV}) = +500$ eV.

The Principle of Superposition for Electric Potential

The formula $\phi = kQ/r$ tells us how to find the potential due to a single point source charge, Q. To find the potential in an electric field that's created by more than one charge, we use the principle of superposition. In fact, applying this principle is even easier here than for electric forces and fields because potential is a scalar. When we add up individual potentials, we're simply adding numbers; we're not adding vectors.

Let's illustrate with an example. In the figure below, the source charges $Q_1 = +10$ nC and $Q_2 = -5$ nC are fixed in the positions shown; the charges and the two points, A and B, form the vertices of a rectangle. What is the potential at Point A? At Point B?

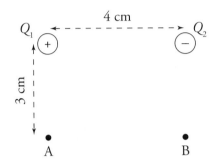

The potential at Point A due to Q_1 alone (ignoring the presence of Q_2) is

$$\phi_{A1} = k_0 \frac{Q_1}{r_{A1}} = (9 \times 10^9 \ \text{N} \cdot \text{m}^2 / \text{C}^2) \frac{+10 \times 10^{-9} \ \text{C}}{3 \times 10^{-2} \ \text{m}} = 3000 \ \text{V}$$

Since Point A is 5 cm from Q_2 (it's the hypotenuse of a 3-4-5 right triangle), the potential at Point A due to Q_2 alone (ignoring the presence of Q_1) is

$$\phi_{A2} = k_0 \frac{Q_2}{r_{A2}} = (9 \times 10^9 \ \text{N} \cdot \text{m}^2 / \text{C}^2) \frac{-5 \times 10^{-9} \ \text{C}}{5 \times 10^{-2} \ \text{m}} = -900 \ \text{V}$$

Therefore, the total electric potential at Point A, due to both source charges, is

$$\phi_A = \phi_{A1} + \phi_{A2} = (3000 \ \text{V}) + (-900 \ \text{V}) = 2100 \ \text{V}$$

Similarly, the total electric potential at Point B is

$$\phi_B = \phi_{B1} + \phi_{B2} = k_0 \frac{Q_1}{r_{B1}} + k_0 \frac{Q_2}{r_{B2}}$$

$$= (9 \times 10^9 \ \text{N} \cdot \text{m}^2 / \text{C}^2) \frac{+10 \times 10^{-9} \ \text{C}}{5 \times 10^{-2} \ \text{m}} + (9 \times 10^9 \ \text{N} \cdot \text{m}^2 / \text{C}^2) \frac{-5 \times 10^{-9} \ \text{C}}{3 \times 10^{-2} \ \text{m}}$$

$$= (1800 \ \text{V}) + (-1500 \ \text{V})$$

$$= 300 \ \text{V}$$

Example 8-24: A charge $q = 1$ nC is moved from position A to position B, along the path labeled *a* in the figure below. Find the work done by the electric field. How would your answer change if *q* had been moved from position A to position B, along the path labeled *b*?

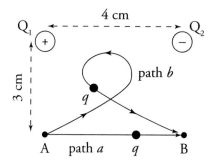

Solution: Path *a* begins at Point A, where $\phi_A = 2100\,\text{V}$, and ends at Point B, where $\phi_B = 300\,\text{V}$, so $\Delta\phi_{A\to B} = \phi_B - \phi_A = 300\,\text{V} - 2100\,\text{V} = -1800\,\text{V}$. Therefore, the change in potential energy of the charge *q* is

$$\Delta PE = q\Delta\phi = (1\times10^{-9}\,\text{C})(-1800\,\text{V}) = -1.8\times10^{-6}\,\text{J}$$

This means that the work done by the electric field, $W_{\text{by E}}$, is equal to $-\Delta PE = 1.8\times10^{-6}\,\text{J}$. If *q* had followed path *b*, the change in potential energy and the work done by the electric field would have been the same as for path *a*. The shape or length of the path is irrelevant; all that matters is the initial point and the ending point, and both paths begin at Point A and end at Point B.

We can't use the formula "work = force × distance" here, because the force is not constant during the object's displacement. To calculate work in an electric field, we use electric potential and the formula $W_{\text{by E}} = -\Delta PE_{\text{elec}}$.

Example 8-25: The figure below shows two source charges, $+2Q$ and $-Q$. What is the minimum amount of work that must be done by some outside force against the electric field to move a negative charge, $-q$, from position A to position B along the semicircular path shown?

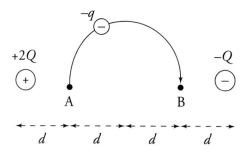

Solution: First, remember that neither the shape nor the length of the path matters; the fact that the path is a semicircle is irrelevant. All that matters is the initial point and the ending point of the path. Using the principle of superposition, the potentials at Points A and B are

$$\phi_A = \frac{k(+2Q)}{d} + \frac{k(-Q)}{3d} = \frac{5kQ}{3d} \quad \text{and} \quad \phi_B = \frac{k(+2Q)}{3d} + \frac{k(-Q)}{d} = -\frac{kQ}{3d}$$

Therefore, the change in potential energy of the charge $-q$ as it's moved from A to B is

$$\Delta PE = (-q)(\phi_B - \phi_A) = (-q)\left(\frac{-kQ}{3d} - \frac{5kQ}{3d}\right) = \frac{2kQq}{d}$$

Since the change in *PE* is positive, we know that the charge $-q$ is not moving as it would naturally on its own (after all, we can see from the figure that it's being moved from a point near a positive source charge, to which it's attracted, to a point near a negative charge, from which it's repelled). Therefore, some outside force is pushing this charge, doing work against the electric field. Since the work done *by* the electric field is $-\Delta PE = -2kQq/d$, the work done *against* the electric field by some outside force must be the opposite of this: $2kQq/d$.

Example 8-26: An electric dipole consists of a pair of equal but opposite charges, $+Q$ and $-Q$, separated by a distance d. What is the electric potential at the point (call it P) that's midway between these source charges?

Solution: The potential at P due to the positive charge alone is $k(+Q)/\left(\frac{1}{2}d\right)$, and the potential at P due to the negative charge alone is $k(-Q)/\left(\frac{1}{2}d\right)$. Adding these, we get zero, which is the potential at P due to both charges. (Notice that although the potential at P is zero, the electric field at P is *not* zero. We can have the "opposite" situation as well; that is, it's possible to have a point where the electric field is zero, but the potential is not. For example, if we had two equal source charges of the *same* sign, say $+Q$ and $+Q$, separated by a distance d, then the potential at the point that's midway between them would not be zero [it would be $2k(+Q)/\left(\frac{1}{2}d\right)$] but the electric field there *would* be zero.)

Example 8-27: An electric dipole consists of a pair of equal but opposite charges, $+Q$ and $-Q$, separated by a distance d. The dashed curves in the figure below are equipotentials. (Notice that the equipotentials are always perpendicular to the electric field lines, wherever they intersect. This is true for *any* electrostatic field, not just for the field created by a dipole.)

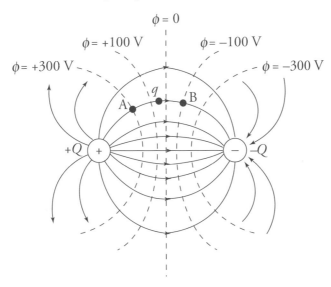

If a particle of mass $m = 1 \times 10^{-6}$ kg and charge $q = 5$ nC starts from rest at Point A and moves to Point B,

a) How much work is done by the electric field?

b) What is the speed of the particle when it reaches Point B?

Solution:

a) The work done by the electric field is equal to the opposite of the change in the particle's electrical potential energy $W_{by\,E} = -\Delta PE_{elec}$. Since the potential at Point A is $\phi_A = +300$ V (because A lies on the $\phi = +300$ V equipotential) and the potential at Point B is $\phi_B = -100$ V (because B lies on the $\phi = -100$ V equipotential), the change in potential from A to B is $\phi_B - \phi_A = (-100\,\text{V}) - (300\,\text{V}) = -400$ V. Therefore,

$$W_{by\,E} = -\Delta PE_{elec} = -q\Delta\phi = -(5 \times 10^{-9}\,\text{C})(-400\,\text{V}) = 2 \times 10^{-6}\,\text{J}$$

b) Since the total work done on the particle is equal to its change in kinetic energy (the Work-Energy Theorem), we have $\Delta KE = 2 \times 10^{-6}$ J. Because the particle started from rest at Point A, we have $KE_{at\,B} = \Delta KE_{A \to B} = 2 \times 10^{-6}$ J, so

$$\frac{1}{2}mv_B^2 = 2 \times 10^{-6}\,\text{J} \to v_B = \sqrt{\frac{2(2 \times 10^{-6}\,\text{J})}{1 \times 10^{-6}\,\text{kg}}} = 2\text{ m/s}$$

Example 8-28: The figure below shows several point source charges, $+Q_1$, $+Q_2$, $-Q_3$, and $-Q_4$, and the electric potential at various points (A, B, C, Z, Y, and Z) in the electric field they produce:

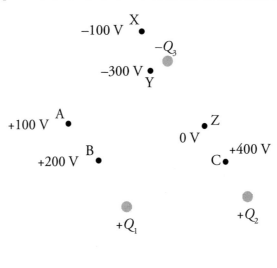

The difference in electric potential between two points is called the **voltage**, V. That is, $V = \Delta\phi$. For example, the voltage from Point A to Point B is $\phi_B - \phi_A = (+200\,\text{V}) - (+100\,\text{V}) = +100\,\text{V}$, and the voltage from X to Y is $V = (-300\,\text{V}) - (-100\,\text{V}) = -200\,\text{V}$.

a) How much work does the electric field do on a charge $q = +2\,\mu\text{C}$ as q is moved from Point X to Point C?

b) True or false? If the charge q is placed at Point Z, it will remain at this point because the electric potential is 0 V.

Solution:

a) The work done by the electric field is equal to the opposite of the change in the electrical potential energy $W_{by\,E} = -\Delta PE_{elec}$. Since $\Delta\phi = V$, the fundamental equation $\Delta PE = q\Delta\phi$ becomes simply

$$\Delta PE = qV$$

Since $V_{X\to C} = \phi_C - \phi_X = (+400\,\text{V}) - (-100\,\text{V}) = +500\,\text{V}$, we have
$$\Delta PE = qV = (2\times10^{-6}\,\text{C})(5\times10^2\,\text{V}) = 1\times10^{-3}\,\text{J}$$

Therefore, $W_{by\,E} = -1\times10^{-3}\,\text{J}$. (Does it make sense that ΔPE is positive and $W_{by\,E}$ is negative? *Yes*, because a positive charge q would have to be pushed by some outside force from Point X (which is near a negative charge) to Point C (which is near a positive charge). When an external force has to do positive work against the electric field, the electrical potential energy increases and the work done by the electric field is negative.)

b) False. If q were placed at a point where the *electric field* was zero, *then* it would feel no force and remain there. However, if q is placed at a point where the electric potential is zero, it will be accelerated toward a point where the potential is lower (because q is positive; recall Example 8-21). In this case, q would be accelerated by the electric field toward the negative source charge $-Q_3$.

Summary of Formulas

Elementary charge: $e = 1.6 \times 10^{-19}$ C

    charge of proton = +e; charge of electron = –e

Charge is quantized: $e = 1.6 \times 10^{-19}$ C

Coulomb's Law: $F_{elec} = k \dfrac{Qq}{r^2}$

    Opposite charges attract, like charges repel.

Coulomb's constant: $k_0 = 9 \times 10^9$ N·m^2/C^2

Principle of Superposition:

The net force, electric field, or electric potential on a charge q (for force) or point P (for electric field or electric potential) due to a collection of other charges (Qs) is equal to the sum of individual effects of each Q.

Electric field due to point charge Q: $E = k \dfrac{Q}{r^2}$

Direction of electric field:

    Positive charges want to move in the direction of the electric field (E).

    Negative charges want to move opposite the direction of the electric field (E).

Electric force and field: $\mathbf{F} = q\mathbf{E}$

Electric potential: $\phi = k \dfrac{Q}{r}$ (a scalar, not a vector)

Positive charges want to move to regions of lower potential.

Negative charges want to move to regions of higher potential.

Change in electrical PE: $\Delta PE_{elec} = q\Delta\phi = qV$

Work done by electric field: $W_{by\,E} = -\Delta PE_{elec}$

Change in KE: $\Delta KE = -\Delta PE$

For conductors, charge rests on the outer surface and the electric field inside is zero.

Chapter 9
D.C. Circuits

9.1 ELECTRIC CIRCUITS

An electric circuit is a pathway for the movement of electric charge, consisting of a voltage source, connecting wires, and other components.

Current

Current can be defined as the movement of charge, but for the purposes of analyzing an electric circuit, we need a more precise definition. For example, imagine picking up a metal paper clip and untwisting it to make it relatively straight. If we could look inside this piece of metal wire at the individual atoms, we would see a lattice with about one electron per atom free to roam freely, unbound to any particular atom. These free electrons are known as **conduction electrons**. (Recall the discussion of metallic bonding in OAT General Chemistry.) The conduction electrons in a metal are zooming around throughout the lattice at very high speeds. However, we only have a current when there is a *net* movement of charge. Let's look at this a little more closely.

The figure below shows an imagined magnified view inside a metal wire. The conduction electrons move at an average speed on the order of a million meters per second ($v \sim 10^6$ m/s). If we chose any cross-sectional slice of the wire, we would see that these conduction electrons cross from left to right as often as they cross from right to left. So, while there is movement of charge, there's no *net* movement of charge; that is, there's no current.

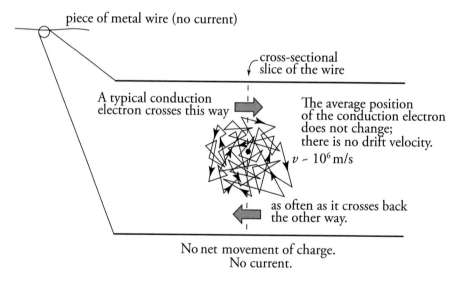

piece of metal wire (no current)

cross-sectional slice of the wire

A typical conduction electron crosses this way

The average position of the conduction electron does not change; there is no drift velocity.

$v \sim 10^6$ m/s

as often as it crosses back the other way.

No net movement of charge.
No current.

So how would this same piece of wire look if there *were* current in it? Superimposed on the conduction electrons' going-nowhere-fast zooming, we would see that there's a slight drift in one particular direction. This is known as the electrons' **drift velocity** (v_d). If we chose any cross-sectional slice of the wire, we'd see that these conduction electrons move across it from, say, left to right more often than they cross back. Thus, the average positions of the conduction electrons do change and there is a *net* movement of charge (in the case pictured below, negative charge to the right). This is **current**.

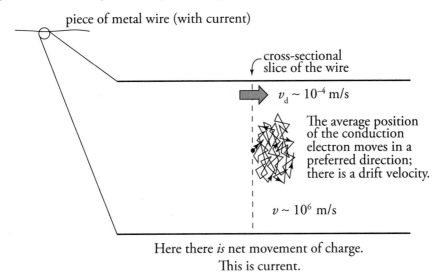

piece of metal wire (with current)

cross-sectional slice of the wire

$v_d \sim 10^{-4}$ m/s

The average position of the conduction electron moves in a preferred direction; there is a drift velocity.

$v \sim 10^6$ m/s

Here there *is* net movement of charge.
This is current.

In the first figure, there was no drift velocity and, therefore, no preferred direction for the movement of charge and no current. In the figure above, however, there is a drift velocity, so there is a flow of charge: a current.

Now, how do we measure current? Since current is the flow of charge, it makes sense to measure current as the amount of charge that moves past a certain point per unit time. Current is denoted by the letter I, and is equal to charge (Q) divided by time (t):

Current

$$I = \frac{Q}{t}$$

The unit of current is the coulomb per second (C/s), which has its own special name: the **ampere** (or just **amp**, for short), abbreviated **A**. Thus, 1 A = 1 C/s. Since we know that one coulomb is a lot of charge (recall Example 8-4 in the preceding chapter), we would expect that one amp is a lot of current. The following table shows that even a small fraction of a coulomb is enough to kill you.

<u>Current</u>	<u>Physiological Effect</u>
~ 0.01 A	slight tingling
~ 0.02 A	painful; muscles may contract around source (can't let go)
~ 0.05 A	painful; can't let go; breathing difficult
~ 0.1 to 0.2 A	ventricular fibrillation (potentially fatal arrhythmia)
> 0.2 A	severe burning; breathing stops; heart stops (may be restarted)

Example 9-1: Within a metal wire, 5×10^{17} conduction electrons drift past a certain point in 4 seconds. What is the magnitude of the current?

Solution: The magnitude of charge that passes the point in $t = 4$ seconds is

$$Q = ne = (5 \times 10^{17})(1.6 \times 10^{-19}\,\text{C}) = 8 \times 10^{-2}\,\text{C}$$

Therefore, the value of the current is

$$I = \frac{Q}{t} = \frac{8 \times 10^{-2}\,\text{C}}{4\,\text{s}} = 0.02\,\text{A}$$

Voltage

Now that we know how to measure current, the next question is, *What causes it?* Look back at the picture of the wire in which there was a current. What would make an electron drift to the right? One answer is to say that there's an electric field inside the wire, and since negative charges move in the direction opposite to the electric field lines, electrons would be induced to drift to the right if the electric field pointed to the left:

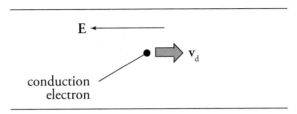

Another (equivalent) answer to the question, "What would make an electron drift to the right?" is that there's a potential difference (a voltage) between the ends of the wire. Because we know that negative charges naturally move toward regions of higher electric potential, electrons would be induced to drift to the right if the right end of the wire were maintained at a higher potential than the left end.

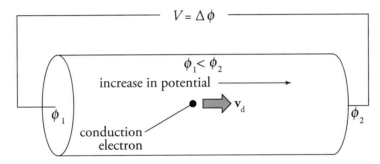

For our purposes in analyzing circuits, this second interpretation of the answer will be the one we use: that is, *it is a voltage that creates a current.* If there's no voltage (no potential difference), then the conduction electrons will just zoom around their original positions, going essentially nowhere; without a potential difference, they'd have no reason to do anything differently.

It is not uncommon to see the voltage that creates a current referred to as **electromotive force** (**emf**), since it is the cause that sets the charges into motion in a preferred direction. Notice, however, that calling it a "force" really isn't correct; it's a voltage.

Resistance

Now that we know what current is, how to measure it, and what causes it, the next question is, *How much do we get?* The answer is, *It depends.* If we took a paper-clip wire and touched its two ends to the terminals of a battery, we'd get a measurable current. Now imagine picking up a rubber band and cutting it, so that it becomes essentially a straightened out "wire" of rubber. If we took this rubber wire and touched its two ends to the terminals of the same battery, we'd get essentially zero current. What's the difference? The metal wire and the rubber wire have very different **resistances**. Metals are conductors and rubber is an insulator. That is, metals have a very low intrinsic resistance, while insulators (like rubber) have a very high intrinsic resistance to the flow of charge. Since insulators have very few free electrons, there's going to be virtually no current, even with an applied voltage, which is why we got essentially zero current with our rubber wire.

Let V be the voltage applied to the ends of an object, and let I be the resulting current. By definition, the resistance of the object, R, is given by this equation:

Resistance

$$R = \frac{V}{I}$$

The unit of resistance is the volt per amp (V/A), which has its own special name: the **ohm**, abbreviated Ω (the Greek letter capital *omega*—get it? "<u>ohm</u>ega"). Thus, $1\ \Omega = 1$ V/A. Notice from the definition that for a given voltage, a large I means a small R, and a small I means a big R; that is, for a fixed voltage, resistance and current are inversely proportional.

Example 9-2: When the potential difference between the ends of a wire is 12 V, the current is measured to be 0.06 A. What's the resistance of the wire?

Solution: Using the definition of resistance, we find that

$$R = \frac{V}{I} = \frac{12\,\text{V}}{0.06\,\text{A}} = 200\ \Omega$$

There's another way to calculate the resistance, using a formula that does not depend on V or I. Instead, it expresses the resistance in terms of the material's *intrinsic* resistance, which is known as its **resistivity** (and denoted by ρ, not to be confused with the material's density):

Resistance and Resistivity

$$R = \rho \frac{L}{A}$$

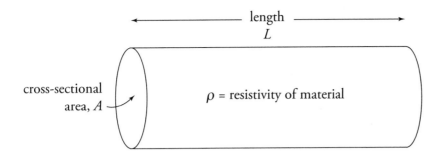

Notice that resistance and resistivity are not the same thing. Each material has its own resistivity; its *intrinsic* resistance. However, the resistance R depends on how we shape the material. For example, if we had two aluminum wires, one that was long and thin and another that was short and thick, both would have the same resistivity (because they're both made of the same material, aluminum), but the wires would have different resistances. The long, thin wire would have the greater resistance because R is proportional to L and inversely proportional to A.

Example 9-3: Consider two copper wires. Wire #1 has three times the length and twice the diameter of Wire #2. If R_1 is the resistance of Wire #1 and R_2 is the resistance of Wire #2, then which of the following is true?

A. $R_2 = (2/3)R_1$
B. $R_2 = (4/3)R_1$
C. $R_2 = 6R_1$
D. $R_2 = 12R_1$

Solution: We're told that $L_1 = 3L_2$, and since $d_1 = 2d_2$, we know that $A_1 = 4A_2$ (because area is proportional to the *square* of the diameter). Since both wires have the same resistivity (because they're both made of the same material), we find that

$$\frac{R_2}{R_1} = \frac{\rho L_2 / A_2}{\rho L_1 / A_1} = \frac{L_2}{L_1} \cdot \frac{A_1}{A_2} = \frac{1}{3} \cdot 4 = \frac{4}{3} \rightarrow R_2 = \frac{4}{3}R_1$$

Thus, the answer is (B).

Example 9-4: The wire used for lighting systems is usually No. 12 wire, in the American Wire Gauge (AWG) system. The diameter of No. 12 wire is just over 2 mm (which means a cross-sectional area of 3.3×10^{-6} m²). What would be the resistance of half a mile (800 m) of No. 12 copper wire, given that the resistivity of copper is 1.7×10^{-8} Ω·m?

Solution: Using the equation $R = \rho L / A$, we get

$$R = \rho \frac{L}{A} = (1.7 \times 10^{-8} \text{ Ω m}) \frac{8 \times 10^2 \text{ m}}{3.3 \times 10^{-6} \text{ m}^2} \approx 4\Omega$$

If we wanted to give a more precise formula for the resistance in terms of resistivity, we would have to include the temperature dependence. The resistivity of conductors generally increases slightly with temperature. However, unless specifically mentioned otherwise, assume that the OAT will treat resistivity as a constant.

Ohm's Law

The definition of resistance, $R = V/I$, is usually written more simply as $V = IR$, and known as **Ohm's Law**.

> **Ohm's Law**
>
> $$V = IR$$

However, the actual statement of Ohm's Law isn't $V = IR$; rather, it's a statement about the behavior of certain conductors, and it isn't true for all materials. A material is said to obey Ohm's Law if its resistance, R, remains constant as the voltage is varied; another requirement is that the current must reverse direction if the polarity of the voltage is reversed.[1] On the OAT, you can assume that materials are "ohmic" unless you are specifically told otherwise.

Resistors

A resistor is a component in an electric circuit that has a specific (and usually known) resistance. When we analyze a circuit, we generally ignore the resistance of the connecting metal wires and think of the resistance as being concentrated solely in the resistors placed in the circuit. We can do this because metal wires are such good conductors, i.e., their resistance is very low. Recall that in Example 9-4, we calculated that even half a mile of household wire has a resistance of only 4 Ω.

In the real world, a resistor is typically a little cylinder filled with an alloy (of carbon or of nickel and copper) and often encircled by colored bands to indicate the numerical value of its resistance, like this:

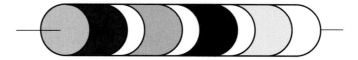

In circuit diagrams, however, a resistor is denoted by the following symbol:

Electric circuits on the OAT may contain just one resistor, but it's more likely that they'll have two or more. There are two ways the OAT will combine resistors: in series or in parallel. Two or more resistors are said to be in **series** if each follows the others along a single connection in a circuit. For example, these two resistors are in series, because R_2 directly follows R_1 along a single path.

---

[1] Some materials don't behave this way, and the relationship between voltage and current is more complex; on the OAT, however, it's safe to assume that $V = IR$ applies unless you're told otherwise.

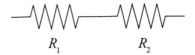

Resistors in Series

On the other hand, two or more resistors are said to be in **parallel** if they provide alternate routes from one point in a circuit to another. For example, the following two resistors are in parallel, because we get from Point P to Point Q in the circuit *either* by traveling through R_1 *or* by traveling through R_2; we don't go through both resistors like we would if they were in series.

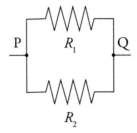

Resistors in Parallel

Typically, we analyze a circuit by first transforming it into a simpler one, one that contains just a single resistor. Therefore, we need a way to turn combinations of resistors (series combinations and parallel combinations) into a single, equivalent resistor; that is, one resistor that provides the same overall resistance as the combination. Here are the formulas:

resistors in series   single equivalent resistor

$R_{eq} = R_1 + R_2$

resistors in parallel

$R_{eq} = \dfrac{R_1 R_2}{R_1 + R_2}$

So, for resistors in series, we simply add the resistances. For example, if a 20 Ω resistor is in series with a 30 Ω resistor, this combination is equivalent to a single 50 Ω resistor, because 20 + 30 = 50. Notice that for a series combination, the equivalent resistance is always greater than the largest resistance in the combination; that's why the "*R*" is bigger in the figure above for the series combination.

For resistors in parallel, the formula is a little more complicated. If we have two resistors in parallel, we get the equivalent resistance by taking the product of the resistances ($R_1 R_2$) and dividing this by their sum ($R_1 + R_2$). For example, if a 3 Ω resistor is in parallel with a 6 Ω resistor, this combination is equivalent to a single 2 Ω resistor, because (3 × 6) divided by (3 + 6) is equal to 2. For a parallel combination, the equivalent resistance is always less than the smallest resistance in the combination; that's why the "R_{eq}" is smaller in the figure above for the parallel combination.

The "product over sum" formula for parallel resistors only works for *two* resistors. If you have three or more resistors in parallel, do them two at a time. Here's an example:

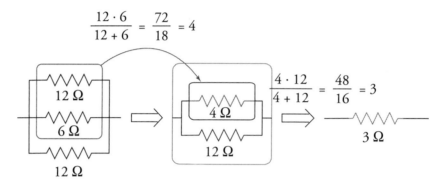

We could have also found the same answer this way:

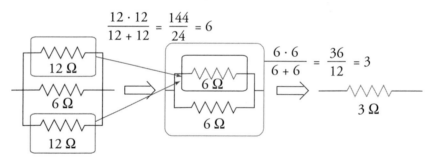

For resistors in series, we just add the individual resistances, no matter how many we have in a row. For example, if we have the following four resistors in series: 10 Ω, 20 Ω, 30 Ω, and 40 Ω, then we can reduce this combination of four series resistors to a single equivalent resistance of 100 Ω, because 10 + 20 + 30 + 40 = 100.

The formula for calculating the equivalent resistance, R, for a parallel combination of resistors R_1, R_2, ... is usually given as:

$$\frac{1}{R_{eq}} = \frac{1}{R_1} + \frac{1}{R_2} + \ldots$$

This formula works for any number of resistors in parallel, not just two. If you prefer this formula, that's perfectly okay. However, you may find adding the fractions to be messier than the "product over sum" rule above. Also, be sure to avoid the common error of forgetting to take the reciprocal of the left-hand side to get your final answer.

Example 9-5: Show that the equivalent resistance of two identical resistors in series is twice the resistance of either resistor, but the equivalent resistance of two identical resistors in parallel is half the resistance of either resistor.

Solution: Let the resistance of each resistor be R. Then, if two such resistors are in series, the equivalent resistance is $R_{eq} = R + R = 2R$. However, if two such resistors are in parallel, then their equivalent resistance is

$$R_{eq} = \frac{R \cdot R}{R + R} = \frac{R^2}{2R} = \frac{R}{2}$$

Example 9-6: What is the equivalent or total resistance of the following combination of resistors?

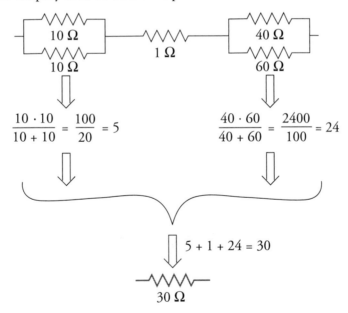

Solution: Here we have a mixture of parallel *and* series combinations. There's a parallel combination (the pair of 10 Ω resistors) that's in series with both a 1 Ω resistor and another parallel combination (the 40 Ω and 60 Ω resistors). To simplify this, we work in steps:

Therefore, the given combination of resistors is equivalent to a single 30 Ω resistor.

DC Circuits

Now that we know how to simplify series and parallel combinations of resistors, we're ready to analyze circuits. The simplest circuit consists of a voltage source (most commonly, it's a battery), a connecting wire between the terminals of the voltage source, and a resistor. As an example, imagine hooking up a light bulb to a typical flashlight battery; one wire connects the positive terminal of the battery to one of the "leads" on the light bulb, and another wire connects the other lead on the bulb to the negative terminal of the battery. This completes the circuit. The diagram on the right below shows the way this real-life circuit would be drawn schematically.

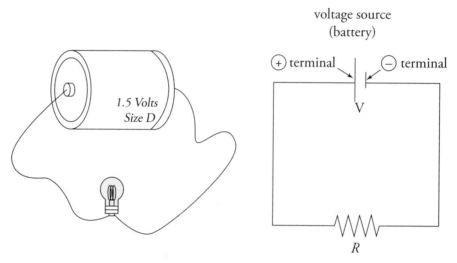

The pair of adjacent parallel lines denotes the voltage source. The job of the voltage source is to maintain a potential difference (a voltage) between its terminals; the value of this voltage is denoted by V or sometimes by ε, for emf (electromotive force). Remember that a voltage is needed to create a current. The terminal that's at the higher potential is denoted by the longer line and called the **positive terminal**; the terminal that's at the lower potential is denoted by the shorter line and called the **negative terminal**.

Once the circuit is set up, we know what will happen inside the metal wires: conduction electrons will drift toward the higher potential terminal; that is, they'll drift away from the negative terminal, toward the positive terminal. The direction of the flow of conduction electrons would be clockwise in the diagram as drawn. However, there is a convention that is followed when discussing the direction of the current. *The direction of the current is taken to be the direction that <u>positive</u> charge carriers would flow, even though the actual charge carriers that do flow might be negatively charged.* (Sounds like the convention for defining the direction of the electric field, doesn't it? "The direction of the electric field is taken to be the direction of the force that a positive charge would feel, even if the actual charge that gets placed in the field isn't positive." In fact, that's the reason for the convention about the direction of the current; to keep things consistent.) Even though we know electrons are drifting clockwise in this circuit, we'd say that the current, I, flows counterclockwise from the positive terminal around to the negative terminal.

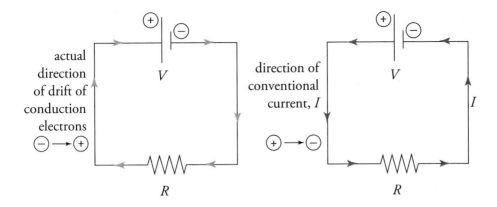

If we were asked for the value of the current in this circuit, this question would be easy to answer. We know V and R, and we want I. Using the equation $V = IR$, we'd say that

$$I = \frac{V}{R}$$

For example, if $V = 1.5$ V and $R = 150$ Ω, then $I = 0.01$ A. So, what made this problem so easy? The answer: there was only one resistor. This will usually be our goal: to simplify a circuit with multiple resistors into a circuit with just a single equivalent resistor. (We say "usually" because there are some question types that can be answered without changing the circuit into one with just a single resistor; we'll show you some examples of those too.)

In order to simplify a circuit with multiple resistors, we first need a way to turn resistors in series and resistors in parallel into a single equivalent resistor; this we already know how to do. However, there are two other important quantities in circuits besides R; namely, I and V. We also need to know what happens to these other quantities when we convert a series or parallel combination of resistors into a single resistor. The following figure contains this needed information:

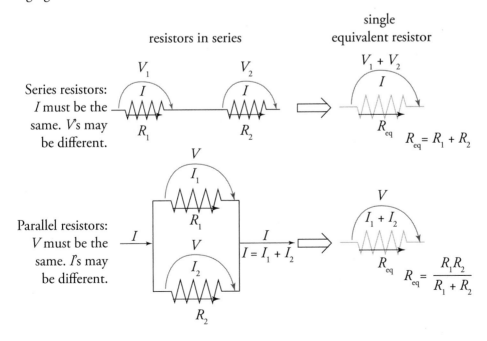

Resistors in series always share the same current, and resistors in parallel always share the same voltage drop. However, the voltage drops across series resistors will be different (and the currents through parallel resistors will be different) if the resistances are different.

With all this information at hand, we're ready to tackle an example. Consider the following circuit:

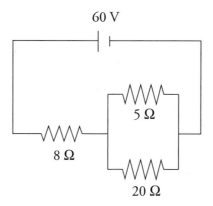

We'll find the current in the circuit, the current through each resistor, and the voltage across each resistor. The first stage of the solution involves simplifying this multiple-resistor circuit into a circuit with just a single equivalent resistor, like this:

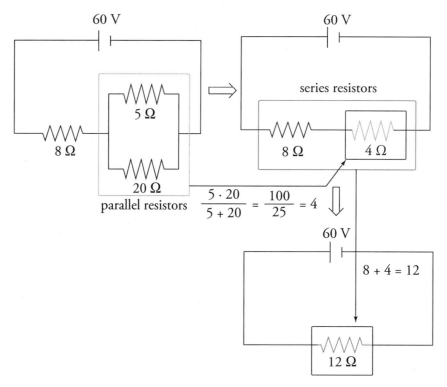

Now that we have an equivalent circuit with just one resistor, we can find the current:

$$I = \frac{V}{R} = \frac{60\,V}{12\,\Omega} = 5\,A$$

If we want to find the currents through (and the voltages across) the individual resistors in the original circuit, we have to work backward. The key to "working backward" is to ask at each stage: "What am I going back to?" If the answer is, "a *series* combination," then the value you bring back is the *current*, because series resistors share the same current. If the answer is, "a *parallel* combination," then the value you bring back is the *voltage*, because parallel resistors share the same voltage.

going back to series combination → bring *I*

going back to parallel combination → bring *V*

Let me illustrate this "working backward" technique with our circuit above. You should read this figure starting at the bottom, then up, then to the left...in other words, in the *reverse* order from what we did before because now we're working backward:

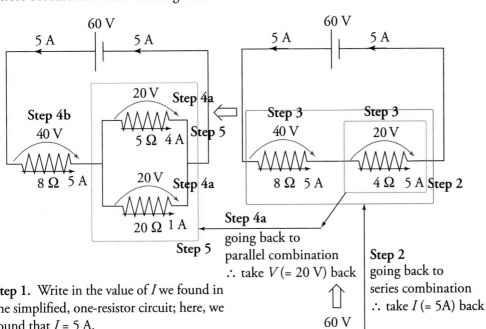

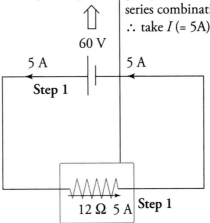

Step 1. Write in the value of *I* we found in the simplified, one-resistor circuit; here, we found that *I* = 5 A.

Step 2. Since we're going back to a series combination, we bring back the value of the current, *I* = 5 A.

Step 3. Use *V* = *IR* to find the voltage across each individual series resistor; here, we get *V* = (5 A)(8 Ω) = 40 V for the first resistor, and *V* = (5 A)(4 Ω) = 20 V for the second resistor.

Step 4a. Since we're going back to a parallel combination, we bring back the value of the voltage, *V* = 20 V.

Step 4b. Simply copy the information for the 8 Ω resistor, since that resistor doesn't change when we go back.

Step 5. Use *I* = *V/R* to find the current across each individual parallel resistor; here, we get *I* = (20 V)/(5 Ω) = 4 A for the top resistor, and *I* = (20 V)/(20 Ω) = 1 A for the bottom resistor.

Now that we have found all the information for the original circuit,

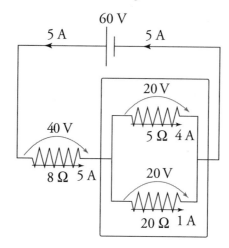

there are a couple of important things to notice, things that will hold true in any circuit. They are conse-quences of **Kirchhoff's laws** (pronounced "Keer-koff").

- *For a circuit containing one battery as the voltage source, the sum of the voltage drops across the resistors in any complete path starting at the (+) terminal and ending at the (−) terminal matches the voltage of the battery.*

For our circuit above, we have 40 V + 20 V = 60 V. (We don't add the 20 V twice, because these resistors are in parallel; each charge carrier moving through the circuit would go *either* across the 20 V voltage as it drifts through the top resistor in the parallel combination *or* across the 20 V voltage as it drifts through the bottom resistor; it doesn't go through both resistors.)

- *The amount of current entering the parallel combination is equal to the sum of the currents that pass through all the individual resistors in the combination.*

For our circuit above, we have 5 A = 4 A + 1 A.

Besides asking about resistance, current, and voltage, the OAT can also ask about power. When current passes through a resistor, the resistor gets hot: it dissipates heat. The rate at which it dissipates heat energy is the **power dissipated by the resistor**. The formula used to calculate this power, P, is known as the **Joule Heating Law**.

Power Dissipated by a Resistor: Joule Heating Law

$$P = I^2 R$$

So, for our circuit above, we find that:

the power dissipated by the 8 Ω resistor is $I^2R = (5 \text{ A})^2(8 \ \Omega)$ $\quad = 200 \text{ W}$
the power dissipated by the 5 Ω resistor is $I^2R = (4 \text{ A})^2(5 \ \Omega)$ $\quad = \ \ 80 \text{ W}$
the power dissipated by the 20 Ω resistor is $I^2R = (1 \text{ A})^2(20 \ \Omega)$ $\quad = \underline{\ \ 20 \text{ W}}$
the total power dissipated by all resistors is the sum: $\qquad\qquad 300 \text{ W}$

The power *supplied* to the circuit by the voltage source (like a battery) is given by this formula: $P = IV$. So, for our circuit above, we find that

power supplied by the 60 V battery is $P = IV = (5 \text{ A})(60 \text{ V}) = 300 \text{ W}$

Notice that these answers match:

power dissipated by all resistors = 300 W = power supplied by the battery

This is simply a consequence of Conservation of Energy, so it will be true in general:

- *The total power dissipated by the resistors is equal to the power supplied by the battery.*

Sometimes, a circuit may contain more than one battery, and in some of these cases, the battery with the lower voltage will be *absorbing* power from the battery with the higher voltage (that is, from the "boss battery" that supplies the power to the circuit). The power *absorbed* by a battery is also given by the formula $P = IV$, and the italicized statement above should then read:

- *The total power dissipated by the resistors and absorbed by other voltage sources (i.e., the total power used by the circuit) is equal to the power supplied to the circuit by the highest-voltage power source.*

One more note: The Joule Heating Law, $P = I^2R$, can be written as $P = I(IR) = IV$, so, in fact, we need just one formula for the power dissipated or supplied by *any* component in a circuit:

Power

$$P = IV$$

However, if you use the formula $P = IV$ to find the power dissipated by a resistor, *be careful* that you only use the *V for that resistor*, and not the *V* for the entire circuit. So, for our circuit above, we'd find that:

the power dissipated by the 8 Ω resistor is $\quad IV = (5 \text{ A})(40 \text{ V}) = 200 \text{ W}$
the power dissipated by the 5 Ω resistor is $\quad IV = (4 \text{ A})(20 \text{ V}) = \ \ 80 \text{ W}$
the power dissipated by the 20 Ω resistor is $\quad IV = (1 \text{ A})(20 \text{ V}) = \ \ 20 \text{ W}$

giving us the same answers we found before when we used the formula $P = I^2R$.

Along with questions about power, there could also be questions about energy. Simply remember the definition: power = energy/time, so

$$energy = power \times time$$

For example, how much energy is dissipated in 5 seconds by the 5-ohm resistor in the circuit above? We calculated that the power dissipated by this resistor is $P = 80$ W $= 80$ J/s; so the energy dissipated in $t = 5$ seconds is $Pt = (80$ J/s$)(5$ s$) = 400$ J.

In some circuits (in practice, most of them), one or more of the resistors are actually doing something useful besides just heating up. However, the circuit diagrams and the calculations we do will be the same. For example, a motor will be shown as a resistor in an OAT circuit; so will a light bulb (which is really just a resistor that happens to get so hot that some of the energy dissipated is emitted as light rather than heat). In either case, the calculations for these components are the same as treating each as a regular resistor. Notice that if you want to calculate the work that can be done by a motor, you'll wind up multiplying power by time.

Finally, a common and useful model/analogy for an electric circuit is a stream of water traveling down a series of waterfalls, with a pump in the collecting pool at the bottom to take the water back up to the top again. The battery (voltage source) is like the pump, and the voltage of the battery is the height it lifts the water. The current is the water, and each resistor is a waterfall. Resistors in series share the same current, because however much water drops down one waterfall must drop down the next one in the line (it has nowhere else to go); the heights of these waterfalls can of course be different, which is why the voltage drops for series resistors may be different. Parallel resistors are parallel waterfalls: they provide different paths for the water to drop from one point in the stream to a lower point. Because such waterfalls connect the same higher point to the same lower point, their heights must be the same; this is why parallel resistors always share the same voltage drop. One waterfall in parallel might be very narrow and only allow a small amount of water to flow down, while another waterfall in the same parallel (side-by-side) combination might be wide and thus allow more water to flow down; this is why resistors in parallel may have different currents. However, the total amount of water entering the top of the parallel waterfall combination must go down all the waterfalls in that combination (again, the water has nowhere else to go); this illustrates why the amount of current entering the parallel combination is equal to the total amount of current that passes through all the resistors in the combination. Finally, the total height of the waterfalls must be the same as the height through which the pump lifts the water from the collecting pool at the bottom; this illustrates why the total voltage drop across the resistors matches the voltage of the battery.

circuit	stream of water flowing down waterfalls with pump at the bottom
current	the flow rate of the water
resistor	waterfall
series	one waterfall after another
parallel	side-by-side waterfalls
voltage	for resistor: height of waterfall (distance water falls)
	for battery: total height the pump lifts the water to start a new cycle
resistance	relative width of channel in the water circuit (narrower width = higher resistance; wider = lower resistance)

Here's a diagram of the water stream and waterfalls that would be analogous to the circuit we analyzed above.

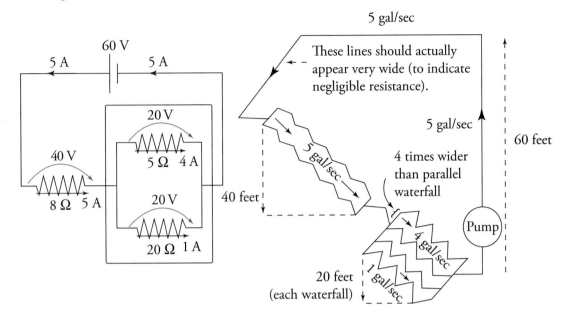

Example 9-7: Verify that the formulas $P = IV$ and $P = I^2R$ are dimensionally correct by showing that the product of current and voltage (IV) and the product of current squared and resistance (I^2R), both have the units of power.

Solution: First, because $[I] = C/s$ and $[V] = J/C$, we have

$$[IV] = [I][V] = \frac{C}{s} \cdot \frac{J}{C} = \frac{J}{s} = W = watt = [P]$$

Next, because $[I] = C/s$ and $[R] = \Omega = V/A$, we have

$$[I^2R] = [I]^2[R] = \left(\frac{C}{s}\right)^2 \cdot \frac{V}{A} = \frac{C^2}{s^2} \cdot \frac{\frac{J}{C}}{\frac{C}{s}} = \frac{C^2}{s^2} \cdot \frac{J \cdot s}{C^2} = \frac{J}{s} = W = watt = [P]$$

Example 9-8: A portion of a circuit is shown below:

$$\overbrace{\text{\textemdash}\!\!\!\!\!\text{\textemdash}}^{} \quad 10\,\Omega \;\; ^{1A} \quad 40\,\Omega \quad 20\,\Omega$$

If the current through the 10-ohm resistor is 1 A, what is the current through the 20-ohm resistor?

   A.   0.25 A
   B.   0.5 A
   C.   1 A
   D.   2 A

Solution: Because these resistors are in series, they all share the same current. If the current in the first resistor is 1 A, then the current through each of the other resistors is also 1 A. The answer is (C).

Example 9-9: A portion of a circuit is shown below:

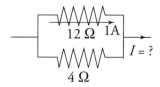

If the current through the 12-ohm resistor is 1 A, what is the value of the current I?

Solution: The voltage drop across the top resistor is $V = IR = (1\ A)(12\ \Omega) = 12$ V. Because the resistors are in parallel, the voltage drop across the bottom resistor must also be 12 V. Using $I = V/R$, we find that the current through the bottom resistor is $(12\ V)/(4\ \Omega) = 3$ A. Therefore, the total amount of current passing through the parallel combination is 1 A + 3 A = 4 A.

Example 9-10: With the information given in the circuit diagram below, what is the voltage of the battery?

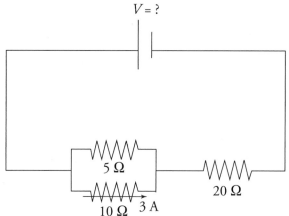

A. 150 V
B. 210 V
C. 240 V
D. 300 V

Solution: The voltage drop across the bottom resistor in the parallel combination is $V = IR = (3\ A)(10\ \Omega) = 30$ V. Because the top and bottom resistors in this combination are in parallel, the voltage drop across the top resistor must also be 30 V. Using $I = V/R$, we find that the current through the top resistor is $(30\ V)/(5\ \Omega) = 6$ A. Therefore, the total amount of current passing through the parallel combination is 6 A + 3 A = 9 A. Since this much current flows through the 20-ohm resistor, the voltage drop across the 20-ohm resistor is $V = IR = (9\ A)$ $(20\ \Omega) = 180$ V. Because the total voltage drop across the resistors must match the voltage of the battery, we have $V = 30$ V + 180 V = 210 V, so the answer is (B). (Remember, don't add the 30 V voltage drop twice here; (C) is a trap.)

Example 9-11: A portion of a circuit is shown below:

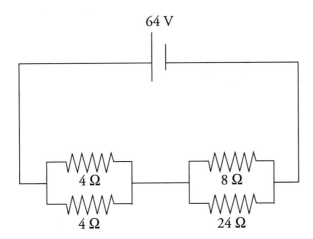

If the current entering the parallel combination is 12 A, how much current flows through the 120-ohm resistor?

Solution: Because the 60-ohm bottom resistor has half the resistance of the 120-ohm top resistor, twice as much current will flow through the bottom resistor as through the top one. So, if we let X stand for the current in the top resistor, then the current in the bottom resistor is $2X$. Because 12 A enters the parallel combination, we must have $X + 2X = 12$ A, so $X = 4$ A. Therefore, the current in the top resistor is 4 A (and the current in the bottom resistor is 8 A). Notice that the voltage drop across the top resistor is $V = IR = (4 \text{ A})(120 \ \Omega) = 480$ V, and the voltage drop across the bottom resistor is $V = IR = (8 \text{ A})(60 \ \Omega) = 480$ V. The fact that these voltages match (as they must for parallel resistors) verifies that our answer is correct.

Example 9-12: How much energy is dissipated in 10 seconds by the 24-ohm resistor in the following circuit?

64 V

4 Ω

4 Ω

8 Ω

24 Ω

- A. 480 J
- B. 640 J
- C. 720 J
- D. 960 J

Solution: The pair of parallel 4-ohm resistors is equivalent to a single 2-ohm resistor [because $(4 \times 4)/(4 + 4) = 2$], and the parallel 8-ohm and 24-ohm resistors are equivalent to a single 6-ohm resistor [because $(8 \times 24)/(8 + 24) = 192/32 = 6$]. These equivalent resistors are in series, so the overall equivalent resistance for the circuit is $2 \ \Omega + 6 \ \Omega = 8 \ \Omega$. This means the current in the circuit is $I = V/R_{eq} = 64/8 = 8$ A. When these 8 amps enter the second parallel combination (the one with the 8-ohm and 24-ohm resistors), it must split up in such a way that the current through the 8-ohm resistor is 3 times the current through the 24-ohm resistor. (Because the 8-ohm resistor has 1/3 the resistance of the 24-ohm resistor, it will get 3 times the current.)

So, if we let X stand for the current in the 24-ohm resistor, then the current through the 8-ohm resistor is $3X$; this gives $X + 3X = 8$ A, so $X = 2$ A. Thus, the current in the 24-ohm resistor is 2 A. [The current in the 8-ohm resistor is $3X = 6$ A. The voltage drop across the 8-ohm resistor is (6 A)(8 Ω) = 48 V, and the voltage drop across the 24-ohm resistor is (2 A)(24 Ω) = 48 V; the fact that these match verifies that our calculation is correct.] Since the current in the 24-ohm resistor is 2 A, the power dissipated by this resistor is $P = I^2R =$ $(2^2)(24) = 96$ W. Therefore, the energy dissipated by this resistor in 10 seconds is (96 W)(10 s) = 960 J, and the answer is (D).

Example 9-13: What is the current in the 100-ohm resistor shown below?

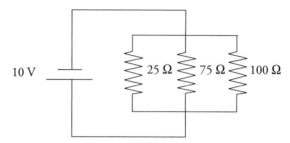

Solution: For this question, we don't need to begin by finding the single equivalent resistance of the given parallel combination, because we already know the voltage across the 100-ohm resistor. The parallel combination is attached directly to the terminals of the battery, so the voltage across each of the resistors must be 10 V. Because we know both V and R, we can find I in one step: $I = V/R = (10$ V$)/(100$ Ω$) = 0.1$ A.

Example 9-14: What is the current in the circuit below?

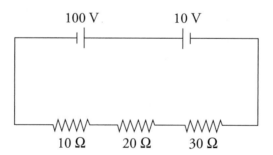

Solution: This circuit contains two batteries. The 100-volt battery wants to send current clockwise. (Remember: We consider current as the directed motion of positive charge, and positive charge carriers would move away from the positive terminal, around the circuit to the negative terminal.) However, the 10-volt battery would want to send current the opposite way: counterclockwise. Since the 100-volt battery has the higher voltage (or, equivalently, the greater emf), it's the "boss" battery. Therefore, current will flow clockwise, but the effective emf will be reduced to $100 - 10 = 90$ V, because the 10-volt battery is opposing the 100-volt boss battery. The equivalent resistance is $10 + 20 + 30 = 60$ Ω (the resistors are in series), so the current in the circuit will be $I = V/R_{eq} = (90$ V$)/(60$ Ω$) = 1.5$ A. (Note: The 10-volt battery is being charged by the 100-volt boss battery.)

Example 9-15: A toaster oven is rated at 720 W. If it draws 6 A of current, what is its resistance?

Solution: Here, we're given P and I, and asked for R. Since $P = I^2 R$, we find that

$$R = \frac{P}{I^2} = \frac{720 \text{ W}}{(6 \text{ A})^2} = 20 \ \Omega$$

Example 9-16: Current passes through an insulated resistor of resistance R, mass m, and specific heat c. The voltage across this resistor is V. If the resistor absorbs all the heat it generates, find an expression for the increase in temperature of the resistor after a time t. (All values are expressed in SI units.)

Solution: The amount of heat energy generated (and absorbed) by the resistor is $q = Pt$, where $P = IV = (V/R)$ $V = V^2/R$. (Here, q stands for "heat energy," not "charge.") Now, using the fundamental equation $q = mc\Delta T$ (from general chemistry), we have

$$\Delta T = \frac{q}{mc} = \frac{Pt}{mc} = \frac{\frac{V^2}{R}t}{mc} = \frac{V^2 t}{Rmc}$$

All real batteries have **internal resistance**, which we denote by r. Let ε denote the emf of the battery; this is its "ideal" voltage (i.e., the voltage between its terminals when there's no current). Once a current is established, the internal resistance causes the voltage between the terminals to be different from ε. If the battery is supplying current I to the circuit, then the **terminal voltage**, V, is less than ε and given by $V = \varepsilon - Ir$. (On the other hand, if the circuit is *supplying* current to the battery [charging it up], then the terminal voltage is greater than ε and given by the equation $V = \varepsilon + Ir$.) The internal resistance is actually *between* the terminals in a real battery, but in circuit diagrams, the internal resistance is drawn next to the battery, like this:

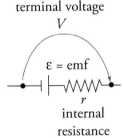

terminal voltage
V

$\varepsilon = $ emf

r
internal
resistance

However, unless you are told otherwise, you may assume that all batteries are ideal and have no internal resistance.

Example 9-17: The battery shown in the circuit below has an emf of 100 V and an internal resistance of 5 Ω. What is its terminal voltage in this circuit? (*Note:* It's not uncommon to see a dashed box drawn around the battery and its internal resistance; this emphasizes that *r* is actually inside the battery.)

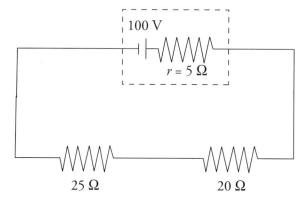

A. 80 V
B. 90 V
C. 100 V
D. 110 V

Solution: The three resistors in this circuit are in series, so the equivalent resistance for the circuit is 5 + 25 + 20 = 50 Ω. Because the emf is 100 V, the current in the circuit is

$$I = \varepsilon \,/\, R = (100 \text{ V})/(50 \text{ }\Omega) = 2 \text{ A}$$

The terminal voltage is therefore

$$V = \varepsilon - Ir = (100 \text{ V}) - (2 \text{ A})(5 \text{ }\Omega) = 90 \text{ V}$$

The answer is (B). (*Note:* You could eliminate (C) and (D) immediately; the terminal voltage must be *less* than the emf because the battery is supplying current to the circuit.)

Example 9-18: A device used to measure the current in a circuit is called an **ammeter** (denoted by Ⓐ in a circuit diagram). It has a very small internal resistance, so that it only negligibly affects the current it's trying to measure; for most purposes, we ignore the resistance of an ammeter. What would an ammeter read if it were placed as shown in the following circuit?

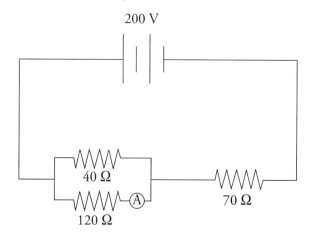

Solution: (The symbol for the battery in this circuit consists of two pairs of parallel lines, rather than the usual one pair. Batteries can be denoted by one *or more* pairs of parallel lines, as long as one "end" is a long line (representing the positive terminal) and the opposite "end" of the battery is a short line (representing the negative terminal). The two parallel resistors are equivalent to a single 30 Ω resistor (because $(40 \times 120)/(40+120) = 4800/160 = 30$). This, in series with the 70 Ω resistor, means the overall resistance of the circuit is $30 + 70 = 100$ Ω, so the current is $I = V/R_{eq} = (200 \text{ V})/(100 \text{ Ω}) = 2$ A. The voltage drop across the 30 Ω equivalent resistance is therefore $(2 \text{ A})(30 \text{ Ω}) = 60$ V, so this is the voltage across each of the individual parallel resistors. The ammeter is placed in the branch with the 120 Ω resistor, so it will measure a current of $V/R = (60 \text{ V})/(120 \text{ Ω}) = 0.5$ A.

Example 9-19: A device used to measure the voltage between two points in a circuit is called a **voltmeter** (denoted by V in a circuit diagram). It has a very large internal resistance so that it won't draw much current and thus affect the voltage it's trying to measure. What would a voltmeter read if it were placed as shown in the following circuit?

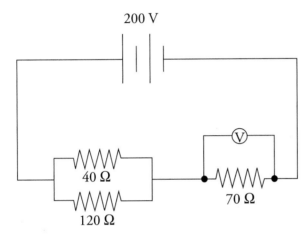

Solution: This is the same circuit we analyzed in the preceding example. Because the current in the circuit is 2 A, the voltage across the 70 Ω resistor will be $V = IR = (2 \text{ A})(70 \text{ Ω}) = 140$ V.

Example 9-20: The diagram below shows a point X held at a potential of $\phi = 60 \text{ V}$ connected by a combination of resistors to a point (denoted by G) that is **grounded**. *The ground is considered to be at potential zero.* What is the current through the 100-ohm resistor?

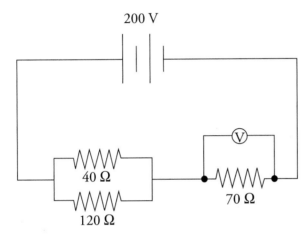

Solution: The parallel resistors are equivalent to a single 20 Ω resistor, which is then in series with the 100 Ω resistor, giving an overall equivalent resistance of $20 + 100 = 120$ Ω. Since the potential difference between points X and G is $V = \phi_X - \phi_G = 60 - 0 = 60$ V, the current in the circuit (and through the 100-ohm resistor) is

$$I = V / R_{eq} = (60 \text{ V})/(120 \text{ Ω}) = 0.5 \text{ A}$$

Example 9-21: The diagram below shows a battery with an emf of 100 V connected to a circuit equipped with a switch, S.

    a)   What is the current in the circuit when the switch is open?

    b)   What is the current in the circuit when the switch is closed?

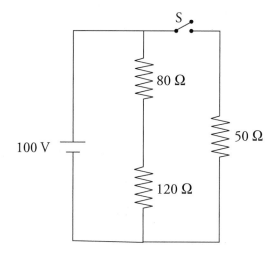

Solution:

    a)   With the switch open (as pictured above) the 50 Ω resistor is effectively taken out of the circuit; no current will flow in that branch. Current will flow only in the part of the circuit shown below:

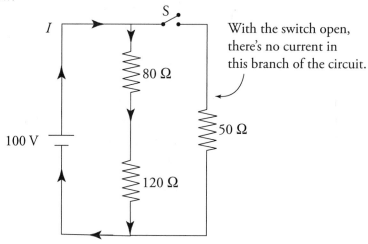

        The two resistors that *are* in the circuit when the switch is open are in series, so the total equivalent resistance is 80 + 120 = 200 Ω; thus, the current is

$$I = V / R_{eq} = (100 \text{ V})/(200 \text{ Ω}) = 0.5 \text{ A}$$

b)   With the switch closed, all the resistors are part of the circuit, and there will be current in all the branches. Let's find the equivalent resistance. The 80 Ω and 120 Ω resistors are in series, so they're equivalent to a single 80 + 120 = 200 Ω resistor, which is then in parallel with the 50 Ω resistor. This gives an overall equivalent resistance of 40 Ω because $(200 \times 50)/(200 + 50)$ is equal to 40. Therefore, the current supplied to the circuit in this case is $I = V/R_{eq} = (100 \text{ V})/(40 \text{ }\Omega) = 2.5 \text{ A}$.

Example 9-22: Three identical light bulbs are connected to a battery, as shown:

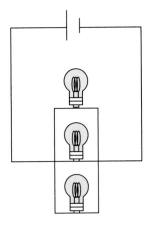

What will happen if the middle bulb burns out?

   A.   The other two bulbs will go out.
   B.   The light intensity of the other two bulbs will decrease, but they won't go out.
   C.   The light intensity of the other two bulbs will increase.
   D.   The light intensity of the other two bulbs will remain the same.

Solution: Let V be the voltage of the battery, and let R be the resistance of each light bulb. The current through each light bulb (that is, through each resistor) is $I = V/R$. If the middle bulb burns out, then the middle branch of the parallel combination is severed; but current can still flow through the top and bottom bulbs, and the current through each will still be $I = V/R$. Because the intensity of the light is directly related to the power each one dissipates, the fact that the current doesn't change means that $P = I^2R$ won't change, so the light intensity of the other two bulbs will remain the same. The answer is (D). [What *will* change if the middle bulb burns out? Before the middle bulb burns out, the current through each of the three bulbs is $I = V/R$, so the battery must be providing a total current of $3I = 3V/R$. After the middle bulb burns out, the current through each of the other two bulbs is still $I = V/R$, so the battery need only provide a total current of $2I = 2V/R$. That is, the total current through the circuit will decrease (since, after all, there are only two bulbs to light, not three). In addition, the power supplied by the battery will also decrease, from $P = (3I)(V) = 3V^2/R$ to $P = (2I)(V) = 2V^2/R$, and the battery will last longer. Finally, notice that if the three bulbs were wired in *series* rather than in parallel, then if any one of the bulbs burned out, they'd all go out because the circuit would be broken.]

9.2 CAPACITORS

A pair of conductors that can hold equal but opposite charges is known as a **capacitor**. The conductors can be of any shape, but the most common capacitor consists of a pair of parallel metal plates; it's known as a **parallel-plate capacitor**:

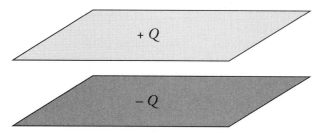

Notice that one plate carries a positive charge and the other plate carries an equal amount of negative charge. Therefore, the *net* charge on a capacitor is zero. However, whenever we talk about the "charge on a capacitor," we always mean the magnitude of charge on either plate, which is $+Q$.

In circuit diagrams, a capacitor is denoted by either of these two symbols:

$$|| \quad \text{or} \quad |($$

The first question we'll answer is, "How do we create a charged capacitor?" Take an uncharged parallel-plate capacitor, and hook the plates to the terminals of a battery. Conduction electrons in the connecting wires will be repelled from the negative terminal and flow to one plate, while electrons from the other plate will be attracted toward the positive terminal of the battery. The current rises quickly at first, but it gradually dies out as the plates acquire charge. The plate that's connected to the positive terminal becomes positively charged, and the plate that's connected to the negative terminal becomes negatively charged. Since the positive plate has a higher potential than the negative plate, the potential difference between the plates opposes the potential difference of the battery. Charge will stop flowing when the potential difference between the plates matches the voltage of the battery because at that point the circuit will look like one that has two opposing voltage sources.

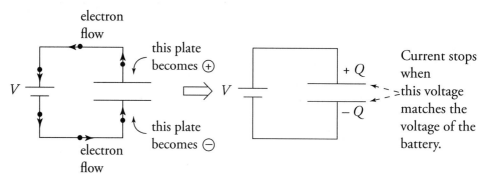

If V is the potential difference between the plates of a charged capacitor, and Q is the charge on the capacitor, then Q and V are proportional. The proportionality constant, C, is called the **capacitance**:

Charge on a Capacitor

$$Q = CV$$

From this equation we can see that the unit of capacitance is coulomb per volt (C/V), which has its own name: the **farad**, abbreviated F. Therefore, 1 C/V = 1 F. Because a coulomb is a lot of charge, we'd expect a farad to be a lot of capacitance. Most real-life capacitors have capacitances that are on the order of a few microfarads.

The capacitance is determined only by the sizes of the plates and how far apart they are (and, as we'll see a little later, whether there's anything between the plates). For a parallel-plate capacitor with empty space between the plates, C is given by the following equation:

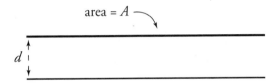

Capacitance of a Parallel Plate Capacitor

$$C = \varepsilon_0 \frac{A}{d}$$

---

where A is the area of each plate, d is their separation, and ε_0 is a fundamental constant of nature. (The constant ε_0 is known as the **permittivity of free space**; it's equal to $1/(4\pi k_0)$, where k_0 is Coulomb's constant, so the approximate numerical value of ε_0 is 8.85×10^{-12} F/m.)

The capacitance C depends only on A and d. Although $Q = CV$, the capacitance C does not depend on either Q or V; it only tells us how Q and V will be related. If you were given an uncharged capacitor, you could determine C without charging it up, by using the formula $C = \varepsilon_0 A/d$.

Intuitively, capacitance measures the plates' "capacity" for holding charge at a certain voltage. Let's say we had two capacitors with different capacitances, and we wanted to store as much charge as we could while keeping V low. We'd choose the capacitor with the greater capacitance because it would be able to hold more charge per volt.

Example 9-23: A capacitor has a capacitance of 2 nF. How much charge can it hold at a voltage of 150 V?

Solution: We're given C and V, and asked for Q. Using the equation $Q = CV$, we find that

$$Q = CV = (2 \times 10^{-9} \text{ F})(150 \text{ V}) = 3 \times 10^{-7} \text{ C}$$

(This means that the positive plate will have a charge of $+Q = 3 \times 10^{-7}$ C, and the negative plate will have a charge of $-Q = -3 \times 10^{-7}$ C.)

Example 9-24: A charged capacitor has charge Q, and the voltage between the plates is V. What will happen to C if Q is doubled?

Solution: Nothing. For a given capacitor, C is a constant. Because $Q = CV$, we see that Q is proportional to V. Doubling Q will not affect C; what *will* happen is that V will double.

Example 9-25: What will happen to the capacitance of a parallel-plate capacitor if the plates were moved closer together, halving the distance between them?

Solution: From the equation $C = \varepsilon_0 A/d$, we see that C is inversely proportional to d. Thus, if d is decreased by a factor of 2, then C will increase by a factor of 2.

Example 9-26: How big would the plates of a parallel-plate capacitor need to be in order to make the capacitance equal to 1 F, if $d = 8.85$ mm?

Solution: We'll start with the equation $C = \varepsilon_0 A/d$ and solve for A:

$$A = \frac{Cd}{\varepsilon_0} = \frac{(1 \text{ F})(8.85 \times 10^{-3} \text{ m})}{8.85 \times 10^{-12} \frac{\text{F}}{\text{m}}} = 10^9 \text{ m}^2$$

(If the plates were squares, they'd have to be nearly 20 miles on each side to make $A = 10^9$ square meters! Now you can see that 1 F is a *lot* of capacitance.)

Now that we know the basic equation for capacitance ($Q = CV$) and how to calculate it ($C = \varepsilon_0 A/d$), the next question is, "What's a capacitor used for?" For OAT purposes, a parallel-plate capacitor has two main uses:

1. to create a uniform electric field, and
2. to store electrical potential energy.

Let's go over each one.

When we studied electric fields in the preceding chapter, we noticed that the electric field created by one or more point source charges varied, depending on the location. For example, as we move farther from the source charges, the field gets weaker. Even if we stay at the same distance from, say, a single source charge, the direction of the field changes as we move around. Therefore, we could never obtain an electric field that was constant in both magnitude and direction throughout some region of space from point-source charges. However, the electric field that's created between the plates of a charged parallel-plate capacitor *is* constant in both magnitude and direction throughout the region between the plates; in other words, a charged parallel-plate capacitor can create a *uniform* electric field. The electric field, E, always points from the positive plate toward the negative plate, and it's the same magnitude at every point between the plates, whether we choose a point closer to the positive plate, closer to the negative plate, or right in the middle between them.

Because E is so straightforward (it's the same everywhere between the plates), the equation for calculating it is equally straightforward. The strength of E depends on the voltage between the plates, V, and their separation distance, d. We call the equation "Ed's formula":

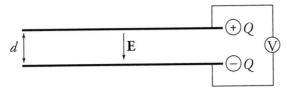

> ### Ed's Formula
>
> $$V = Ed$$

The equation $F = qE$ showed us that the units of E are N/C (because $E = F/q$). Ed's formula now tells us that the units of E are V/m (because $E = V/d$). You'll see both newtons-per-coulomb and volts-per-meter used as units for the electric field; it turns out that these units are exactly the same.

Example 9-27: The charge on a parallel-plate capacitor is 4×10^{-6} C. If the distance between the plates is 2 mm and the capacitance is 1 μF, what's the strength of the electric field between the plates?

Solution: Since $Q = CV$, we have $V = Q/C = (4 \times 10^{-6} \text{ C})/(10^{-6} \text{ F}) = 4$ V. Now, using the equation $V = Ed$, we find that

$$E = \frac{V}{d} = \frac{4 \text{ V}}{2 \times 10^{-3} \text{ m}} = 2000 \tfrac{\text{V}}{\text{m}}$$

Example 9-28: The plates of a parallel plate capacitor are separated by a distance of 2 mm. The device's capacitance is 1 μF. How much charge needs to be transferred from one plate to the other in order to create a uniform electric field whose strength is 10^4 V/m?

Solution: Because $Q = CV$ and $V = Ed$, we find that

$$Q = CEd = (1 \times 10^{-6} \text{ F})(10^4 \tfrac{\text{V}}{\text{m}})(2 \times 10^{-3} \text{ m}) = 2 \times 10^{-5} \text{ C}$$

Example 9-29: A proton (whose mass is m) is placed on top of the positively charged plate of a parallel-plate capacitor, as shown below.

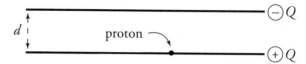

The charge on the capacitor is Q, and the capacitance is C. If the electric field in the region between the plates has magnitude E, which of the following expressions gives the time required for the proton to move up to the other plate?

A. $d\sqrt{\dfrac{eQ}{mC}}$

B. $d\sqrt{\dfrac{m}{eQC}}$

C. $d\sqrt{\dfrac{2eQ}{mC}}$

D. $d\sqrt{\dfrac{2mC}{eQ}}$

Solution: Once we find the acceleration of the proton, we can use Big Five #3, with $v_0 = 0$ (namely, $y = \frac{1}{2}at^2$) to find the time it will take for the proton to move the distance $y = d$. The acceleration of the proton is F/m, where $F = qE = eE$ is the force the proton feels; this gives $a = eE/m$. (We're ignoring the gravitational force on the proton because it is so much weaker than the electric force.) Now, since $E = V/d$ and $V = Q/C$, the expression for a becomes $a = eQ/mdC$. Substituting eQ/mdC for a, and d for y, Big Five #3 gives us

$$y = \frac{1}{2}at^2 \;\rightarrow\; d = \frac{1}{2}\cdot\frac{eQ}{mdC}t^2 \;\rightarrow\; t = d\sqrt{\frac{2mC}{eQ}}$$

The answer is (D). Another way we could have attacked this question is to look at the answer choices and see if they make sense. If (A) were correct, then it would imply that a greater charge Q would *increase* the time required for the proton to move to the top plate. This doesn't make sense because a greater Q would create a greater force on the proton, giving it a greater acceleration, thus making it move faster, and causing t to decrease. We can also see that (C) can't be correct, for the same reason. Choice (B) could be eliminated because the units don't work out to be seconds, as shown below; therefore, the answer *had* to be (D).

$$[d]\sqrt{\frac{[m]}{[e][Q][C]}} = m\sqrt{\frac{kg}{C\cdot C\cdot \frac{C}{V}}} = m\sqrt{\frac{kg}{C\cdot C\cdot \frac{C}{J/C}}} = \frac{m}{C^2}\sqrt{kg\cdot J} = \frac{m}{C^2}\sqrt{kg\cdot \frac{kg\cdot m^2}{s^2}} = \frac{kg\cdot m^2}{C^2\cdot s} \neq s$$

Example 9-30: An electron is projected horizontally into the space between the plates of a parallel-plate capacitor, as shown below, where the electric field has a magnitude of 56 V/m. The initial velocity of the electron is horizontal and has a magnitude of $v_0 = 5 \times 10^6$ m/s.

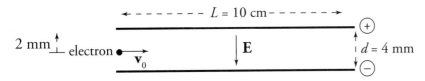

a) What is the force on the electron while it's in the region between the plates? (Neglect gravity.) What's the acceleration of the electron in this region? (Note: electron mass $\approx 9 \times 10^{-31}$ kg.)
b) How long would it take the electron to cover the horizontal distance L through the capacitor?
c) Describe the electron's trajectory through this region.

Solution:

a) Because the electric field **E** is constant between the plates, the force on the electron is also constant and given by $\mathbf{F} = q\mathbf{E} = -e\mathbf{E}$; this force points upward, in the direction opposite to the electric field (because q is negative), toward the positively charged top plate. Substituting in the numerical values gives $F = eE = (1.6 \times 10^{-19}$ C$) \times (56$ N/C$) = 9 \times 10^{-18}$ N. If the mass of the electron is m, then its acceleration, **a**, is **F**/m. Like **F**, the acceleration is uniform and vertical, pointing upward, toward the top plate. The magnitude of **a** is $a = F/m = (9 \times 10^{-18}$ N$)/(9 \times 10^{-31}$ kg$) = 10^{13}$ m/s^2.

b) Because the acceleration of the electron is vertical, the electron's horizontal velocity will not change. Because v_{0x} is always equal to v_{0x}, the time required to traverse the 10 cm horizontal distance through the region between the plates is

$$x = v_x t \;\rightarrow\; t = \frac{x}{v_x} = \frac{x}{v_{0x}} = \frac{L}{v_{0x}} = \frac{10 \times 10^{-2}\ \text{m}}{5 \times 10^6\ \text{m/s}} = 2 \times 10^{-8}\ \text{s}$$

c) Because the acceleration is constant, we can use the Big Five to describe the motion of the electron. In fact, the motion of the electron between the plates is just like the motion of a projectile whose initial velocity is horizontal. The only difference is that while a projectile would curve downward in a half-parabola, the electron in the figure above will curve upward. Adapting Big Five #3 to vertical motion (in the y direction), we have $y = v_{0y}t + \frac{1}{2}a_y t^2$. Because $v_{0y} = 0$, this equation simplifies to $y = \frac{1}{2}a_y t^2$. Now, in the time t that the electron moves through the region between the plates (which we found in part b) its vertical displacement will be $y = \frac{1}{2}(10^{13}\,\text{m/s}^2)(2 \times 10^{-8}\,\text{s})^2 = 2 \times 10^{-3}\,\text{m} = 2\text{mm}$. Therefore, the electron will just hit the right edge of the top plate.

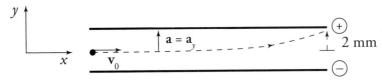

Now let's look at the second important use of a capacitor: as a storage device for electrical potential energy. We can think of the process of charging a capacitor as a transferal of electrons from one plate to the other. The plate that the electrons are taken from is left positively charged, and the plate the electrons are transferred to becomes negatively charged. Also, because we're simply transferring charge from one plate to the other, we are always assured at each moment that the plates carry equal but opposite charges.

During this charging process, an outside agent (the voltage source) must do work against the electric field that's created between the plates of the capacitor. Once we begin the process of transferring electrons from one plate to the other, it becomes increasingly difficult to transfer more. After all, it takes effort to remove more electrons from the plate that is left positively charged, *and* it takes effort to place them on the plate that is negatively charged. The fact that we have to "fight" against the system means we're storing potential energy.

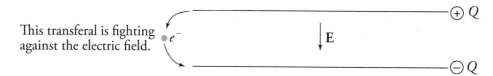

To increase the charge on the capacitor, work is required to remove extra electrons from the positive plate and move them to the negative plate. This work against the electric field is stored as electrical potential energy.

Because it requires more work to transfer more charge, we'd expect that the amount of potential energy stored should depend on Q, the final charge on the capacitor; that is, as Q increases, so should the PE. We'd also expect that the amount of stored PE should depend on the voltage between the plates. After all, we defined potential difference, V, by the equation $\Delta PE = qV$, where q was the charge that moved between the points whose potential difference was V. Hence, the higher voltage V leads to an increase in stored potential energy. If the final charge on the capacitor is Q and the final resulting voltage is V, then PE is proportional to both Q and V. Here's how we can intuitively find the formula for PE in this case: we transferred a total amount of charge equal to Q, fighting against the voltage that prevailed at each stage. If the final voltage is V, then the average voltage during the charging process is $\frac{1}{2}V$. Since ΔPE is equal to charge times voltage, we get $\Delta PE = Q \cdot \left(\frac{1}{2}V\right) = \frac{1}{2}QV$. At the beginning of the charging process, when there was no charge on the capacitor, we had $PE_i = 0$, so $\Delta PE = PE_f - PE_i = PE_f - 0 = PE_f$. Therefore, we have $PE_f = \frac{1}{2}QV$:

Electrical PE Stored in a Capacitor

$$PE = \tfrac{1}{2}QV$$

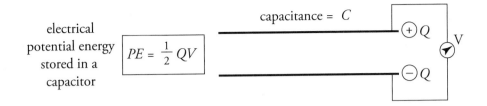

electrical potential energy stored in a capacitor

$$PE = \frac{1}{2}QV$$

capacitance = C

Using the fundamental equation $Q = CV$, we can rewrite this equation in terms of C and V, or in terms of Q and C:

$$PE = \frac{1}{2}QV = \frac{1}{2}CV^2 = \frac{Q^2}{2C}$$

If you lift a rock off the ground, you do work against the gravitational field of the Earth, and, as a result, you store gravitational potential energy. To recapture this stored energy, you let the rock fall back to the ground, transferring the gravitational potential energy into mechanical kinetic energy. Similarly, if you transfer electrons from one plate of a capacitor to the other, you do work against the electric field of the capacitor, and, as a result, you store electrical potential energy. To recapture this stored electrical energy, you let the electrons go back to their original plate, effectively **discharging** the capacitor. The movement of electrons can be used in a productive manner by providing a path for them and placing some electrical devices along the way. As a result, the electrons that return to the plate end up passing through, say, a light bulb, and the current causes the bulb to light. We've been able to tap into the energy stored in the capacitor to do useful work. When we connect the charged capacitor plates by a wire with some resistor(s) along it, the charge drains off rapidly at first, but the rate at which the charge leaves gradually decreases as time goes on. The same is true of the resulting current; it too starts off high and then gradually drops to zero as the capacitor discharges.

Discharging a Capacitor

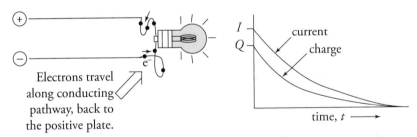

Electrons travel along conducting pathway, back to the positive plate.

9.2

Example 9-31: A defibrillator contains a circuit whose primary components are a battery, a capacitor, and a switch. When the heart is undergoing ventricular fibrillation, the normally ordered electrical signals that organize the heart's pumping behavior are out of sync. The strong current delivered by the conducting paddles of the defibrillator can depolarize the entirety of the heart and potentially reset its orderly pumping triggered by the SA node. The defibrillator circuit first charges the capacitor with the battery. During the application and discharging of the circuit, a switch is closed to allow the capacitor to discharge through the paddles and the patient's tissue. Which of the following graphs best illustrates the voltage between the capacitor plates during this latter process?

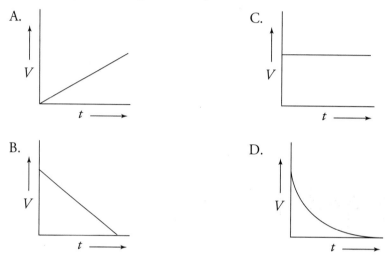

Solution: As the capacitor loses charge, Q decreases. Since $V = Q/C$, we know that V must decrease too. This eliminates (A) and (C). The charge drains off rapidly at first, but the rate at which the charge leaves gradually decreases as time goes on; therefore, the decrease in Q (and therefore in V also) is not linear. Thus, the best graph is the one in (D). (The defibrillator circuit will also feature an *inductor* or *solenoid*, described later in this chapter. This has the effect of slowing the discharge of the capacitor and prolonging the application of current sufficiently to completely depolarize the heart.)

Dielectrics

If the plates of a capacitor were touching at the start of the charging process, then we'd effectively have a single conductor, not a pair, and no transferal of electrons from one plate to the other could begin; it wouldn't work as a capacitor. And if the plates were ever allowed to touch during the charging process, the capacitor would discharge almost immediately, since the transferred electrons would have a direct route back to the positive plate. All the electrical potential energy that had been stored would be lost in an instant, without any useful work being done by the stored energy. So for a capacitor to be useful, we need to keep the plates from touching.

Let's consider ways to do that. One way would be to mount them on separate insulating handles, like this:

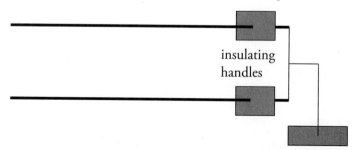

insulating
handles

That could work, but the way it's typically done is to sandwich a slab of insulating material between the plates. Such an insulator is known as a **dielectric**:

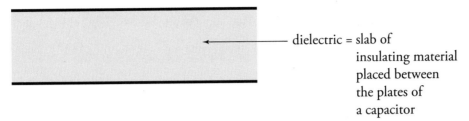

dielectric = slab of insulating material placed between the plates of a capacitor

Not only does a dielectric keep the plates from touching, but there's also a bonus: *the presence of a dielectric always increases the capacitance.* For the capacitor whose plates are mounted on insulating handles, with vacuum (or, for all practical purposes, air) between the plates, the capacitance is given by the equation we gave earlier: $C = \varepsilon_0 A/d$. However, if the capacitor is fitted with a dielectric, the capacitance is multiplied by a factor of K, where K is known as the **dielectric constant** of the insulating material. For example, wax paper is a dielectric, with a dielectric constant of about 3.5. If a parallel-plate capacitor were fitted with wax paper as a dielectric, the capacitance would be multiplied by 3.5. Other common dielectrics are Teflon and certain plastics and ceramics.

Here's the formula for the capacitance of a parallel-plate capacitor with a dielectric:

Capacitance of a Parallel-Plate Capacitor with a Dielectric

$$C_{\substack{\text{with} \\ \text{dielectric}}} = K \cdot C_{\substack{\text{without} \\ \text{dielectric}}} = K \varepsilon_0 \frac{A}{d}$$

The value of K for vacuum is exactly 1, which makes sense since having empty space between the plates means there's *no* dielectric. The OAT will assume that $K = 1$ for air as well because the actual value of K for air (~1.0005) is so close to 1. A capacitor with just air between its plates is known simply as an *air capacitor*. K is never less than 1, which is the reason dielectrics always increase capacitance.

Example 9-32: The area, A, of each plate of a parallel-plate capacitor satisfies the equation $\varepsilon_0 A = 10^{-10}$ F·m. If the plates are separated by a distance of 2 mm and this space is filled by a sheet of mica with a dielectric constant of 6, what is the capacitance of this capacitor?

Solution: The presence of the mica increases the capacitance by a factor of 6, so:

$$C_{\substack{\text{with} \\ \text{dielectric}}} = K \cdot C_{\substack{\text{without} \\ \text{dielectric}}} = K \varepsilon_0 \frac{A}{d} = 6 \cdot \frac{10^{-10} \text{ F·m}}{2 \times 10^{-3} \text{ m}} = 3 \times 10^{-7} \text{ F}$$

Example 9-33: The inner and outer surfaces of a cell membrane act as plates in a parallel-plate capacitor. Consider a 1 μm² section of an axon: the dielectric constant of the membrane is 8 and the membrane is 6 nm thick. If the voltage across the membrane is 70 mV, what is the approximate magnitude of charge that resides on each side of this 1 μm² section? (*Note:* $\varepsilon_0 = 8.85 \times 10^{-12}$ C²/N·m²)

Solution: The capacitance is $C_{\text{with dielectric}} = K\varepsilon_0 A / d$, with $K = 8$, so

$$Q = CV = K\varepsilon_0 \frac{A}{d} \cdot V = (8)(8.85 \times 10^{-12} \tfrac{\text{C}^2}{\text{N·m}^2}) \cdot \frac{1\ \mu\text{m}^2 \cdot \left(\frac{1\ \text{m}}{10^6\ \mu\text{m}}\right)^2}{6 \times 10^{-9}\ \text{m}} \cdot (70 \times 10^{-3}\ \text{V}) \approx 1 \times 10^{-15}\ \text{C}$$

Example 9-34: The capacitance of a certain air capacitor whose plates are separated by a distance of 1 mm is 4 pF. If the plates are moved apart to a distance of 2.2 mm to accommodate a slab of porcelain of thickness 2.2 mm that is then inserted between them, the capacitance becomes 12 pF. What is the dielectric constant of porcelain?

Solution: The capacitance without the porcelain is $C_{\text{without dielectric}} = \varepsilon_0 A / d_1$, and the capacitance with the porcelain is $C_{\text{with dielectric}} = K\varepsilon_0 A / d_2$. The ratio of these values is

$$\frac{C_{\text{with dielectric}}}{C_{\text{without dielectric}}} = \frac{K\varepsilon_0 A / d_2}{\varepsilon_0 A / d_1} = K\frac{d_1}{d_2} = K\frac{1\ \text{mm}}{2.2\ \text{mm}} = \frac{K}{2.2}$$

Now, because the capacitance increased by a factor of 3, we have

$$\frac{K}{2.2} = 3 \rightarrow \quad \therefore K = 6.6$$

The presence of a dielectric can affect other properties of a capacitor besides capacitance. However, the ways a dielectric affects the charge, voltage, and electric field depend on whether the capacitor is connected or disconnected from the battery that charged it.

Let's begin by looking at the case in which a capacitor without a dielectric is charged by a battery and then disconnected from it. What happens if we then insert a dielectric between the plates? First, since the capacitor is disconnected from the battery, the charge that exists on the plates is trapped and cannot change. Therefore, Q remains constant. Because the capacitance C increases, the equation $Q = CV$ tells us that the voltage will decrease; in fact, because Q stays constant and C increases by a factor of K, we see that V will decrease by a factor of K. Next, using the equation $V = Ed$, we see that because V decreases by a factor of K, so does E. Finally, using the equation $PE = \frac{1}{2}QV$, we conclude that since Q stays constant and V decreases by a factor of K, the stored electrical potential energy decreases by a factor of K.

We can look at this a little more closely: First, why does the electric field strength, E, decrease in this case? The dielectric is an insulator, so although the field between the plates won't move any free electrons through the material, it will polarize the molecules. That is, the electric field will create tiny dipole moments in the molecules of the insulator, with the negative (δ^-) ends closer to the positive plate and the positive (δ^+) ends closer to the negative plate. As a result, we'll have a layer of negative charge at the surface of the dielectric that's near the positive plate and a layer of positive charge at the surface of the dielectric that's near the negative plate. These layers of induced charge on the opposite surfaces of the dielectric are the source of a new electric field through the dielectric, E_{induced}, a field that points in the opposite direction from the electric field created by the charged capacitor plates themselves (because electric fields always point from positive and toward negative source charges).

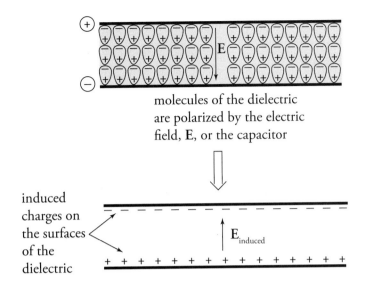

molecules of the dielectric
are polarized by the electric
field, **E**, or the capacitor

induced
charges on
the surfaces
of the
dielectric

$\mathbf{E}_{\text{induced}}$

The total electric field between the plates is then the sum of the field created by the plates, **E**, and the field created by the layers of induced charge on the surfaces of the dielectric, $\mathbf{E}_{\text{induced}}$. Because $\mathbf{E}_{\text{induced}}$ points in the direction *opposite* to **E**, the *net* field strength is reduced to $E - E_{\text{induced}}$. This is the physical reason why the electric field magnitude is reduced in this case.

We also found that the potential energy would be reduced if we inserted a dielectric after disconnecting the capacitor from the charging battery. Where did this energy go? Most of it is stored as electrical potential energy inside those induced dipoles in the dielectric. (Unfortunately, that stored energy is hard to recapture in a useful way.) You would notice that as you began to place the dielectric between the plates, the electric field would actually pull it in; thus, some of the stored potential energy turns into kinetic energy of the dielectric as it was pulled into the space between the capacitor plates. Finally, there would be some heat production (the usual OAT answer to "Where did the energy go?").

Now let's examine the case in which a capacitor without a dielectric is first charged up and then while it's still connected to its voltage source, we insert a dielectric between its plates. First, since the capacitor is still connected to the battery, the voltage between the plates must match the voltage of the battery. Therefore, V will not change.[3] Because the capacitance C increases, the equation $Q = CV$ tells us that the charge Q must increase; in fact, because V doesn't change and C increases by a factor of K, we see that Q will increase by a factor of K. Next, using the equation $V = Ed$, we see that because V doesn't change, neither will E. Finally, using the equation $PE = \frac{1}{2}QV$, we conclude that since V doesn't change and Q increases by a factor of K, the stored electrical potential energy increases by a factor of K. An important point to notice is that V doesn't change because the battery will transfer additional charge to the capacitor plates. This increase in Q offsets any momentary decrease in the electric field strength when the dielectric is inserted (because the molecules of the dielectric are polarized, as above) and brings the electric field strength back to its original value. Furthermore, as more charge is transferred to the plates, more electrical potential energy is stored.

---

[3] This analysis assumes that the circuit has no resistance, so the newly increased capacitance can be "filled up" instantaneously. In practice, voltage in the capacitor would drop at first but then rise quickly until it was again equal to the battery's voltage.

The following figure summarizes the effects on the properties of a capacitor with the insertion of a dielectric in the two cases:

charge capacitor
to voltage *V*

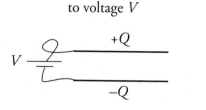

$+Q$

$-Q$

charge capacitor
to voltage *V*

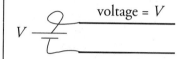

voltage = *V*

then disconnect battery
and insert dielectric

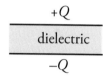

$+Q$

dielectric

$-Q$

keep battery connected
and insert dielectric

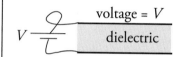

voltage = *V*

dielectric

- *C* increases by factor of *K*
- *Q* stays the same
- *V* decreases by a factor of *K*
- *E* decreases by a factor of *K*

- *C* increases by factor of *K*
- *Q* increases by factor of *K*
- *V* stays the same
- *E* stays the same

Example 9-35: An air capacitor is charged and disconnected from the battery. The electric field between the plates is **E**. Now, a dielectric with dielectric constant $K = 4$ is inserted between the plates. What is the electric field created by the layers of induced charges on the surfaces of the dielectric?

A. $3E/4$ opposite the direction of **E**
B. $E/4$ opposite the direction of **E**
C. $E/4$ in the same direction of **E**
D. $3E/4$ in the same direction of **E**

Solution: The question is asking for $\mathbf{E}_{induced}$. First, $\mathbf{E}_{induced}$ points in the *opposite* direction from **E**, so the answer must be either (A) or (B). To find the magnitude of $\mathbf{E}_{induced}$, we use the fact that $E - E_{induced} = E/K$; since $K = 4$, we see that $E_{induced} = 3E/4$. Thus, the answer is (A).

Example 9-36: A parallel-plate capacitor, with air between the plates, is charged to a voltage of $V = 1000$ V by a battery. The values of Q, E, and PE are also measured. The battery is then disconnected from the capacitor and a dielectric with dielectric constant $K = 4$ is inserted between the plates. The values of V, Q, E, and PE are measured again. Which of these values did *not* change?

A. V
B. Q
C. E
D. PE

Solution: Since the battery was disconnected from the capacitor after charging, the value of Q does not change: there's nowhere for charges to go and no source of new charges. The values of V, E, and PE will all decrease by a factor of K. The answer is (B).

Example 9-37: Cell membranes have a dielectric number of about 9. If the internal potential of the cell is about 70 mV lower than the external potential, how much charge could accumulate on a square micrometer of phospholipid layer with a thickness of 8 nanometers ($\varepsilon_0 \approx 9 \times 10^{-12}$ F/m)?

Solution:

$$C = \frac{K\varepsilon_0 A}{d} = \frac{9(9 \times 10^{-12}\text{ F/m})(10^{-6}\text{ m})^2}{8 \times 10^{-9}} \approx 10^{-14}\text{ F}$$

Now the charge this cell membrane capacitor can hold at the given voltage is $Q = CV = (10^{-8}$ F$)$ $(70 \times 10^{-3}$ V$) = 7 \times 10^{-16}$ C. This may not seem like much, but considering that the charge of one sodium or potassium ion is 1.6×10^{-19} C, this amounts to about 4 billion ions. This is NOT what actually happens to a living cell, mind you, because a living cell is not a passive participant in its local environment (and there are chemical considerations in addition to electrical ones).

Combinations of Capacitors

Like resistors, capacitors can also be placed in series and in parallel within a circuit. In this section, we'll see how to find the equivalent capacitance for each of these cases.

Capacitors in **parallel** all have the same voltage (like *resistors* in parallel), but the equivalent capacitance is the sum of the individual capacitances (like resistors in *series*):

equivalent capacitance
for capacitors in parallel
$$\boxed{C_{eq} = C_1 + C_2 + C_3 + \cdots}$$

For example, in the figure below, the equivalent capacitance, C_{eq}, is 2 μF + 3 μF + 4 μF = 9 μF:

capacitors in parallel

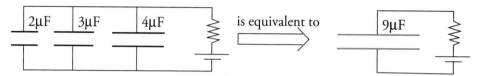

Capacitors in **series** all have the same charge (similar to *resistors* in series all having the same current), but the equivalent capacitance is found from the same formula that we used for resistors in *parallel*:

equivalent capacitance
for capacitors in series

$$\frac{1}{C_{eq}} = \frac{1}{C_1} + \frac{1}{C_2} + \frac{1}{C_3} + \dots$$

Equivalently, we could simplify the capacitors two at a time using the expression *product/sum*. For example, in the figure below, the equivalent capacitance, C_{eq}, is 2 μF, because 1/12 + 1/6 + 1/4 = 1/2. (We could also calculate it as (12 × 6)/(12 + 6) = 4 and (4 × 4)/(4 + 4) = 2.)

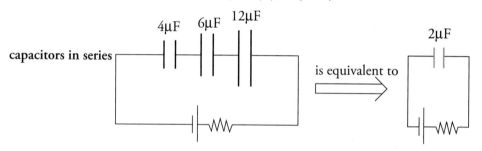

Example 9-38: Three uncharged capacitors are arranged in a circuit as shown.

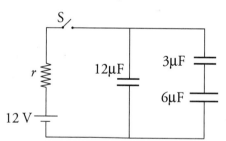

After the switch S has been closed for a long time and electrostatic equilibrium is reached, how much charge is on the 6 μF capacitor?

Solution: The 3 μF and 6 μF capacitors are in series, so they're equivalent to a single 2 μF capacitor, because $(3 \times 6)/(3 + 6) = 2$. Therefore, the circuit shown above is equivalent to

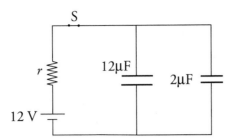

These two capacitors are in parallel, so both will have the same voltage: 12 V, since the plates of each are connected to the terminals of a 12 V battery. Now, using the equation $Q = CV$, we see that the charge on the 2 μF capacitor will be

$$Q = (2\ \mu F)(12\ V) = 24\ \mu C$$

Since the 2 μF capacitor is equivalent to the series combination consisting of the 3 μF and 6 μF capacitors, the charge on each of these capacitors must be the same, 24 μC. (For extra practice, you may wish to verify the final voltages and charges on each of the three capacitors in the original circuit; the answers are shown below.)

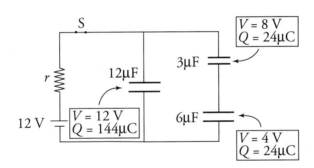

Summary Of Formulas

CIRCUITS

Current: $I = \dfrac{Q}{t}$

- in the direction of "flow of positive charge"

- actual flow of electrons is in the opposite direction

Resistance: $R = \rho \dfrac{L}{A}$ (ρ = resistivity, not density)

Ohm's Law: $V = IR$ (where R is constant as V varies)

Resistors in series: $R_{eq} = R_1 + R_2 + \ldots$

Resistors in parallel: $\dfrac{1}{R_{eq}} = \dfrac{1}{R_1} + \dfrac{1}{R_2} + \ldots$ or $R_{eq} = \dfrac{R_1 R_2}{R_1 + R_2}$ (two at a time)

Current is the same for resistors in series; voltage is the same for resistors in parallel.

Kirchhoff's Rules:

- The sum of the voltage-drops across the resistors in any complete path is equal to the voltage of the battery.

- The amount of current entering a parallel combination of resistors is equal to the sum of the currents that pass through the individual resistors.

Power of circuit element: $P = IV = I^2 R = \dfrac{V^2}{R}$

Total power supplied by a battery equals the total power dissipated by the resistors.

The ground is at potential zero (potential = 0).

PARALLEL PLATE CAPACITORS

Charge on a capacitor: $Q = CV$

- The capacitance does not depend on voltage or charge. It is determined by the formula below.

Capacitance:

no dielectric: $C = \varepsilon_0 \dfrac{A}{d}$

with dielectric: $C_{\text{with dielectric}} = KC_{\text{without dielectric}} = K\varepsilon_0 \dfrac{A}{d}$ [K = dielectric constant]

- Inserting a dielectric always increases the capacitance. If the battery remains attached, V is constant; if the battery is taken away Q is constant.

Electric field in parallel-plate capacitor:

$$V = Ed$$

Stored potential energy in capacitor:

$$PE = \frac{1}{2}QV = \frac{1}{2}CV^2 = \frac{Q^2}{2C}$$

- The work done by the battery to charge the capacitor = PE.

Capacitors in series: $\dfrac{1}{C_{eq}} = \dfrac{1}{C_1} + \dfrac{1}{C_2} + \ldots$ or $C_{eq} = \dfrac{C_1 C_2}{C_1 + C_2}$ [two at a time]

Capacitors in parallel: $C_{eq} = C_1 + C_2 + \ldots$

Chapter 10
Simple Harmonic
Motion and Waves

10.1 SIMPLE HARMONIC MOTION (SHM)

The spring in the series of diagrams below is fixed at its left-hand end and has a block attached to its right-hand end. When the spring is neither stretched nor compressed (i.e., when it's at its natural length, as shown in Diagram 1 below), we say the spring is at its **equilibrium position**. In general, the point at which the net force on the block is zero, which in this case is when the spring is at its natural length, is called the equilibrium position, and we label it the zero position.

Now, imagine that we stretch the spring (Diagram 1 to Diagram 2), and let go. Once released, the spring pulls back to the left, going through its equilibrium position and then to the point of maximum compression. From here, the spring pushes back to the right, passing again through its equilibrium position, and returning to the point of maximum extension. If friction is negligible, this back-and-forth motion (the **oscillations**) will continue indefinitely, and the time it takes for the block to go through one oscillation, for example, from Diagram 2 to Diagram 6, is a constant. The oscillations of the block at the end of this spring provide us with a physical example of **simple harmonic motion** (often abbreviated SHM).

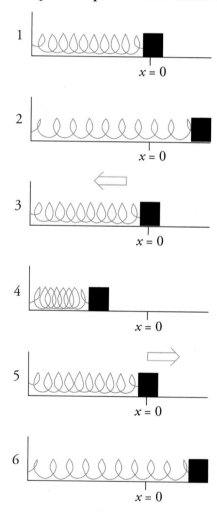

The Dynamics of SHM

Force

Let's first describe the motion of the block attached to the spring from the point of view of the force it feels. The spring exerts a force on the block that's proportional to its displacement. If we call the equilibrium position $x = 0$, then the force exerted by the spring is given by

Hooke's Law

$$\mathbf{F} = -kx$$

The proportionality constant, k, called the **spring constant**, tells us how strong the spring is; the greater the value of k, the stiffer (and stronger) the spring.

What is the role of the minus sign in Hooke's Law? Look back at the diagrams on the previous page. Since we're calling the equilibrium position $x = 0$, when the block is to the right of equilibrium, its position, x, is positive. At this point, the stretched spring wants to pull back to the left; because the direction of the force of the spring is to the left, we indicate this direction by calling it negative. Similarly, when the block is to the left of equilibrium, its position, x, is negative. At this point, the compressed spring wants to push back to the right; because the direction of the force of the spring is to the right, we indicate this direction by calling it positive. We see that the direction of the spring force is always directed opposite to its displacement from equilibrium, and for this reason, the minus sign is needed in Hooke's Law. Furthermore, because the spring is always trying to restore the block to equilibrium, we say that the spring provides the **restoring force**; it's this force that maintains the oscillations.

Energy

Unfortunately, knowing an equation for the force doesn't allow us to solve directly for other things, such as the speed of the block at some later time: The force changes as the block moves, so acceleration is not uniform. However, there is a way to figure out how fast the block moves using Conservation of Energy. When we pull on the spring to get the oscillations started, we're exerting a force over a distance; that is, we're doing work. Because we're doing work against the spring, the spring stores potential energy, called **elastic potential energy**. If we once again call the equilibrium position of the spring $x = 0$, then the potential energy of a stretched or compressed spring is given by this equation:

Elastic Potential Energy

$$PE_{\text{elastic}} = \tfrac{1}{2}kx^2$$

When we release the block from rest in Diagram 2 above, the spring is stretched and the block isn't moving, so all the energy is in the form of elastic potential energy. This potential energy turns into kinetic energy, until at $x = 0$ (equilibrium), all the energy has been converted to kinetic energy. As the block rushes past equilibrium, this kinetic energy gradually turns back into elastic potential energy until the point where the spring is at maximum compression and it's all transformed back to potential energy. The compressed spring then pushes outward, converting its potential energy back to kinetic; the block rushes through equilibrium again, and kinetic energy is transformed back to potential energy, until it reaches its starting point (Diagram 6 above) at maximum extension. At this instant, we're back to our full reserve of elastic potential energy (and no kinetic energy), and the process is ready to repeat.

As a result, we can look at the motion of the block from the point of view of the back-and-forth transfer between elastic potential energy and kinetic energy.

The maximum displacement of the block from equilibrium is called the **amplitude**, denoted by A. This positive number tells us how far to the left and right of equilibrium the block will travel. So, in the series of diagrams above, the block's position at maximum extension is $x = +A$, and its position at maximum compression is $x = -A$.

We can summarize the dynamics of the oscillations in this table:

	at $x = -A$	at $x = 0$	at $x = +A$
magnitude of restoring force	max	0	max
magnitude of acceleration	max	0	max
$PE_{elastic}$ of spring	max	0	max
KE of block	0	max	0
speed (v) of block	0	max	0

Because we're ignoring any frictional forces during the oscillations of the block, total mechanical energy will be conserved. That is, the sum of the block's kinetic energy, $\frac{1}{2}mv^2$, and the spring's potential energy, $\frac{1}{2}kx^2$, will be a constant. We can use this fact to figure out the maximum speed of the block. At the instant the block is passing through equilibrium, all the potential energy of the spring has been transformed into kinetic energy of the block. If the amplitude of the oscillations is A, then the maximum elastic potential energy, $\frac{1}{2}kA^2$ (the value of $\frac{1}{2}kx^2$ when $x = \pm A$), is completely converted to maximum kinetic energy at $x = 0$. This gives us:

$$PE_{elastic,\ max} \rightarrow KE_{max}$$

$$\tfrac{1}{2}kA^2 = \tfrac{1}{2}mv_{max}^2$$

$$\therefore v_{max} = A\sqrt{\frac{k}{m}}$$

Example 10-1: A block of mass 200 g is oscillating on the end of a horizontal spring of spring constant 100 N/m and natural length 12 cm. When the spring is stretched to a length of 14 cm, what is the acceleration of the block?

Solution: When the spring is stretched by 2 cm, Hooke's Law tells us that the force exerted by the spring has a magnitude of $F = kx = (100$ N/m$)(0.02$ m$) = 2$ N. Therefore, by Newton's Second Law, the acceleration of the block will have a magnitude of $a = F/m = (2$ N$)/(0.2$ kg$) = 10$ m/s^2.

Example 10-2: If the block in Example 10-1 above were replaced with a block of mass 800 g, how would its maximum speed change?

Solution: The equation derived above, $v_{max} = A\sqrt{k/m}$, tells us that v_{max} is inversely proportional to the square root of the mass of the oscillator. Therefore, if m increases by a factor of 4, v_{max} will decrease by a factor of 2.

So far, we have examined the simple harmonic motion of a horizontal spring. However, SHM can be demonstrated with a vertical spring that is fixed at one end. Consider a horizontal spring with a natural length of l_0 and a block of mass m attached to one end. When turned 90° to make the spring oscillate in the vertical dimension, the spring will stretch/compress to establish a new "natural length." To find this new equilibrium point, we apply Newton's First Law to balance the restoring force (caused by the spring) with the force of gravity being exerted on the block. Once this equilibrium is established, a new applied force can initiate simple harmonic motion with $x = 0$ at the newly established natural length point.

The Kinematics of SHM

Period

An oscillation of the block is known as a **cycle**. One cycle is one *round trip*. For example, in the series of diagrams shown earlier, as the block moves from Diagram 2 through to Diagram 6, it completes one round trip; this is one cycle. The amount of time required for the block to complete one cycle is called the **period** of the motion, denoted by T. The period T is measured in seconds, and the longer the period, the slower the oscillations.

Frequency

Rather than timing one cycle (to give the period), we can instead count the number of cycles that take place in one second. This is known as the **frequency**, denoted by f. The units of f are cycles per second, and 1 cycle/second is renamed 1 **hertz** (Hz). The lower the frequency, the slower the oscillations.

Now the first thing we notice is that period and frequency are reciprocals. After all, the period is "the number of seconds per cycle," and the frequency is "the number of cycles per second." So, we have these fundamental relationships:

Period and Frequency

$$f = \frac{1}{T} \text{ and } T = \frac{1}{f}$$

What isn't so obvious is that both the frequency and the period can be figured out (using calculus) just from the spring constant, k, and the mass of the block, m. Here are the formulas:

$$f = \frac{1}{2\pi}\sqrt{\frac{k}{m}} \text{ and } T = 2\pi\sqrt{\frac{m}{k}}$$

Notice that neither f nor T depends on A, the amplitude. This is why we call the motion of the block on the spring *simple* harmonic motion. It turns out that this follows from the fact that the restoring force is directly proportional to the displacement (from Hooke's Law).

It's possible for a system to oscillate because of a restoring force that is not directly proportional to the displacement. If this were the case, the frequency and period would depend on the amplitude; we'd still call the motion *harmonic*, which just means back-and-forth, but we wouldn't call it *simple* harmonic.

Example 10-3: Suppose that the block shown in the series of diagrams on the first page of this chapter requires 0.25 sec to move from Diagram 4 to Diagram 6. What is the frequency of the oscillations?

Solution: The interval from Diagram 4 to Diagram 6 represents *half* a cycle, which requires *half* a period to complete. If half a period is 0.25 sec, then the period is 0.5 sec. Therefore, the frequency, f, is $1/T$ = 1/(0.5 s) = 2 Hz.

Pendulums

Besides the spring-block simple harmonic oscillator, there's another oscillator that the OAT will expect you to know about: the simple pendulum. If the connecting rod or string between the suspension point and the object at the end of a pendulum has negligible mass (so that all the mass is in the object at the end of the rod or string), and if there is no friction at the suspension point during oscillation, we say the pendulum is a **simple pendulum**.

The displacement of the mass is not taken as a distance from equilibrium (as in the spring-block case), but rather as the angle it makes with the vertical. The vertical (shown as a dashed line in the figure below) is the equilibrium position, $\theta = 0$. The restoring force here is gravity; specifically, it's equal to $mg \sin \theta$, which is the component of the object's weight in the direction toward equilibrium.

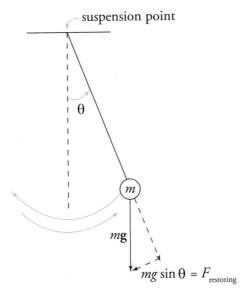

Strictly speaking, a pendulum does not undergo simple harmonic motion because the restoring force is not proportional to the displacement ($mg \sin \theta$ is not exactly proportional to θ). However, if the angle is small, then $\sin \theta \approx \theta$ (in radians), so the restoring force can be approximated as $mg\theta$, which is proportional to θ.[1] In this case, we can treat the motion as simple harmonic, and the frequency and period are given by the following equations:

$$f = \frac{1}{2\pi}\sqrt{\frac{g}{l}} \text{ and } T = 2\pi\sqrt{\frac{l}{g}}$$

where l is the length of the pendulum and g is the acceleration due to gravity. Observe that in the case of simple harmonic motion of a simple pendulum, the mass of the swinging object does not affect the frequency or period of oscillation.

---

[1] The conversion between degrees and radians is as follows: 180 degrees = π radians. If the angle is given in degrees, the restoring force is approximately $mg\theta(\pi/180°)$, which is still proportional to θ.

Example 10-4: The bob (mass = m) of a simple pendulum is raised to a height h above its lowest point and released. Find an expression for the maximum speed of the pendulum.

Solution: When the bob is at height h above its lowest point, it has gravitational potential energy equal to mgh (relative to its lowest point). As it passes through the equilibrium position, all this potential energy is converted to kinetic energy. Therefore, $mgh = \frac{1}{2}mv_{max}^2$, and we get $v_{max} = \sqrt{2gh}$. This is the speed of the bob as it passes through equilibrium, which is where it attains its maximum speed.

10.2 WAVES

A **wave** is a disturbance in a medium that transfers energy from one place to another. The medium itself is not transported, just the disturbance.

Transverse Waves

Perhaps the simplest example of a wave is one we can create by wiggling one end of a long rope:

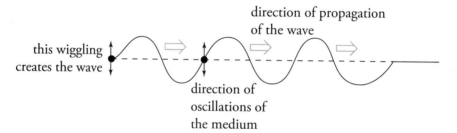

This wave uses the rope as the medium, traveling from one end to the other. Notice that the wave is moving horizontally, but the rope itself is moving up and down. That's why this is called a **transverse** wave: the wave travels (propagates) in a direction that's *perpendicular* to the direction in which the medium is vibrating.

Frequency and Period

The most fundamental characteristic of a wave is its frequency. If we pick a spot on the rope and count how many times it moves up and down (the number of round trips it makes) in one second, we've just measured the **frequency**, f, which we express in hertz (cycles per second).

The **period** of a wave, T, is the reciprocal of the frequency, and is the amount of time it takes any spot on the rope to complete one cycle (in this case, one up-and-down round trip).

Wavelength and Amplitude

The figure below identifies the **crests (peaks)** and **troughs** of the wave. The distance from one crest to the next (i.e., the length of one cycle of the wave) is called the **wavelength**, denoted by λ, the Greek letter lambda. We can also measure the wavelength by measuring the distance from one trough to the next, or, in fact, between any two consecutive corresponding points along the wave.

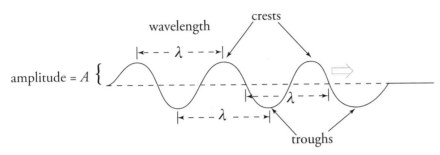

The **amplitude** of a wave, A, is the maximum displacement from equilibrium that any point in the medium makes as the wave goes by. In the case of a wave on a rope, the amplitude is the distance from the original horizontal position of the rope up to a crest; it's also the distance from the horizontal position down to a trough.

Wave Speed

To figure out how fast the wave travels, we just notice that the wave travels a distance of λ in time T; that is, λ is the length of one wave cycle, and T, the period, is the time required for one wave cycle to go by. Since distance = rate × time, we get $\lambda = vT$. Solving this for v gives us $\lambda(1/T) = v$, and since $f = 1/T$, the equation becomes $v = \lambda f$. *This is the most important equation for waves and one of the most important equations for the OAT.*

Wave Equation

$$v = \lambda f$$

For a transverse wave on a rope, there's another equation we can use to figure out the wave speed:

$$v = \sqrt{\frac{\text{tension}}{\text{linear density}}}$$

The linear density of a rope is its mass per unit length.

10.2

Two Big Rules for Waves

Notice that the second equation for the wave speed shows that v does not depend on f (or λ). While this may seem to contradict the first equation, $v = \lambda f$, it really doesn't. The speed of the wave depends on the characteristics of the rope; how tense it is, and what it's made of. We can wiggle the end at any frequency we want, and the speed of the wave we create will be a constant. However, because $\lambda f = v$ must always be true, a higher f will mean a shorter λ (and a lower f will mean a longer λ). Thus, changing f doesn't change v: It changes λ. This brings up our first big rule for waves:

> **Big Rule 1:** The speed of a wave is determined by the type of wave and the characteristics of the medium, *not* by the frequency.

Notice that two different types of wave can move with different speeds through the same medium; for example, sound and light move through air with very different speeds. There are exceptions to Big Rule 1, but the only one the OAT will expect you to know about is *dispersion*, which is discussed in the last physics chapter, on Optics. Any other exception would be discussed in the passage; otherwise, you can assume the rule applies.

Our second big rule for waves concerns what happens when a wave passes from one medium into another. Because wave speed is determined by the characteristics of the medium, a change in the medium implies a change in wave speed, but the frequency won't change.

> **Big Rule 2:** When a wave passes into another medium, its speed changes, but its frequency does *not*.

Because f is constant, Rule 2 tells us that the wavelength is proportional to wave speed.

Notice that Rule 1 applies to different waves in one medium, while Rule 2 applies to a single wave in different media. Memorize these rules. The OAT loves waves.

Example 10-5: A transverse wave of frequency 4 Hz travels at a speed of 6 m/s along a rope. What would be the speed of a 12 Hz wave along this same rope?

Solution: Big Rule 1 for waves says that the speed of a wave is determined by the type of wave and the characteristics of the medium, not by the frequency. If all we do is change the frequency, the wave speed will not change: the wave speed will still be 6 m/s. (What *will* change? The wavelength. Because $\lambda = v/f$, a change in f with no change in v will change λ.)

Example 10-6: Which one of the following statements is true concerning the amplitude of a wave?

    A. Amplitude increases with increasing frequency.
    B. Amplitude increases with increasing wavelength.
    C. Amplitude increases with increasing wave speed.
    D. None of the above.

Solution: The amplitude is determined by how much energy we put into the wave to get it started. If we wiggle the rope up and down through a large distance (a large amplitude), this takes more energy on our part, and as a result, the wave carries more energy. However, the amplitude doesn't depend on f, λ, or v. The answer is (D).

Example 10-7: A wave of frequency 12 Hz has a wavelength of 3 m. What is the speed of this wave?

Solution: Using the equation $v = \lambda f$, we find that v = (3 m)(12 Hz) = 36 m/s.

Example 10-8: The horizontal distance between each crest and the closest trough of a transverse traveling wave along a long horizontal rope is 2 m. If the wave speed is 8 m/s, what is the period of this wave?

Solution: If the horizontal distance between each crest and the closest trough for a transverse traveling wave is 2 m, then the wavelength is 4 m. Now, using $v = \lambda f$, we find that $f = v/\lambda$ = (8 m/s)/(4 m) = 2 Hz, so $T = 1/f = 1/(2 \text{ Hz})$ = 0.5 sec.

Example 10-9: What happens when the wave shown below passes from the thick, heavy rope into the thinner, lighter rope?

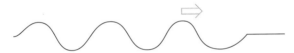

Solution: According to Big Rule 2 for waves, when a wave passes into another medium, its speed changes, but its frequency does not. How does the speed change? Because the rope is lighter (i.e., it has a lower linear density), the equation for wave speed on a string (given above) tells us that v will *increase*. So, if v increases but f doesn't change, then λ will also increase because $\lambda = v/f$.

Example 10-10: A certain rope transmits a 2 Hz transverse wave of amplitude 10 cm with a speed of 1 m/s. What would be the wavelength of a 5 Hz transverse wave of amplitude 8 cm on this same rope?

Solution: First, ignore the amplitudes; they're included in the question only to make things seem more complicated than they are. The amplitude of a wave indicates how much energy the wave transports, but it has nothing to do with wavelength, period, frequency, or wave speed (recall Example 10-6 above). Now, if a 2 Hz transverse wave has a speed of 1 m/s on this rope, then a transverse wave of *any* frequency will have a speed of 1 m/s on this rope; that's what Big Rule 1 for waves tells us. Thus, if f = 5 Hz and v = 1 m/s, then

$$\lambda = \frac{v}{f} = \frac{1 \text{ m/s}}{5 \text{ Hz}} = 0.2 \text{ m}$$

Example 10-11: How long will it take a wave of wavelength λ and period T to travel a distance d?

A. $\lambda\,Td$

B. $\dfrac{\lambda d}{T}$

C. $\dfrac{Td}{\lambda}$

D. $\dfrac{\lambda T}{d}$

Proven Techniques

Solution: First, let's see if we can eliminate any choices because the units don't work out correctly. We're being asked for an amount of time, so the answer must have the dimension (and units) of time. Choice (A) can't be correct, since it has units of $[\lambda][T]$ $[d]$ = m·sec·m = m²·sec. Notice that both λ and d have units of meters, which we don't want in the answer, so these units must cancel. Therefore, (B) can't be correct either since λ and d are multiplied by each other, rather than being divided as they should to make their units cancel.

One difference between the two remaining choices is that in (C), the distance d is in the numerator, while in (D), the distance d is in the denominator. Now, let's think about this: more time will be required for the wave to travel a greater distance. In other words, the bigger d is, the greater the travel time should be. Therefore, we can eliminate (D); after all, since d is in the denominator in choice (D), a larger d will result in a smaller amount of time, which doesn't make sense. Thus, the answer must be (C).

Here's an alternate solution using equations. Because *distance = speed × time* ($d = vt$), we know that $t = d/v$. We can find v using the wave equation $v = \lambda f$, and since $f = 1/T$, we find that

$$t = \frac{d}{v} = \frac{d}{\lambda f} = \frac{d}{\lambda} \times \frac{1}{f} = \frac{d}{\lambda} \times T = \frac{Td}{\lambda}$$

The answer is indeed (C), just as we figured out by checking units and using logic.

Longitudinal Waves

Longitudinal waves don't propagate in the same manner as transverse waves. Instead, the direction in which the particles of the conducting medium oscillate is parallel to the direction of wave propagation. Sound waves, also known as compression waves, are longitudinal waves in gas, liquid, or solid; when a compression wave's frequency is between 20 Hz and 20 kHz, humans can perceive it as sound. Sound frequencies below 20 Hz are known as infrasound, and sound frequencies above 20 kHz are known as ultrasound.

Let's take a closer look at sound waves. As a stereo speaker, vocal fold, or tuning fork vibrates, it creates regions of high pressure (**compressions**) that alternate with regions of low pressure (**rarefactions**). These pressure waves are transmitted through the air (or some other medium) and can eventually reach our ears and brain, which translate the vibrations into sound.

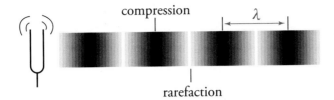

Like other waves, a longitudinal compression wave has a wavelength, a speed, a frequency, a period, and an amplitude. The equation $v = \lambda f$ holds, as do the two Big Rules for waves. Sound can travel in any medium: gas, liquid, or solid. In general, *sound travels slowest through gases, faster through liquids, and fastest through solids*. The speed of sound in air is about 340 m/s (that's about 760 miles per hour), but it varies slightly with temperature, pressure, and humidity.

10.3 INTERFERENCE OF WAVES

When two or more waves are superimposed on each other, they will combine to form a single resultant wave. This is called **interference**. The amplitude of the resultant wave will depend on the amplitudes of the combining waves *and* on how these waves travel relative to each other.

If crest meets crest, and trough meets trough, we say that the waves are **in phase** with each other. Their amplitudes will *add*, and we say the waves interfere **constructively**. However, if the crest of one wave coincides with the *trough* of the other (and vice versa), we say that the waves are exactly **out of phase** with each other. In this case, their amplitudes *subtract*, and we say that the waves interfere **destructively**.

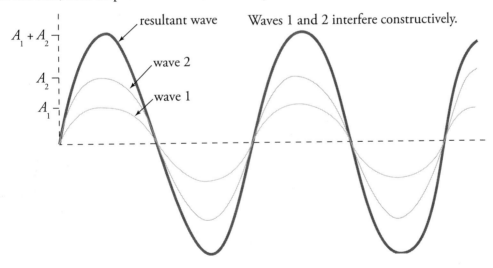

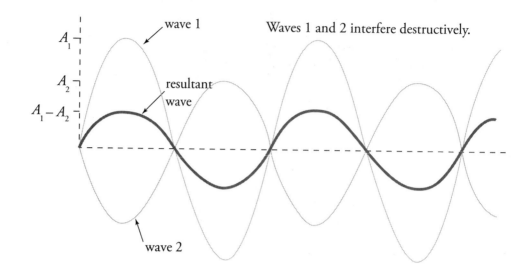

A passage might also say that waves that are directly opposite each other in amplitude are *180 degrees out of phase*, or *π radians out of phase*; it is common to refer to a whole cycle or wave as being 360 degrees or 2π radians, as if it were a circle. If the waves aren't exactly in phase ($0°$, $360°$, or 2π radians) or exactly out of phase ($180°$ or π radians), the amplitude of the resultant wave will be somewhere between the difference and the sum of the amplitudes of the interfering waves.

The interfering waves may also have different wavelengths. These waves will produce a more complicated-looking resultant wave, but we'd still say the waves interfere constructively where they reinforce each other, and destructively where they tend to cancel each other out.

Summary of Formulas

Simple Harmonic Motion (SHM) requires:

- dynamics condition: restoring force is directly proportional to displacement from equilibrium ($x = 0$) and points towards that equilibrium point

- kinematics condition: frequency and period are independent of the amplitude of oscillations

Hooke's Law (spring): $\mathbf{F} = -k\mathbf{x}$

Elastic potential energy (spring): $PE_{\text{elastic}} = \frac{1}{2}kx^2$

Spring-block oscillator frequency: $f = \dfrac{1}{2\pi}\sqrt{\dfrac{k}{m}}$

Simple pendulum frequency (small oscillations): $f = \dfrac{1}{2\pi}\sqrt{\dfrac{g}{l}}$

Period/frequency
(all harmonic motion and waves): $T = 1/f$

Wave equation: $v = \lambda f$

Two Big Rules for Waves to be used with wave equation:

1) Wave speed v depends on wave type and the medium, not on frequency

2) A single wave passing between media maintains a constant frequency

Chapter 11
Optics

11.1   ELECTROMAGNETIC WAVES

We've seen that if we oscillate one end of a long rope, we generate a wave that travels down the rope and whose frequency is the frequency with which we oscillate.

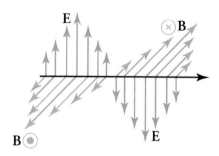

You can think of an electromagnetic wave in a similar way: an oscillating electric charge generates an **electromagnetic (EM)** wave, which is composed of oscillating electric and magnetic fields. These fields oscillate with the same frequency at which the electric charge that created the wave oscillated. The fields oscillate in phase with each other, perpendicular to each other and to the direction of propagation. For this reason, electromagnetic waves are transverse waves. The direction in which the wave's electric field oscillates is called the direction of **polarization** of the wave.

Most EM waves have electric fields oscillating in all perpendicular directions to propagation equally and are thus *unpolarized*.

Unlike waves on a rope or sound waves, electromagnetic waves do not require a material medium to propagate; they can travel through empty space (vacuum). When an EM wave travels through a vacuum, its speed is a constant. It is one of the fundamental constants of nature and a value you should memorize for the OAT:

Speed of Light in Vacuum

$$c = 3 \times 10^8 \, \text{m/s}$$

All electromagnetic waves, regardless of frequency, travel through a vacuum at this speed.

The most important equation for waves, $v = \lambda f$, is also true for electromagnetic waves. For EM waves traveling through a vacuum, $v = c$, so the equation becomes $\lambda f = c$.

The frequencies for electromagnetic waves span a huge range, and different ranges have been given specific names. This assignment of names to specific regions based on frequency (or wavelength) is known as the **electromagnetic spectrum** and is shown here.

Notice that visible light occupies only a small part of the electromagnetic spectrum. When waves from all over the visible spectrum are mixed together, the resulting light is perceived as white. You should memorize the order of the colors of the visible spectrum from lowest frequency (longest wavelength) to highest frequency (shortest wavelength): ROYGBV ("Roy-Gee-Biv"), which stands for red, orange, yellow, green, blue, and violet. In terms of wavelengths, violet light has a wavelength (in vacuum) of about 400 nm and red light has a wavelength of about 700 nm; the other colors are in between.

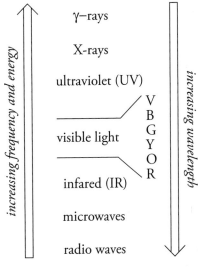

Photons

When electromagnetic radiation interacts with matter (absorption and emission), we find that it carries energy, and that the energy is quantized. That is, the energy associated with EM radiation is absorbed or emitted by matter in "packets"; individual bundles. Each such bundle of energy is called a **photon**, and the energy of a photon is directly proportional to the frequency:

Photon Energy

$$E = hf = h\frac{c}{\lambda}$$

The constant of proportionality, h, is called **Planck's constant**. (In SI units, its value is about 6.6×10^{-34} J·s. Don't worry about memorizing this constant; it would be given to you on the OAT if it were needed.)

The fact that electromagnetic radiation carries energy in packets (photons), which we can think of as "particles of light," gives rise to the idea of **wave-particle duality** for electromagnetic radiation: EM radiation travels like a wave but interacts with matter like a particle. One peculiarity of this duality is that, for waves, energy is proportional to the square of amplitude (recall the intensity relation from the previous chapter), whereas for particles (photons), energy is proportional to frequency. In Chapter 9, we noted that these two properties were independent of one another. Thus, the wave and particle models for light differ significantly in their predictions, and yet each is sometimes true.

Example 11-1: Which one of the following statements is true regarding red photons and blue photons traveling through a vacuum?

A. Red light travels faster than blue light and carries more energy.
B. Blue light travels faster than red light and carries more energy.
C. Red light travels at the same speed as blue light and carries more energy.
D. Blue light travels at the same speed as red light and carries more energy.

Solution: All electromagnetic waves, regardless of frequency, travel through vacuum at the same speed, *c*. This eliminates (A) and (B). Now, because blue light has a higher frequency than red light (remember ROYGBV, which lists the colors in order of increasing frequency), photons of blue light have higher energy than photons of red light. Therefore, the answer is (D).

11.2 REFLECTION AND REFRACTION

When a beam of light strikes the boundary between two transparent media, some of the light will be reflected from the surface. In the figure below, some of the sunlight will be reflected off the water in the tank.

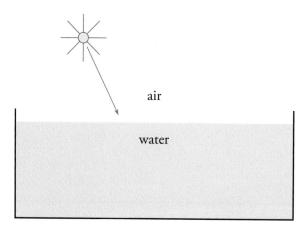

When a ray of light passing through one medium is reflected from the surface of another, the angle at which it bounces off the new medium is equal to the angle at which it strikes. In other words, *the angle of reflection is equal to the angle of incidence*. This fact is known as the **Law of Reflection**. Notice that, by definition, the angles of incidence and reflection are measured with reference to a line that's perpendicular to the plane of interface between the two media; that is, the angle of incidence and the angle of reflection are the angles that the incident and reflected rays make with *the normal*, not with the surface.

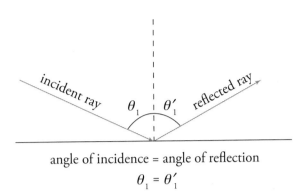

angle of incidence = angle of reflection

$$\theta_1 = \theta_1'$$

Example 11-2: In the figure above, assume that a ray of sunlight strikes the water, making an angle of 60° with the surface. What is the angle of reflection?

A. 15°
B. 30°
C. 60°
D. 90°

Solution: Be careful. If the incident ray makes an angle of 60° with the surface, then it makes an angle of 30° with the normal. Therefore, the angle of incidence is 30°. By the Law of Reflection, the angle of reflection is 30° also. Choice (B) is the answer.

In the figure below, not all of the sunlight that encounters the surface of the water is reflected; some is transmitted into the water. Unless the angle of incidence is 0°, the light will be *bent* as it enters the water. The bending is called **refraction**. The **angle of refraction** is the angle that the **transmitted** (or **refracted**) ray makes with the line that's perpendicular to the plane of interface between the two media.

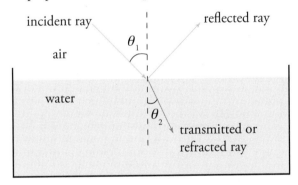

If $\theta_1 = 0°$ (that is, if the incident ray is perpendicular to the boundary), then $\theta_2 = 0°$. However, if θ_1 is any other angle, then θ_2 will be different from θ_1; that is, the ray bends as it's transmitted. In order to figure out the angle of refraction, we first need to discuss a medium's index of refraction.

Index of Refraction

Light travels at speed $c = 3 \times 10^8$ m/s when traveling in a vacuum. However, when light travels through a material medium such as water or glass, its transmission speed is less than c. Every medium, in fact, has an **index of refraction** that tells us how much slower light travels through that medium than through empty space.

Index of Refraction

$$\text{index of refraction} = \frac{\text{speed of light in vacuum}}{\text{speed of light in medium}}$$

$$n = \frac{c}{v}$$

The index of refraction of vacuum is, by definition, exactly equal to 1. Because the index for air is very close to 1, we simply use $n = 1$ for air as well. (The OAT will use this approximation unless otherwise specified.) Notice that n has no units, it's never less than 1, and the greater the value of n for a medium, the slower light travels through that medium. For most materials, the value of n is between 1 and 2.5. Glass has an index of refraction of about 1.5 (but varies depending on the type of glass), while a diamond has a particularly high value of n, about 2.4. Values of n above 2.5 are rare.

Example 11-3: Light travels through water at an approximate speed of 2.25×10^8 m/s. What is the refractive index of water?

    A.   0.75
    B.   1.33
    C.   1.50
    D.   2.25

Solution: First, eliminate (A): the index of refraction is never less than 1. Now, by definition,

$$n = \frac{c}{v} = \frac{3 \times 10^8 \text{ m/s}}{2.25 \times 10^8 \text{ m/s}} = \frac{3}{2.25} = \frac{3}{2\frac{1}{4}} = \frac{3}{\frac{9}{4}} = 3 \cdot \frac{4}{9} = \frac{4}{3} \approx 1.33$$

Therefore, the answer is (B).

Now that we know about the index of refraction, we can state the rule that's used to figure out the angle of refraction. It's called the Law of Refraction, or Snell's Law:

Law of Refraction (Snell's Law)

$$n_1 \sin\theta_1 = n_2 \sin\theta_2$$

In this equation, n_1 is the refractive index of the medium through which the incident ray is traveling, and n_2 is the refractive index of the medium through which the transmitted (or refracted) ray is traveling.

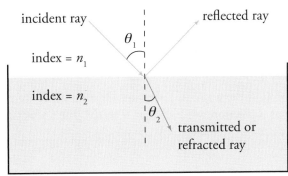

It follows from Snell's Law that if $n_2 > n_1$, then $\theta_2 < \theta_1$. That is, if the transmitting medium has a higher index of refraction than the incident medium, then the ray will bend *toward* the normal. Similarly, if $n_2 < n_1$, then $\theta_2 > \theta_1$. That is, if the transmitting medium has a lower index of refraction than the incident medium, then the ray will bend *away from* the normal. You should memorize both of these facts.

Example 11-4: A ray of light traveling through air is incident on a piece of glass whose refractive index is 1.5. If the sine of the angle of incidence is 0.6, what's the sine of the angle of refraction?

Solution: Using the Law of Refraction, we find that

$$n_1 \sin\theta_1 = n_2 \sin\theta_2 \rightarrow (1)(0.6) = (1.5)(\sin\theta_2) \rightarrow \sin\theta_2 = \frac{0.6}{1.5} = \frac{\frac{3}{5}}{\frac{3}{2}} = \frac{2}{5} = 0.4$$

Notice that $\sin\theta_2$ is less than $\sin\theta_1$; this immediately tells us that $\theta_2 < \theta_1$. The light is traveling from air ($n_1 = 1$) into glass, whose refractive index is higher. If the transmitting medium (i.e., the second one) has a higher index of refraction than the incident medium (i.e., the first one), then θ_2 *will* be less than θ_1; that is, the ray will bend toward the normal.

Example 11-5: Consider the diagram below, showing an incident ray, reflected ray, and transmitted ray:

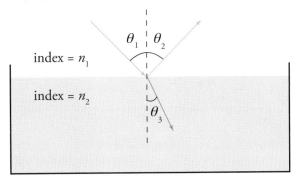

What information is needed to find θ_2?

    A. n_1, n_2, and θ_1
    B. n_1, n_2, and θ_3
    C. n_1 only
    D. θ_1 only

Solution: The angle labeled θ_2 is the angle of reflection. To find it, all we need to know is the angle of incidence, θ_1. (By the Law of Reflection, we find that $\theta_2 = \theta_1$.) The answer is (D). (This unconventional labeling of the angles is a common OAT tactic, by the way.)

Total Internal Reflection

When a light ray traveling in a medium of high refractive index approaches a medium of lower refractive index (for example, a light ray traveling in water towards the interface with the air), it may or may not escape into the second medium. If the ray's angle of incidence exceeds a certain **critical angle**, the light ray will undergo **total internal reflection**: All of the incident ray's energy will be reflected back into its original medium; there will be no refracted ray.

Critical Angle for Total Internal Reflection

$$\sin \theta_{\text{crit}} = \frac{n_2}{n_1}$$

In this equation, n_1 is the refractive index of the medium through which the incident ray is traveling, and n_2 is the refractive index of the medium on the other side of the boundary. The angle θ_{crit} is the critical angle. What this means is that if the angle of incidence, θ_1, is greater than θ_{crit}, then total internal reflection will occur.[1] However, if θ_1 is less than θ_{crit}, then total internal reflection will not occur. (If θ_1 just happens to equal θ_{crit}, then the refracted beam skims along the boundary with $\theta_2 = 90°$.)

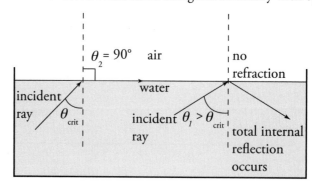

---

[1] If you forget the formula for the critical angle, there's another way to know that total internal reflection occurs: If you plug numbers into the Law of Refraction and find that $\sin \theta > 1$ (which is impossible), that tells you there is no angle of refraction, so there must be total internal reflection.

Notice that there can be a critical angle for total internal reflection *only if n_1 is greater than n_2*. For example, a beam of light incident in the air and striking the surface of the water can never experience total internal reflection because $n_1 < n_2$. In other words, there'll be some reflection and some refraction, as usual. In this case, some of the light's intensity will always be transmitted into the water.

Example 11-6: A beam of light is incident on the boundary between air and a piece of glass whose index of refraction is $\sqrt{2}$. When would total internal reflection (TIR, for short) of this beam occur?

Solution: First, in order to have TIR, the beam would have to start in the glass, trying to exit into the air. (If the beam were traveling in the air and incident on the glass, then TIR could not occur.) Furthermore, the angle of incidence would have to be greater than the critical angle, which we calculate as follows:

$$\sin \theta_{crit} = \frac{n_2}{n_1} = \frac{1}{\sqrt{2}} = \frac{\sqrt{2}}{2} \rightarrow \theta_{crit} = 45°$$

11.3 WAVE EFFECTS

Diffraction

Simply put, waves, whether they're water waves, sound waves, EM waves, etc., don't always travel in a single direction when they encounter an obstruction. This redistribution of the wave's intensity is known as **diffraction**. Water waves bend around a rock sticking up out of the water, for example. The "obstruction" can even be a hole. For example, water or light incident on a hole in a barrier will pass through and *spread out* beyond the barrier. These effects are observed when the size of the object or opening is comparable to the wavelength of the waves.

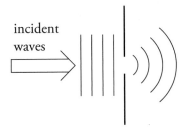

Dispersion

When light moves from one medium to another, some wavelengths are bent more than others. The reason for this is that electromagnetic waves of different frequencies travel at slightly different speeds when traveling through a material medium like glass or water. Although Big Rule 1 for waves states that the speed of a wave is determined by the medium, not by the wave's frequency, light waves traveling through a material medium are an exception to this rule.[2] (In fact, they're the only exception that's at all likely to appear on the OAT.) When light travels through a material (not vacuum), different frequencies will have different speeds. Thus, when we say that the index of refraction for a piece

---

[2] This isn't the case when electromagnetic waves travel through vacuum, where *all* frequencies travel at the same speed, c.

of glass is 1.5, what is really true is that the index varies slightly as the color of the light varies. For example, the index of refraction of the glass could be 1.47 for red light but 1.54 for violet light.[3] Because different colors have different refractive indexes, they will have different angles of refraction. This is why when white light passes through a prism, the beam is broken into its component colors. Each color leaves the prism at its own angle of refraction.[4] We call this variation in wave speed for different frequencies (and the effects this variation produces) **dispersion**.

Polarization

Normally, the electric-field components of the waves in a beam of light vibrate in *all* planes. **Polarized** light is light whose direction of polarization has been restricted somehow. For example, all the waves in a beam of **plane-polarized** light have their electric-field components vibrating in a single plane.

It is possible to transform unpolarized light into polarized light by several methods. One method is the use of a *polarizing filter.* The filter has a polarization axis, so that when unpolarized light strikes the filter, only the portion of the waves vibrating in that direction pass through while the portion of the waves vibrating perpendicular to the axis is absorbed. The light that emerges is now polarized in in direction of the axis and has half the intensity of the original unpolarized light.

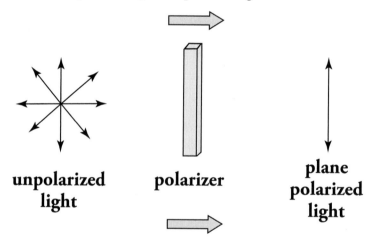

unpolarized light   **polarizer**   **plane polarized light**

If polarized light passes through a second polarizer, the amount of light that passes through or is absorbed depends on the angle between the direction of polarization of the incident light and the axis of the polarizer. As an example, if vertically polarized light is incident upon a horizontally polarizing filter, none of the light will pass through.

---

[3] In general, as in this example, the higher the frequency of the light, the lower the speed. However, there are complicated exceptions to this rule of thumb, and there's no need to memorize it or learn about the exceptions for the OAT.

[4] The greater the index of refraction, the more the light will be bent on entering the medium from air or vacuum, so high-frequency violet light will generally bend more than red light.

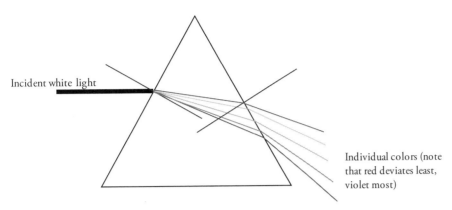

Incident white light

Individual colors (note
that red deviates least,
violet most)

It's worth mentioning here that polarization can't be applied to longitudinal waves like sound. After all, if polarization is the filtering or selection of the direction of wave oscillation, but longitudinal waves only oscillate in one direction (parallel to the direction of wave propagation), then a longitudinal wave can't be made to oscillate in a different manner. For example, if a sound wave propagates to the right, then its wave oscillations will be in the left-right direction; they can't be in the up-down direction as the wave continues to propagate to the right.

Also note that light can be filtered by color. If white light is passed through a blue filter, then blue light comes out the other side, i.e., the filter only allows blue light to pass through it. The other colors (wavelengths) are absorbed by the filter. Furthermore, if a blue filter is placed in front of a red filter, no color will be transmitted; it will appear black.

11.4 MIRRORS

A **mirror** is a surface, usually made of glass or metal, that forms an image of an object by *reflecting* light.

Plane Mirrors

A **plane** mirror is an ordinary flat mirror. If you put an object in front of a plane mirror, the image will appear to be behind the mirror. The image will be the same size as the object and will appear to be as far behind the mirror's surface as the object is in front of it. The image will also appear upright; it won't be inverted.

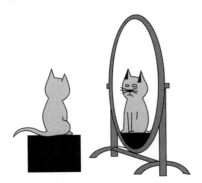

Curved Mirrors

We all have experience with plane mirrors, but a **curved** mirror presents us with images that are less familiar. The purpose of this section is to find a systematic way to describe the images formed by curved mirrors.

There are essentially two types of curved mirrors: concave and convex. The shiny (reflecting) surface of a **concave** mirror appears like the entrance to a "cave" from the point of view of the object. The reflecting surface of a **convex** mirror bends away from the object. As a simple demonstration of the difference, imagine holding a polished spoon. If you look into the spoon, you're looking at a concave surface; if you turn it around and look at the back of the spoon, you're looking at a convex surface.

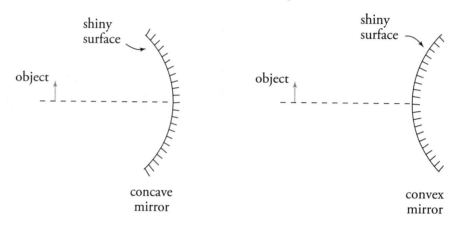

The curved mirrors we'll consider could be termed **spherical** mirrors, because near the center of the mirror, the surface is spherical (that is, part of a sphere).

When light parallel to the central **axis** of a concave mirror strikes the surface, it's reflected through a point called the **focus** (or **focal point**), denoted by F. This point is halfway to the **center of curvature**, C, of the mirror, which is the center of the sphere that the mirror is "cut from." The distance between the center of curvature and the mirror is called the **radius of curvature**, r. (The radius of curvature is also sometimes denoted by RC.) Because the focal point is halfway between the mirror and C, the distance from the mirror to the focal point, the all-important **focal length**, f, is half the radius of curvature: $f = \frac{1}{2}r$.

When light parallel to the central *axis* of a *convex* mirror strikes the surface, it's reflected directly *away from* the "imaginary" **focal point** behind the mirror.

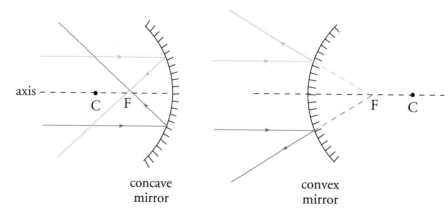

We see an image in a mirror at the point where the rays reflected off the mirror intersect *or* at the point from where the reflected rays seem to intersect (and therefore emanate from) behind the mirror. The following figures illustrate the process of image formation by curved mirrors:

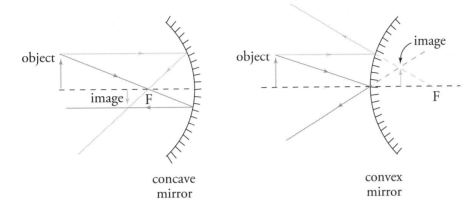

concave
mirror

convex
mirror

The ray diagram for the concave mirror shows two incident rays reflecting off the mirror. One ray, parallel to the axis, is reflected through the focal point. Another ray, which goes through the focal point, is reflected parallel to the axis. The intersection point of these reflected rays determines the location of the image.

The ray diagram for the convex mirror also shows two incident rays reflecting off the mirror. One ray, parallel to the axis, is reflected directly away from the focal point. Another ray, which hits the center of the mirror (the point where its axis of symmetry intersects the mirror surface), is reflected at the same angle below the axis. Following these reflected rays back behind the mirror, their intersection point determines the location of the image.

Ray diagrams (like the ones drawn in the figure above) can be used to determine the approximate location of the image, but they usually can't give precise answers to all the questions we may be asked about the image formed by a mirror. What we want is a systematic way to get precise answers to these four questions:

1. Where is the image?
2. Is the image real *or* is it virtual?
3. Is the image upright or is it inverted?
4. How tall is the image (compared to the object)?

Before we discuss how to answer these questions, let's first define the terms *real* and *virtual*. An image is said to be **real** if light rays actually focus at the position of the image. A real image can be projected onto a surface. An image is said to be **virtual** if light rays don't actually focus at the apparent location of the image. For example, look back at the figure above, showing the formation of images by a concave mirror and by a convex mirror. The image formed by the concave mirror in that diagram is real: light rays actually intersect at the image location. However, the image formed by the convex mirror is virtual: no light rays intersect at its location, they just seem to come from that location.

The Mirror Equation

To answer the first two questions given above, we use the mirror (and lens) equation:

Mirror (and Lens) Equation

$$\frac{1}{o} + \frac{1}{i} = \frac{1}{f}$$

Here, o stands for the object's distance from the mirror, and is always positive. The value of f represents the focal length of the mirror. The value of i that satisfies this equation gives us the image's distance from the mirror. Both f and i are positive if they are on the same side as the human observer in relation to the mirror or lens. In the case of a mirror, the human observer is on the same side as the object. In the case of a lens, the human observer is on the opposite side of the object. Using the mirror (and lens) equation, we can find the location of the image, answering the first question.

The second question is also answered using the mirror equation. If we get a *positive* value for i, that tells us that the image is in front of the mirror and it's *real*; a *negative* value for i means the image is behind the mirror and is *virtual*. For example, let's say that $o = 2$ cm and $f = 6$ cm. Substituting these values into the mirror equation, we find that $i = -3$ cm. Therefore, the image is 3 cm behind the mirror and it's virtual. Note that you can use any unit for the measurement of distance, as long as it is the same unit for o, i, and f.

The Magnification Equation

To answer the last two questions, we then use the magnification equation:

Magnification Equation

$$m = -\frac{i}{o}$$

The value of m is the **magnification factor**; multiplying the height of the object by m gives us the height of the image. The sign of m tells us whether the image is upright or inverted. If m is *positive*, the image is *upright*; if m is *negative*, the image is *inverted*. To illustrate this, let's continue our example above, with $o = 2$ cm and $f = 6$ cm. We found that $i = -3$ cm. Therefore, the magnification factor is $m = -(-3 \text{ cm})/(2 \text{ cm}) = +1.5$. This tells us that the height of the image is 1.5 times the height of the object, and (because m is positive) the image is upright.

The object distance, o, is always positive. If i is positive, then m is negative; if i is negative, then m is positive. In other words,

Real images are inverted, and virtual images are upright.

Now, the only thing that's left to do is to find the way to "tell" the mirror equation whether we have a concave mirror or a convex mirror. The rule is simple: When using the mirror equation, we write the focal length of a *concave* mirror as a *positive* number, and we write the focal length of a *convex* mirror as a *negative* number. Here's a summary of mirrors:

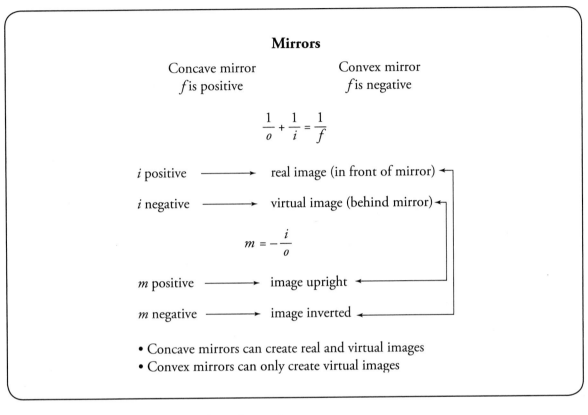

Mirrors

Concave mirror
f is positive

Convex mirror
f is negative

$$\frac{1}{o} + \frac{1}{i} = \frac{1}{f}$$

i positive $\longrightarrow$ real image (in front of mirror)

i negative $\longrightarrow$ virtual image (behind mirror)

$$m = -\frac{i}{o}$$

m positive $\longrightarrow$ image upright

m negative $\longrightarrow$ image inverted

- Concave mirrors can create real and virtual images
- Convex mirrors can only create virtual images

Example 11-7: Describe the image formed in a plane mirror.

A. Real and upright
B. Real and inverted
C. Virtual and upright
D. Virtual and inverted

Solution: First, eliminate (A) and (D); *real* always goes with *inverted*, and *virtual* always goes with *upright*. We know from common experience that the image formed in a flat mirror is upright, so the answer must be (C).

Example 11-8: If an object is placed very far from a concave mirror, where will the image be formed?

A. Halfway between the focal point and the mirror
B. At the focal point
C. At the center of curvature
D. At infinity

Solution: Use the mirror equation. "The object is placed very far from a mirror" means that we take $o = \infty$, so $1/o = 0$. The mirror equation then says $1/i = 1/f$, so $i = f$. That is, the image is formed at the focal point of the mirror, (B).

Example 11-9: An object is placed 40 cm in front of a concave mirror with a radius of curvature of 60 cm. Locate and describe the image.

Solution: Because $f = \frac{1}{2}r$, we know that f = 30 cm. The mirror equation now gives

$$\frac{1}{40\text{ cm}} + \frac{1}{i} = \frac{1}{30\text{ cm}} \rightarrow \frac{1}{i} = \frac{1}{30} - \frac{1}{40} = \frac{4-3}{120} = \frac{1}{120} \rightarrow \therefore i = 120\text{ cm}$$

(Be careful: The OAT often gives the radius of curvature, r. What you want is f, the focal length, which is half of r.) Since i is positive, we know the image is real; also, it's located 120 cm from the mirror on the same side of the mirror as the object. (*Virtual* images are located *behind* the mirror.) Since $m = -i/o = -(120\text{ cm})/(40\text{ cm}) = -3$, we know that the image is 3 times the height of the object and inverted.

Example 11-10: An object is placed 40 cm in front of a convex mirror with a radius of curvature of –60 cm. Locate and describe the image.

Solution: Because $f = \frac{1}{2}r$, we know that f = –30 cm. The mirror equation now gives

$$\frac{1}{40\text{ cm}} + \frac{1}{i} = \frac{1}{-30\text{ cm}} \rightarrow \frac{1}{i} = -\frac{1}{30} - \frac{1}{40} = \frac{-4-3}{120} = \frac{-7}{120} \rightarrow \therefore i = -\frac{120}{7}\text{ cm}$$

Since i is negative, we know the image is virtual; also, it's located $120/7 \approx 17$ cm from the mirror on the opposite side of the mirror from the object. Since $m = -i/o = -(-\frac{120}{7}\text{ cm})/(40\text{ cm}) = +3/7$, we know that the image is 3/7 times the height of the object and upright. Comparing this example to the preceding one, notice how critical the sign of f was. It changed everything about the image.

Example 11-11: A convex mirror forms an upright image 12 cm behind the mirror when an object of height 15 cm is placed 20 cm in front of it. What is the height of the image?

Solution: To find the height of the image, we need the magnification. We're given that o = 20 cm and i = –12 cm. (We know that i is negative because not only do convex mirrors only form virtual images [a good fact to remember, by the way], but the question also says that the image is formed "behind the mirror." Images formed behind the mirror are virtual.) Therefore, $m = -i/o = -(-12\text{ cm})/(20\text{ cm}) = 3/5$. Multiplying the height of the object by the magnification gives the height of the image. Therefore, the height of the image is (3/5)(15 cm) = 9 cm.

11.5 LENSES

A **lens** is a thin piece of clear glass or plastic that forms an image of an object by *refracting* light. The purpose of this section is to find a systematic way to describe the images formed by lenses.

There are essentially two types of lenses: converging and diverging. **Converging** lenses are thicker in the middle than they are at the ends, and they refract light rays that are parallel to the axis *toward* the focal point on the other side of the lens. **Diverging** lenses are thinner in the middle than they are at the ends, and they refract light rays that are parallel to the axis *away from* the "imaginary" focal point that's in front of the lens.

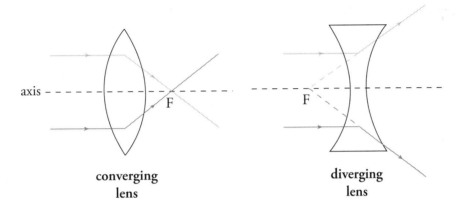

converging lens

diverging lens

We want to be able to answer the same four questions for lenses as we did for mirrors. Fortunately, *virtually everything we did for mirrors carries over unchanged to lenses.* For example, the mirror equation is also the lens equation, and the magnification equation is also the same. The conventions for positive and negative *i* and *m* are also the same for lenses as they are for mirrors.

We distinguish between the two types of lenses in the same way we distinguished between the two types of mirrors. When using the lens equation, we write the focal length of a *converging* lens as a *positive* number, and we write the focal length of a *diverging* lens as a *negative* number.

Here's an important note. The OAT uses the terms *concave* and *convex* to refer to different mirrors and lenses. The diagrams above show us that the surfaces of a converging lens are convex, and the surfaces of a diverging lens are concave. Thus, a concave lens is the same as a diverging lens, and a convex lens is the same as a converging lens. Now for a warning: For a concave *mirror*, *f* is positive; and for a convex *mirror*, *f* is negative. When these terms are applied to lenses, things necessarily switch: For a concave *lens*, *f* is negative; and for a convex *lens*, *f* is positive. *Be careful* when you see the words *concave* or *convex*. Whether these terms describe a mirror or a lens will make a critically important difference in whether you write the focal length as a positive or as a negative number.

Besides the fact the lenses form images by refracting light (rather than by reflecting light, as is the case for mirrors), there's really only one difference: For lenses, *real* images are formed on the *opposite* side of the lens from the object, while *virtual* images are formed on the *same* side of the lens as the object.

Here's a summary of lenses:

Lenses

Converging lens (convex lens) f is positive	Diverging lens (concave lens) f is negative

$$\frac{1}{o} + \frac{1}{i} = \frac{1}{f}$$

i positive $\Rightarrow$ real image (other side of lens)
i negative $\Rightarrow$ virtual image (same side of lens as object)

$$m = -\frac{i}{o}$$

m positive $\Rightarrow$ image upright
m negative $\Rightarrow$ image inverted

- Converging (convex) lenses can create real and virtual images
- Diverging (concave) lenses can only create virtual images

Example 11-12: An object is placed 10 cm in front of a diverging lens with a focal length of −40 cm, then the image will be located:

- A. 5 cm in front of the lens.
- B. 5 cm behind the lens.
- C. 8 cm in front of the lens.
- D. 8 cm behind the lens.

Solution: We use the lens equation to find i:

$$\frac{1}{10 \text{ cm}} + \frac{1}{i} = \frac{1}{-40 \text{ cm}} \rightarrow \frac{1}{i} = -\frac{1}{40} - \frac{1}{10} = \frac{-1-4}{40} = \frac{-5}{40} = -\frac{1}{8} \rightarrow \therefore i = -8 \text{ cm}$$

This eliminates (A) and (B). Because i is negative, the image is virtual, and for lenses, virtual images are formed on the same side of the lens as the object. Therefore, the answer is (C).

Example 11-13: An object of height 10 cm is held 50 cm in front of a convex lens with a focal length of magnitude 40 cm. Describe the image.

Solution: The fact that the lens is convex means that it's a converging lens with a *positive* focal length; therefore, f = +40 cm. The lens equation now gives us i:

$$\frac{1}{50 \text{ cm}} + \frac{1}{i} = \frac{1}{40 \text{ cm}} \rightarrow \frac{1}{i} = \frac{1}{40} - \frac{1}{50} = \frac{5-4}{200} = \frac{1}{200} \rightarrow \therefore i = 200 \text{ cm}$$

Because i is positive, we know the image is real; also, it's located 200 cm from the lens on the *opposite* side of the lens from the object. Because $m = -i/o = -(200 \text{ cm})/(50 \text{ cm}) = -4$, we know that the image is 4 times the height of the object and inverted.

Lens Power

A lens with a short focal length refracts light more (i.e., through larger angles) than a lens with a longer focal length. We say that the lens of short focal length has a greater *power* than a lens with a longer focal length.

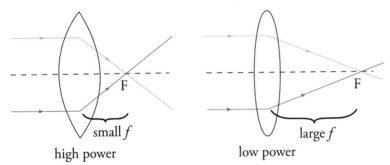

| small f | large f |
| high power | low power |

The **power** of a lens is defined to be the reciprocal of f, the focal length. When f is expressed in *meters*, the unit of lens power is called the **diopter** (abbreviated **D**).

Lens Power

$$P = \frac{1}{f}, \text{ where } f \text{ is in meters}$$

For example, to find the power of a lens whose focal length is 40 cm, we first write f in meters: $f = 0.4$ m. Since $0.4 = 2/5$, the reciprocal of 0.4 is $5/2 = 2.5$. Therefore, the power of this lens is 2.5 diopters. Since the focal length of a converging lens is positive, the power of a converging lens is positive. Similarly, since the focal length of a diverging lens is negative, the power of a diverging lens is negative.

If two (or more) lenses are placed side by side, the power of the lens combination is equal to the sum of the powers of the individual lenses. In the case of two lenses, $P = P_1 + P_2$. For example, if we place a converging lens with a power of 3 D right next to a converging lens with a power of 1 D, then the power of the lens combination will be 4 D.

Example 11-14: A lens has a focal length of –20 cm. Is the lens converging or diverging? What is the power of this lens?

Solution: The fact that the lens has a negative focal length means that it's a diverging (or concave) lens. Rewriting f in meters, we have $f = -\frac{1}{5}$ m. Therefore, the power of this lens is

$$P = \frac{1}{f} = \frac{1}{-\frac{1}{5} \text{ m}} = -5 \text{ D}$$

The Basics of Eyesight Correction

Let's now look at the fundamental use of auxiliary lenses to correct the two most common types of eye defects: myopia and hyperopia. **Myopia** is the technical name for *nearsightedness*; myopic individuals cannot focus clearly on distant objects. **Hyperopia** (or **hypermetropia**) is the technical name for *farsightedness*; in contrast to myopes, hyperopic individuals cannot focus clearly on objects that are near the eye. (As we age, most of us will be afflicted with *presbyopia*, in which the eyes' ability to *accommodate* is compromised by the loss of elasticity in the lens of the eye. **Accommodation** refers to the ability to focus on nearby objects through the action of the ciliary muscles, which essentially squeeze the lens of the eye, increasing its curvature and decreasing its focal length. However, the correction for presbyopia is the same as that for hyperopia.)

Correcting Myopia. Light rays from objects whose distance from the eye is greater than about 6 m are essentially parallel to the axis of the lens of the eye, so a relaxed eye will focus these rays at the focal point. Because the diameter of a myopic eye is greater than the focal length of the lens of the eye, the image of the object is focused not on the retina but in front of it. As a result, a myopic individual receives a blurred image of distant objects. To correct this defect, a lens that "delays" the focusing is required. In essence, what is needed is a lens to diverge the parallel rays before they enter the lens of the eye so that they will focus beyond the focal point of the unaided eye, specifically on the retina. Because diverging lenses have negative focal lengths, they have negative powers (this follows from the definition $P = 1/f$). The greater the distance between the focal point of the lens of the myopic eye and the retina, the more the auxiliary lens must diverge the incoming parallel rays; that is, the more powerful the corrective lens (and the more negative the lens power).

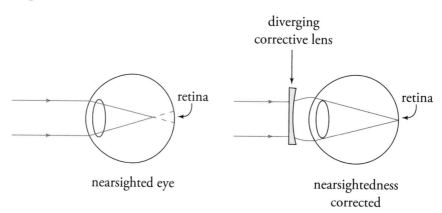

nearsighted eye   nearsightedness corrected

Correcting Hyperopia or Presbyopia. In these cases, light rays would be focused beyond the retina, either due to the diameter of the eye being smaller than the focal length of the lens of the eye or the inability of the ciliary muscles to decrease the focal length of the lens of the eye. To correct this defect, a lens that "accelerates" the focusing is required. In essence, what is needed is a lens to converge the rays before they enter the lens of the eye so that they will focus in front of the focal point of the unaided eye, specifically, on the retina. Because converging lenses have positive focal lengths, they have positive powers. (This follows from the definition $P = 1/f$.) The greater the distance between the focal point of the lens of the hyperopic eye and the retina, the more the auxiliary lens must converge the incoming rays, that is, the more powerful the corrective lens (and the more positive the lens power).

11.5

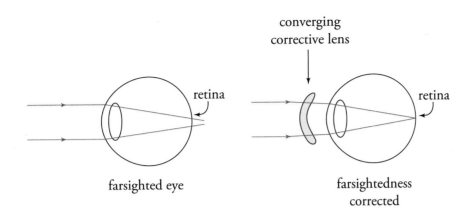

converging
corrective lens

retina

farsighted eye

retina

farsightedness
corrected

If you wear eyeglasses or contacts, check the prescription. If you have trouble seeing faraway objects, then you're nearsighted (myopic), and your corrective lenses are diverging and will have a negative power. On the other hand, if you have trouble seeing objects that are close-up, then you're farsighted (hyperopic), and your corrective lenses are converging and will have a positive power. Also, if the power of your left corrective lens is different from the power of your right corrective lens, the lens with the power of greater *magnitude* corresponds to the weaker eye. For example, if your left eye requires a lens of power -3.5 D while your right eye requires a lens of power -3.25 D, then your left eye is weaker because $3.5 > 3.25$.

Summary of Formulas

Light acts as both a wave and a particle depending on the circumstance. In the former, energy is a function of amplitude; in the latter, energy is a function of frequency.

$$c = 3 \times 10^8 \text{ m/s for light in a vacuum}$$

- All angles for reflection and refraction formulas are measured from the normal to the surface.

Photon energy: $E = hf = h\dfrac{c}{\lambda}$

Law of Reflection: $\theta_1 = \theta_1'$

Index of Refraction: $n = \dfrac{c}{v}, n \geq 1$

Law of Refraction (Snell's Law): $n_1 \sin\theta_1 = n_2 \sin\theta_2$

Total internal reflection: If $n_1 > n_2$ and $\theta_1 > \theta_{crit}$, where $\sin\theta_{crit} = \dfrac{n_2}{n_1}$

Total internal reflection (meaning no light is transmitted from the incident medium through the boundary) can occur for incident angles greater than θ_{crit} and only when the incident medium has a larger index of refraction (n) than that of the medium beyond the boundary.

Mirror/lens equation: $\dfrac{1}{o} + \dfrac{1}{i} = \dfrac{1}{f}$

Magnification: $m = -\dfrac{i}{o}$

Converging mirror or lens (concave mirror or convex lens) $\leftrightarrow$ f positive

Diverging mirror or lens (convex mirror or concave lens) $\leftrightarrow$ f negative

Note o is always positive; the sign for i corresponds to the sign conventions for f.

Real, inverted image $\leftrightarrow$ positive i

Virtual, upright image $\leftrightarrow$ negative i

Lens power: $P = \dfrac{1}{f}$ (P in diopters when f is expressed in meters)

Chapter 12
Thermal Energy and Thermodynamics

12.1 INTRODUCTION

Objects contain **thermal energy**, which is due to the random motion of its molecules. **Heat** is defined to be thermal energy transmitted from one body to another. Note that objects don't *contain* heat; heat is energy that's in *transit*. By contrast, **temperature** is a measure of the intensity of an object's internal thermal energy. The study of the energy transfers involving work and heat, and the resulting changes in internal energy, temperature, volume, and pressure is called **thermodynamics**.

The SI unit for temperature is the **Kelvin**, where *absolute zero* is defined as 0 K and the *triple point* of water (the point where the solid, liquid, and gas phase of water can coexist) is 273.16 K. A Kelvin is the same size as a Celsius degree, and the conversion between the **absolute temperature** T in kelvins and the temperature expressed in Celsius degrees is

$$T = T(\text{in } °C) + 273.15$$

When a substance absorbs or gives off heat, one of two things can happen: (1) the temperature of the substance changes, *or* (2) the substance undergoes a phase change. If (1) occurs, then

$$Q = mc\Delta T$$

where Q denotes the heat transferred, m is the mass of the sample, c is the specific heat, and ΔT is the resulting temperature change. Intuitively, a substance's specific heat measures its ability to absorb heat and resist changes in temperature; that is, the greater the value of c, the smaller ΔT will be for a given amount of heat, Q.

If (2) occurs, then the sample's temperature remains constant throughout the transformation (that is, $\Delta T = 0$, so the previous equation does not apply) and

$$Q = mL$$

Where L denotes the **latent heat of phase transformation**. This equation tells us how much heat must be transferred in order to cause a sample of mass m to completely undergo a phase change. In the case of a phase change from solid to liquid (or vice versa), L is called the **latent heat of fusion**. For a phase change between liquid and vapor, L is called the **latent heat of vaporization**. In general, more energy is required to break the intermolecular bonds in going from liquid to vapor than is required to loosen the intermolecular bonds to go from solid to liquid, so $L_{vaporization} > L_{fusion}$.

12.2   HEAT TRANSFER AND THERMAL EXPANSION

When a substance undergoes a temperature change, it changes in size. Steel beams that form bridges or railroad tracks elongate and can buckle on a hot day; a balloon filled with air shrinks when placed in a freezer. The change in the length of the steel beam or in the volume of the gas in the balloon depends on the amount of the temperature change and on the identity of the substance being affected.

Let's first consider changes in length (of a steel beam, for example). When its initial temperature is T_i, its length is L_i. Then, if the beam's temperature changes to T_f, the length changes to L_f, where

$$L_f - L_i = \alpha L_i (T_f - T_i)$$

Where α is the **coefficient of linear expansion** of the material. This equation is usually remembered in the simpler form

$$\Delta L = \alpha L_i \Delta T$$

Nearly all substances have a positive value of α, which means they expand upon heating. If α is negative, then the substance shrinks when heated.

Example 12-1: A steel beam used in the construction of a bridge has a length of 20 m when the ambient temperature is 10°C. On a very hot day, when the temperature is 35°C, by how much will the beam stretch? (The coefficient of linear expansion for structural steel is +1.2 × 10^{-5}/°C.)

Solution: The change in length of the beam will be

$$\Delta L = \alpha L_i \Delta T = \frac{1.2 \times 10^{-5}}{°C}(20 \text{ m})(35°C - 10°C) = 6 \times 10^{-3} \text{ m} = 6 \text{ mm}$$

Substances also undergo volume changes when heat is lost or absorbed. The change in volume, ΔV, corresponding to a temperature change, ΔT, is given by the equation

$$\Delta V = \beta V_i \Delta T$$

where V_i is the sample's initial volume and β is the **coefficient of volume expansion** of the substance. Nearly all substances have a positive value for β, which means they expand upon heating. If β is negative, then the substance shrinks when heated. An extremely important example of a substance with a negative value of β is liquid water between 0°C and 4°C. Unlike the vast majority of substances, liquid water *expands* as it nears its freezing point and solidifies (which is why ice floats in water).

Example 12-2: A driver fills up a spare tank with 12 gallons of gas near the top of a mountain where the temperature is 2°C. By how much will the volume of the gasoline expand when the temperature is 22°C at the bottom of the mountain? (The coefficient of volume expansion for gasoline is $+9.5 \times 10^{-4}/°C$.)

Solution: The change in the volume of the gasoline will be

$$\Delta V = \beta V_1 \Delta T = \frac{9.5 \times 10^{-4}}{°C}(13 \text{ gal})(22°C - 2°C) = 0.25 \text{ gal}$$

12.3   THE KINETIC THEORY OF GASES

Unlike the condensed phases of matter—solid and liquid—the atoms or molecules that make up a gas do not oscillate around relatively fixed equilibrium positions. Rather, the motion is much more chaotic as the molecules zip around freely. As each gas molecule strikes a wall of its container, it exerts a force on the wall. The average force per unit area exerted by all the molecules is called the **pressure**.

The Ideal Gas Law

Three physical properties—pressure (P), volume (V), and temperature (T)—describe a gas. At low densities, all gases approach *ideal* or *perfect* behavior, which means that these three variables obey the equation

$$PV = nRT$$

where n is the number of moles of gas and R is the **universal gas constant** (equal to 8.31 J/mol·K). This equation is known as the **Ideal Gas Law.**

An important consequence of this equation is the observation that for a fixed volume of gas, an increase in P gives a proportional increase in T. The pressure increases when the gas molecules strike the walls of its container with more force, which occurs if they move more rapidly. We can make this more precise. Using Newton's Second Law (in the form *rate of change of momentum = force*) to find the average force—and, consequently, the pressure—that the gas molecules exert, it can be shown that the product of the pressure exerted by N molecules of gas in a container of volume V is related to the average kinetic energy of the molecules by the equation $PV = \frac{2}{3} NKE_{avg}$. Comparing this to the Ideal Gas Law, we see that

$\frac{2}{3} NKE_{avg} = nRT$. We can rewrite this equation in the form $\frac{2}{3} N_A KE_{avg} = RT$, since, by definition, $N = nN_A$, where N_A is Avogadro's number. The ratio R/N_A is a fundamental constant of nature called **Boltzmann's constant** ($k_B = 1.38 \times 10^{-23}$ J/K), so our equation becomes

$$KE_{avg} = \frac{3}{2} k_B T$$

This equation states that *the average translational kinetic energy of the gas molecules is directly proportional to the temperature of the sample.*

Since the average kinetic energy of the gas molecules is $KE_{avg} = \frac{1}{2} m(v^2)_{avg}$, where m is the mass of each molecule, the equation above becomes $\frac{1}{2} m(v^2)_{avg} = \frac{3}{2} k_B T$, so

$$\sqrt{v^2_{avg}} = \sqrt{\frac{3k_B T}{m}}$$

The quantity on the left-hand side of this equation, the square root of the average of the square of v, is called the **root-mean-square** speed, v_{rms}, so

$$v_{rms} = \sqrt{\frac{3k_B T}{m}}$$

Because $k_B = R/N_A$ and $mN_A = M =$ the mass of one mole of the molecules (the **molar mass**), the equation for v_{rms} is also commonly written in the form

$$v_{rms} = \sqrt{\frac{3RT}{M}}$$

Notice that these last two displayed equations determine only v_{rms}, the molecules in the container have a wide range of speeds, some much slower and other much faster than v_{rms}. The importance of the root-mean-square speed is that it gives us an average speed that is easy to calculate directly from the temperature of the gas.

Example 12-3: Compare the average (root-mean-square) speeds of nitrogen molecules and oxygen molecules at room temperature (20°C = 293 K).

Solution: First, since N_2 has a smaller molar mass than O_2 (28 g/mol for N_2 vs. 32 g/mol for O_2), the nitrogen molecules will move faster on average than the heavier oxygen molecules. The ratio of their root-mean-square speeds is

$$\frac{v_{rms}, N_2}{v_{rms}, O_2} = \sqrt{\frac{3RT / M_{N_2}}{3RT / M_{O_2}}} = \sqrt{\frac{M_{O_2}}{M_{N_2}}} = \sqrt{\frac{32 \text{ g/mol}}{28 \text{ g/mol}}} = \sqrt{\frac{8}{7}}$$

Example 12-4: A 0.2 mol sample of an ideal gas is confined to a container whose volume is 10 L. What will happen to the root-mean-square speed of its molecules if the sample is heated until the pressure doubles?

Solution: Since n and V are fixed, T is proportional to P (this follows from the Ideal Gas Law), therefore, if P doubles, then T doubles. Since v_{rms} is proportional to the square root of T, if T increases by a factor of 2, then v_{rms} will increase by a factor of $\sqrt{2} = 1.4$.

12.4 THE LAWS OF THERMODYNAMICS

The Zeroth Law of Thermodynamics

When two objects are brought into contact, heat will flow from the warmer object to the cooler one until they both reach **thermal equilibrium,** at which point their temperatures are the same. If Objects 1 and 2 are each in thermal equilibrium with Object 3, then Objects 1 and 2 are in thermal equilibrium with each other. The Zeroth Law assures us that the concept of temperature is well-defined and has a physical meaning.

The First Law of Thermodynamics

Simply put, the First Law of Thermodynamics is a statement of the Conservation of Energy that includes heat. To illustrate its use, we'll consider the following example of a system and its surroundings. It's the prototype that's studied extensively in thermodynamics.

An insulated, cylindrical container filled with an ideal gas rests on a heat reservoir that can serve as a heat source or a heat sink. The container is covered by a tight-fitting—but frictionless—weighted piston that can be raised or lowered. The confined gas is the *system*, and the piston and heat reservoir are the *surroundings*.

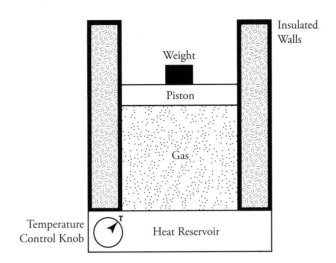

The **state** of the gas is given once the values of its pressure, volume, and temperature are known, and the equation that connects these state variables is the Ideal Gas Law, $PV = nRT$. Different experiments can be performed on the gas, such as heating it or allowing it to cool, increasing or decreasing the weight on the piston, etc., and we can determine not only the energy transfers (work and heat) but also how the state variables are affected. If each experiment is carried out slowly, so that at each moment, the system and its surroundings are in thermal equilibrium, we can plot the pressure (P) vs. the volume (V) on a **P-V diagram**. Each point in the diagram represents a particular value of P and V for the gas, and by following the graph, we can study how the system is affected as it moves from one state to another.

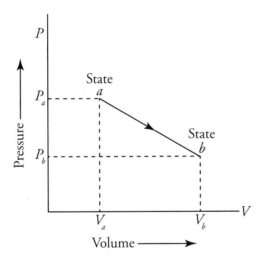

Work is done on or by the system when the piston is moved and the volume of the gas changes. For example, imagine that the gas pushes the piston upward, causing an increase in volume. The work done by the gas during its expansion is $W = F\Delta s$. But since $F = PA$, we have $W = PA\Delta s$, and because $A\Delta s = \Delta V$, we have, finally (assuming P is constant),

$$W = P\Delta V$$

This equation is also true if the piston is pushed down, causing the volume of the gas to decrease. In this case, ΔV is negative, so W is negative. In general, then, W is positive when the system does work pushing against its surroundings, and W is negative when the surroundings push against the system.

The equation $W = P\Delta V$ is valid if the pressure P does not change during the process. If P *does* change, then the work can be evaluated by finding the area under the graph in the P-V diagram; moving left to right gives a positive area (and thus positive work), while moving right to left gives a negative area (and thus negative work).

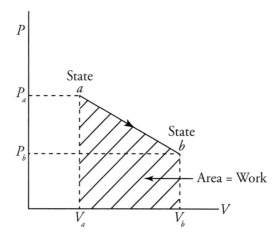

Example 12-5: What's the value of W for the process $a \rightarrow b$ following Path 1 and for the same process following Path 2 shown in the P-V diagram below?

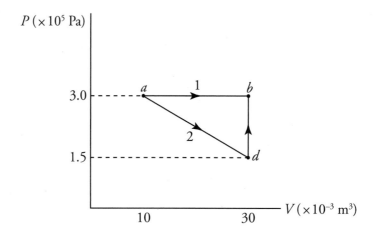

Solution: Along Path 1, P remains constant, so the work done is simply $P\Delta V$:

$$W = P\Delta V = (3 \times 10^5 \text{ Pa})[(30 \times 10^{-3} \text{ m}^3) - (10 \times 10^{-3} \text{ m}^3)] = 6000 \text{ J}$$

If the gas is brought from state a to state b along Path 2, then work is done only along the part from a to d. From d to b, the volume of the gas does not change, so no work can be performed. The area under the graph from a to d is the area of a trapezoid, so

$$W = \frac{1}{2}h(b_1 + b_2) = \frac{1}{2}(\Delta V)(P_a + P_d)$$

$$= \frac{1}{2}(20 \times 10^{-3}\ \text{m}^3)[(3 \times 10^5\ \text{Pa}) + (1.5 \times 10^5\ \text{Pa})]$$

$$= 4500\ \text{J}$$

Notice that $W_{a \to b} = 6000$ J along path 1, but $W_{a \to b} = 4500$ J along path 2.

As the preceding example shows, the value of W depends not only on the initial and final states of the system, but also on the path between the two. In general, different paths give different values for W. The value of Q is also path dependent. However, experiments have shown that the value of $Q - W$ is *not* path dependent; it depends *only* on the initial and final state of the system, so it must describe a change in some fundamental property. This fundamental property is called the system's **internal energy**, denoted U. Therefore, the change in the system's internal energy, $\Delta E_{\text{internal}}$, is equal to $Q - W$, regardless of the process that brought the system from its initial state to its final state. This statement is known as **The First Law of Thermodynamics**:

$$\Delta E_{\text{internal}} = Q - W$$

Example 12-6: A 0.5 mol sample of an ideal gas is brought from state a to state b along the path shown in the P-V diagram below. [Since the pressure remains constant (as we can see since the graph in the P-V diagram is a horizontal line), the process is called *isobaric*.]

a) Compare the temperature at state b to the temperature at state a.
b) Calculate the work done during the process.
c) Given that the gas absorbed 10,000 J of heat from a to b, determine the change in its internal energy.

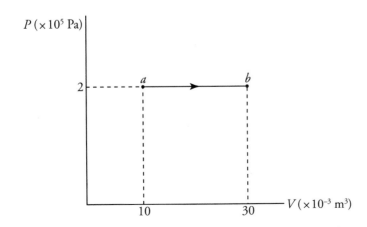

Solution:

a) The Ideal Gas Law tells us that if n and P are constant, then T is proportional to V. Since V increased by a factor of 3, so did the absolute temperature of the gas.

b) Since the pressure remains constant during the process, we can use the equation $W = P\Delta V$. Because $\Delta V = (30 - 10) \times 10^{-3}$ m^3 = 20×10^{-3} m^3, we find that

$$W = P\Delta V = (2 \times 10^5 \text{ Pa})(20 \times 10^{-3} \text{ m}^3) = 4000 \text{ J}$$

The expanding gas did positive work against its surroundings, pushing the piston upward.

c) Since the gas *absorbed* heat, $Q = +10,000$ J, so by the First Law of Thermodynamics,

$$\Delta E_{\text{internal}} = Q - W = 10,000 \text{ J} - 4000 \text{ J} = 6000 \text{ J}$$

We see that the internal energy increased is consistent with the fact that the temperature increased (part a).

Example 12-7: A 0.5 mol sample of an ideal gas is brought from state a to state b along the path shown in the P-V diagram below.

a) Calculate the work done during the process.
b) Determine the change in the internal energy of the gas.
c) How much heat was added to the gas?

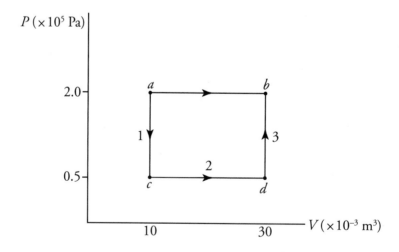

Solution:

a) Notice that the initial and final states of the gas are the same as in the preceding example, but the path is different. Over Paths 1 and 3, the volume does not change, so no work is done. Work is done only over Path 2:

$$W = P\Delta V = (0.5 \times 10^5 \text{ Pa})(20 \times 10^{-3} \text{ m}^3) = 1000 \text{ J}$$

Once again, the expanding gas does positive work against its surroundings, pushing the piston upward.

b) Because the initial and final states of the gas are the same here as they were in the preceding example, the change in internal energy, $\Delta E_{internal}$, must be the same. Therefore, $\Delta E_{internal}$ = 6000 J.

c) By the First Law of Thermodynamics, $\Delta E_{internal} = Q - W$, so

$$Q = \Delta E_{internal} + W = 6000 \text{ J} + 1000 \text{ J} = 7000 \text{ J}$$

Notice that neither Q nor W is the same as its value in the preceding example. Both Q and W are path dependent; change the path, and you will generally change the values of both these variables. But their difference $Q - W$, the change in internal energy ($\Delta E_{internal}$), depends on the initial state and the final state, not the choice of path.

Example 12-8: An *isochoric* process is one that takes place with no change in volume. What can you say about the change in internal energy of the gas if it undergoes an isochoric change of state?

Solution: An isochoric process appears as a vertical line in a P-V diagram. Since no change in volume occurs, $W = 0$. Then by the First Law of Thermodynamics, $\Delta E_{internal} = Q - W = Q$. Therefore, the change in internal energy is entirely due (and equal to) to the heat transferred. If heat is transferred into the system (positive Q), then $\Delta E_{internal}$ is positive; if heat is transferred out of the system (negative Q), then $\Delta E_{internal}$ is negative.

Example 12-9: A 0.5 mol sample of an ideal gas is brought from state a back to state a along the path (cycle) shown in the P-V diagram below. Find

a) the change in the internal energy of the gas
b) the work done on the gas during the cycle
c) the heat added to (or removal from) the gas during the cycle

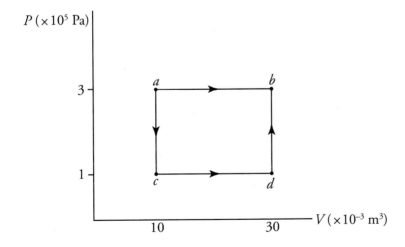

Solution: A process such as this, which begins and ends at the same state, is said to be cyclical.

a) Because the final state is the same as the initial state, the internal energy of the system cannot have changed; therefore, $\Delta E_{internal} = 0$.

b) The total work involved in the process is equal to the work done from c to d plus the work done from b to a, because only along these paths does the volume change. Along these portions of the path, we find that

$$W_{cd} = P_{cd}\Delta V_{cd} = 1 \times 10^5 \text{ Pa})(+20 \times 10^{-3} \text{ m}^3) = +2000 \text{ J}$$
$$W_{ba} = P_{ba}\Delta V_{ba} = (3 \times 10^5 \text{ Pa})(-20 \times 10^{-3} \text{ m}^3) = -6000 \text{ J}$$

so the total work done is $W = -4000$ J. The fact that W is negative means that, overall, work was done *on* the gas by the surroundings. Notice that for a cyclical process, the total work done is equal to the area enclosed by the loop, with clockwise travel taken as positive and counterclockwise travel taken as a negative.

c) The First Law of Thermodynamics states that $\Delta E_{internal} = Q - W$. Since $\Delta E_{internal} = 0$, it must be true that $Q = W$ (which will always be the case for a cyclical process). Therefore, $Q = -4000$ J (and since Q is negative, heat was *removed* from the sample).

Example 12-10: A 0.5 mol sample of an ideal gas is brought from state a to state d along an isotherm, then isobarically to state c and isochorically back to state a, as shown in the P-V diagram below. By definition, the temperature remains constant along an *isotherm*, and a process that takes place with no variation in temperature is said to be *isothermal*. Given that the work done during the isothermal part of the cycle is 3300 J, how much heat is transferred during the isothermal process from a to d?

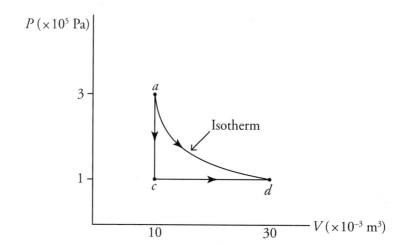

Solution: Be careful not to confuse *isothermal* with *adiabatic*. A process is isothermal if the temperature remains constant; a process is called **adiabatic** if $Q = 0$. Isothermal and adiabatic are two different things. How could a process be isothermal without also being adiabatic at the same time? Remember that the temperature is determined by the internal energy of the gas, which is affected by changes in Q or W or both. Therefore, it's possible for U to remain unchanged even if Q is not 0 (because there can be an equal W to cancel it out). In fact, this is the key to this problem. Since T doesn't change from a to d, neither can the internal energy, which depends entirely on T. Because $\Delta E_{internal} = 0$, it must be true that $Q = W$. Since W equals 3300 J, so must Q. The gas absorbs heat from the reservoir and uses all this energy to do positive work as it expands and pushes the piston upward, leaving none to increase its internal energy.

The Second Law of Thermodynamics

The Second Law of Thermodynamics is called one of the grandest laws of physics, because in one of its many equivalent forms, it defines the direction of time. The form of the second law that we need sounds much less grandiose and deals with heat engines.

Converting work to heat is easy—slamming on your brakes. Even rubbing your hands together shows that work can be completely converted into heat. What we'll look at is the reverse process: How efficiently can heat be converted into work? A device that uses heat to produce useful work is called a **heat engine**. The internal-combustion engine in your car is an example. In particular, we're interested in engines that take its working substance (a mixture of air and fuel in the case of your car engine) through a cyclic process, so that the cycle can be repeated. The basic components of any cyclic heat engine are simple to describe: Energy in the form of heat comes into the engine from a high-temperature source, some of this energy is converted into useful work, the remainder is ejected as exhaust heat into a low-temperature sink, and the system returns to its original state to run through the cycle again.

Since we're looking at cyclic engines only, the system returns to its original state at the end of each cycle, so ΔU must be 0. Therefore, by the First Law of Thermodynamics, $Q_{net} = W$. That is, the net heat absorbed by the system is equal to the work performed by the system. The heat that is absorbed from the high-temperature source is denoted Q_H (H for *hot*), and the heat that is discharged into the low-temperature reservoir is denoted Q_C (C for *cold*). Because heat *in* is positive and heat *out* is negative, Q_H is positive and Q_C is negative, and the net heat absorbed is $Q_H + Q_C$. Instead of writing Q_{net} in this way, it's customary to write it as $Q_H - |Q_C|$, to show explicitly that Q_{net} is less than Q_H. The **thermal efficiency**, e, of the heat engine is equal to the ratio of what we get out—the work, W—to what we have to put in—the heat is absorbed, Q_H. Therefore, $e = W/Q_H$. Since $W = Q_{net} = Q_H - |Q_C|$, this gives

$$e = \frac{Q_H - |Q_C|}{Q_H} = 1 - \frac{|Q_C|}{Q_H}$$

Notice that unless $Q_C = 0$, the engine's efficiency is always less than 1. One of the forms of the **Second Law of Thermodynamics** states that for any cyclic heat engine, some exhaust heat is always produced. Because $Q_C \neq 0$, no cyclic heat engine can operate at 100% efficiency; it is impossible to completely convert heat into useful work.

Example 12-11: A heat engine draws 1000 J of heat from its high-temperature source and discards 600 J of exhaust heat into its cold-temperature reservoir each cycle. How much work does this engine perform per cycle, and what is its thermal efficiency?

Solution: The work output per cycle is equal to the difference between the heat energy drawn in and the heat energy discarded:

$$W = Q_H - |Q_C| = 1000 \text{ J} - 600 \text{ J} = 400 \text{ J}$$

Therefore, the efficiency of this engine is

$$e = \frac{W}{Q_H} = \frac{400\ J}{1000\ J} = 40\%$$

The Carnot Cycle

The Second Law of Thermodynamics tells us that there are no perfect heat engines. But how can we construct, in principle, the best possible heat engine—that is, one with the maximum possible efficiency that doesn't violate the Second Law? Such an engine is called a **Carnot engine**, and the cycle through which its working substance (gas) is carried is called a **Carnot cycle**, a specially-designed series of expansions and compressions. It can be shown that a heat engine utilizing the Carnot cycle has the highest possible efficiency consistent with the Second Law of Thermodynamics. The efficiency of a Carnot engine is given by the equation

$$e_C = \frac{T_H - T_C}{T_H} = 1 = \frac{T_C}{T_H}$$

Notice that the **Carnot efficiency** depends only on the absolute temperatures of the heat source and heat sink. The equation $e_C = 1 - (T_C/T_H)$ gives the maximum theoretical efficiency of any cyclic heat engine. It cannot equal 1 unless $T_C = 0$, that is, unless the temperature of the cold reservoir is absolute zero. But absolute zero can never be reached: the **Third Law of Thermodynamics**.

Summary of Formulas

Heat Transfer with Constant Phase: $Q = mc\Delta T$

Heat Transfer with Phase Change: $Q = mL$

Thermal Expansion: $\quad \Delta L = \alpha L_i \Delta T \qquad\qquad \Delta V = \alpha V_i \Delta T$

Ideal Gas Law: $\quad PV = nRT$

Kinetic Theory of Gases: $\quad KE_{avg} = \dfrac{3}{2} k_B T \qquad\qquad v_{rms} = \sqrt{\dfrac{3RT}{M}}$

Work Done during Isobaric Thermodynamic Process: $\quad W = P\Delta V$

Work Done during any Thermodynamics Process: W = area under the graph in a P-V diagram

First Law of Thermodynamics: $\quad \Delta E_{internal} = Q - W$

Efficiency of Cyclic Heat Engine: $\quad e = \dfrac{Q_H - |Q_C|}{Q_H} = 1 - \dfrac{|Q_C|}{Q_H}$

Chapter 13
Nuclear Physics

The subject matter of the previous chapters was developed in the seventeenth, eighteenth, and nineteenth centuries, but as we delve into the physics of the very small, we enter the twentieth century. Let's first look at the structure of the atom, then travel into the nucleus itself. About 10 percent of the questions on the OAT will cover the field of modern physics.

Although nuclear physics isn't listed by the ADA as part of the physics content to be tested on the OAT, topics within nuclear physics are included in the general chemistry content. Furthermore, nuclear physics used to be covered on the physics portion of the OAT. Therefore, for both of these reasons, we include nuclear physics here in case the odd question appears on test day. However, be judicious on how you distribute your study time. Recall that the majority of questions on physics (and general chemistry) will come from other topics like linear kinematics and optics.

13.1 NUCLEAR PHYSICS

The nucleus of the atom is composed of particles called **protons** and **neutrons**, which are collectively called **nucleons**. The number of protons in a given nucleus is called the atom's **atomic number**, or Z, and the number of neutrons (the **neutron number**) is denoted N. The total number of nucleons, $Z + N$, is called the **mass number** (or **nucleon number**), and is denoted A. The number of protons in the nucleus of an atom defines the element. For example, the element chlorine (abbreviated Cl) is characterized by the fact that the nucleus of every chlorine atom contains 17 protons, so the atomic number of chlorine is 17; however, different chlorine atoms may contain different numbers of neutrons. In fact, about three-fourths of all naturally occurring chlorine atoms have 18 neutrons in their nuclei (mass number = 35), and most of the remaining one-fourth contain 20 neutrons (mass number = 37). Nuclei that contain the same numbers of protons but different numbers of neutrons are called **isotopes**.

> The notation for a **nuclide**—the term for a nucleus with specific numbers of protons and neutrons—is to write Z and A, one above the other, before the chemical symbol of the element.
>
> $$^A_Z \text{X}$$

The isotopes of chlorine mentioned earlier would be written as follows:

$$^{35}_{17}\text{Cl} \quad \text{and} \quad ^{37}_{17}\text{Cl}$$

Example 13-1: How many protons and neutrons are contained in the nuclide $^{63}_{29}\text{Cu}$?

Solution: The subscript (the atomic number, Z) gives the number of protons, which is 29. The superscript (the mass number, A) gives the total number of nucleons. Since $A = 63 = Z + N$, we find that $N = 63 - 29 = 34$.

Example 13-2: The element neon (abbreviated Ne, atomic number 10) has several isotopes. The most abundant isotope contains 10 neutrons, and two others contain 11 and 12. Write symbols for these three nuclides.

Solution: The mass numbers of these isotopes are 10 + 10 = 20, 10 + 11 = 21, and 10 + 12 = 22. So, we'd write them as follows:

$$^{20}_{10}\text{Ne}\,,\quad ^{21}_{10}\text{Ne}\,,\quad \text{and}\quad ^{22}_{10}\text{Ne}$$

Another common notation—which we also use—is to write the mass number after the name of the element. These three isotopes of neon would be written as neon-20, neon-21, and neon-22.

The Nuclear Force

Why wouldn't any nucleus that has more than one proton be unstable? After all, protons are positively charged and would therefore experience a repulsive Coulomb force from each other. Why don't these nuclei explode? And what holds neutrons—which have no electric charge—in the nucleus? These issues are resolved by the presence of another fundamental force, the **strong nuclear force**, which binds together neutrons and protons to form nuclei. Although the strength of the Coulomb force can be expressed by a simple mathematical formula (it's inversely proportional to the square of their separation), the nuclear force is much more complicated; no simple formula can be written for the strength of the nuclear force.

Binding Energy

The masses of the proton and neutron are listed below.

proton: $m_p = 1.6726 \times 10^{-27}$ kg

neutron: $m_n = 1.6749 \times 10^{-27}$ kg

Because these masses are so tiny, a much smaller mass unit is used. With the most abundant isotope of carbon (carbon-12) as a reference, the **atomic mass unit** (abbreviated **amu** or simply **u**) is defined as 1/12 the mass of a ^{12}C atom. The conversion between kg and u is 1 u = 1.6605×10^{-27} kg. In terms of atomic mass units

proton: $m_p = 1.00728$ u

neutron: $m_n = 1.00867$ u

Now consider the **deuteron**, the nucleus of **deuterium**, an isotope of hydrogen that contains 1 proton and 1 neutron. The mass of a deuteron is 2.01356 u, which is a little *less* than the sum of the individual masses of the proton and neutron. The difference between the mass of any bound nucleus and the sum of the masses of its constituent nucleons is called the **mass defect**, Δm. In the case of the deuteron (symbolized **d**), the mass defect is

$$\Delta m = (m_p + m_n) - m_d$$
$$= (1.00728 \text{ u} + 1.00867 \text{ u}) - (2.01356 \text{ u})$$
$$= 0.00239 \text{ u}$$

What happened to this missing mass? It was converted to energy when the deuteron was formed. It also represents the amount of energy needed to break the deuteron into a separate proton and neutron. Since this tells us how strongly the nucleus is bound, it is called the **binding energy** of the nucleus.

> The conversion between mass and energy is given by Einstein's **mass–energy equivalence** equation, $E = mc^2$ (where c is the speed of light); the binding energy, E_B, is equal to the mass defect, Δm
>
> $$E_B = (\Delta m)c^2$$
>
> Using $E = mc^2$, the energy equivalent of 1 atomic mass unit is about 931 MeV.

In terms of electronvolts, then, the binding energy of the deuteron is

$$E_B \text{ (deuteron)} = 0.00239 \text{ u} \times \frac{931 \text{ MeV}}{1 \text{ u}} = 2.23 \text{ MeV}$$

Since the deuteron contains 2 nucleons, the **binding energy per nucleon** is

$$\frac{2.23 \text{ MeV}}{2 \text{ nucleons}} = 1.12 \text{ MeV/nucleon}$$

This is the lowest value of all nuclides. The highest, 8.8 MeV/nucleon, is for an isotope of nickel, ^{62}Ni. Typically, when nuclei smaller than nickel are fused to form a single nucleus, the binding energy per nucleon increases, which tells us that energy is released in the process. On the other hand, when nuclei *larger* than nickel are *split*, binding energy per nucleon again increases, releasing energy.

13.2 RADIOACTIVITY

The stability of a nucleus depends on the ability of the nuclear force to balance the repulsive Coulomb forces between the protons. Many nuclides are ultimately unstable and will undergo spontaneous restructuring to become more stable. An unstable nucleus that will spontaneously change into a lower-energy configuration is said to be **radioactive**. Nuclei that are too large (A is too great) or ones in which the neutron-to-proton ratio is unfavorable are radioactive, and there are several different modes of radioactive decay. We'll look at the most important ones: **alpha** decay, **beta** decay (three forms), and **gamma** decay.

Alpha Decay

> When a nucleus undergoes alpha decay, it emits an alpha particle, which consists of two protons and two neutrons and is the same as the nucleus of a helium-4 atom. An alpha particle can be represented as
>
> $$\alpha \, , \; {}^{4}_{2}\alpha \, , \; \text{or} \; {}^{4}_{2}\text{He}$$

Very large nuclei can shed nucleons quickly by emitting one or more alpha particles, for example, radon-222 (${}^{222}_{86}\text{Rn}$) is radioactive and undergoes alpha decay.

$$ {}^{222}_{86}\text{Rn} \; \rightarrow \; {}^{218}_{84}\text{Po} + {}^{4}_{2}\alpha $$

This reaction illustrates two important features of any nuclear reaction.

> (1) Mass number is conserved (in this case, 222 = 218 + 4).
> (2) Charge is conserved (in this case, 86 = 84 + 2).

The decaying nuclide is known as the **parent**, and the resulting nuclide is known as the **daughter**. (Here, radon-222 is the parent nuclide and polonium-218 is the daughter.) Alpha decay decreases the mass number by 4 and the atomic number by 2. Therefore, alpha decay looks like the following:

$$ {}^{A}_{Z}\text{X} \; \rightarrow \; {}^{A-4}_{Z-2}\text{X}' + {}^{4}_{2}\alpha $$

Beta Decay

There are three subcategories of **beta** (β) decay, called β^-, β^+, and **electron capture (EC)**.

β^- Decay

When the neutron-to-proton ratio is too large, the nucleus undergoes β^- decay, which is the most common form of beta decay. β^- decay occurs when a neutron transforms into a proton and an electron, and the electron is ejected from the nucleus. The expelled electron is called a **beta particle**. The transformation of a neutron into a proton and an electron (and another particle, the **electron-antineutrino**, $\bar{v}_e$) is caused by the action of the **weak nuclear force**, another of nature's fundamental forces. A common example of a nuclide that undergoes β^- decay is carbon-14, which is used to date archaeological artifacts.

$$^{14}_{6}C \rightarrow {}^{14}_{7}N + {}^{0}_{-1}e + \bar{v}_e$$

Notice how the ejected electron is written: The superscript is its nucleon number (which is zero), and the subscript is its charge. The reaction is balanced, since $14 = 14 + 0$ and $6 = 7 + (-1)$.

β^+ Decay

When the neutron-to-proton ratio is too small, the nucleus will undergo β^+ decay. In this form of beta decay, a proton is transformed into a neutron and a **positron**, ${}^{0}_{+1}e$ (the electron's **antiparticle**), plus another particle, the **electron-neutrino**, v_e, which are then both ejected from the nucleus. An example of a positron emitter is fluorine-17.

$$^{17}_{9}F \rightarrow {}^{17}_{8}O + {}^{0}_{+1}e + v_e$$

Electron Capture

Another way in which a nucleus can increase its neutron-to-proton ratio is to capture an orbiting electron and then cause the transformation of a proton into a neutron. Beryllium-7 undergoes this process.

$$^{7}_{4}Be + {}^{0}_{-1}e \rightarrow {}^{7}_{3}Li + v_e$$

Gamma Decay

In each of the decay processes defined above, the daughter was a different element from the parent. Radon becomes polonium as a result of α decay, carbon becomes nitrogen as a result of β^- decay, fluorine becomes oxygen from β^+ decay, and beryllium becomes lithium from electron capture. By contrast, gamma decay does not alter the identity of the nucleus; it just allows the nucleus to relax and shed energy. Imagine that potassium-42 undergoes β^- decay to form calcium-42.

$$^{42}_{19}K \rightarrow {}^{42}_{20}Ca^* + {}^{0}_{-1}e + \bar{v}_e$$

The asterisk indicates that the daughter calcium nucleus is left in a high-energy, excited state. For this excited nucleus to drop to its ground state, it must emit a photon of energy, a **gamma ray**, symbolized by γ.

$$^{42}_{20}\text{Ca}^* \rightarrow {}^{42}_{20}\text{Ca} + \gamma$$

Example 13-6: What's the daughter nucleus in each of the following radioactive decays?

a)   Strontium-90 ($^{90}_{38}\text{Sr}$); $\beta-$ decay

b)   Argon-37 ($^{37}_{18}\text{Ar}$); electron capture

c)   Plutonium-239 ($^{239}_{94}\text{Pu}$); alpha decay

d)   Cobalt-58 ($^{58}_{27}\text{Co}$); $\beta+$ decay

Solution:

a) $^{90}_{38}\text{Sr} \rightarrow {}^{90}_{39}\text{Y} + {}^{0}_{-1}e + \bar{\nu}_e \quad \Rightarrow \quad$ daughter = yttrium-90

b) $^{37}_{18}\text{Ar} + {}^{0}_{-1}e \rightarrow {}^{37}_{17}\text{Cl} + \nu_e \quad \Rightarrow \quad$ daughter = chlorine-37

c) $^{239}_{94}\text{Pu} \rightarrow {}^{235}_{92}\text{U} + {}^{4}_{2}\alpha \quad \Rightarrow \quad$ daughter = uranium-235

d) $^{58}_{27}\text{Co} \rightarrow {}^{58}_{26}\text{Fe} + {}^{0}_{+1}e^{+} + \nu_e \quad \Rightarrow \quad$ daughter = iron-58

Radioactive Decay Rates

Although it's impossible to say precisely when a particular radioactive nuclide will decay, it *is* possible to predict the decay rates of a pure radioactive sample. As a radioactive sample disintegrates, the number of decays per second decreases, but the *fraction* of nuclei that decay per second—the **decay constant**—does not change. The decay constant is determined by the identity of the radioisotope. Boron-9 has a decay constant of 7.5×10^{17} s^{-1} (rapid), while uranium-238 has a decay constant of about 5×10^{-18} s^{-1} (slow).

> The **activity** (A) of a radioactive sample is the number of disintegrations it undergoes per second; it decreases with time according to the equation
>
> $$A = A_0 e^{-\lambda t}$$
>
> where A_0 is the activity at time $t = 0$ and λ is the decay constant (not to be confused with wavelength).

Activity is expressed in disintegrations per second: 1 disintegration per second is one **becquerel (Bq)**. The greater the value of λ, the faster the sample decays. This equation also describes the number (N) of radioactive nuclei in a given sample, $N = N_0 e^{-\lambda t}$, or the mass (m) of the sample, $m = m_0 e^{-\lambda t}$.

The most common way to indicate the rapidity with which radioactive samples decay is to give their **half-life**. Just as the name suggests, the half-life is the time required for half of a given sample to decay.

Half-life, $T_{1/2}$, is inversely proportional to the decay constant, λ, and in terms of the half-life, the exponential decay of a sample's mass (or activity) can be written as

$$m = m_0 \left(\frac{1}{2}\right)^{t/T_{1/2}}$$

A sample's activity or mass can be graphed as a function of time; the result is the **exponential decay** curve, which you should study carefully.

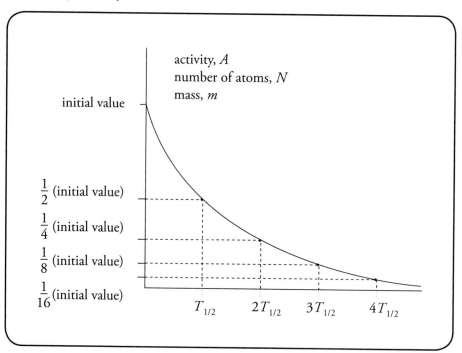

Example 13-7: The half-life of iodine-131 (a β^- emitter) is 8 days. If a sample of ^{131}I has a mass of 1 gram, what will the mass be 40 days later?

Solution: Every 8 days, the sample's mass decreases by a factor of 2. We can illustrate the decay in the following diagram:

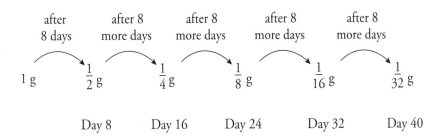

Example 13-8: Home smoke detectors contain a small radioactive sample of americium-241 ($^{241}_{95}$Am), an alpha-particle emitter that has a half-life of 430 years. What is the daughter nucleus of the decay?

Solution: $^{241}_{95}$Am $\rightarrow$ $^{237}_{93}$Np $+ ^{4}_{2}\alpha$ $\Rightarrow$ daughter = neptunium-237

13.3   NUCLEAR REACTIONS

Natural radioactive decay provides one example of a nuclear reaction. Other examples of nuclear reactions include the bombardment of target nuclei with subatomic particles to artificially induce radioactivity (this is **nuclear fission**), and the **nuclear fusion** of small nuclei at extremely high temperatures. In all cases of nuclear reactions that we'll study, nucleon number and charge must be conserved. To balance nuclear reactions, we write $^{1}_{1}$p or $^{1}_{1}$H for a proton and $^{1}_{0}$n for a neutron. Gamma-ray photons can also be produced in nuclear reactions; they have no charge or nucleon number and are represented as $^{0}_{0}\gamma$.

Example 13-9: A mercury-198 nucleus is bombarded by a neutron, which causes a nuclear reaction.

$$^{1}_{0}n + {}^{198}_{80}Hg \rightarrow {}^{197}_{79}Au + {}^{?}_{?}X$$

What's the unknown product particle, X?

Solution: In order to balance the superscripts, we must have 1 + 198 = 197 + A, so A = 2, and the subscripts are balanced if 0 + 80 = 79 + Z, so Z = 1.

$$^{1}_{0}n + {}^{198}_{80}Hg \rightarrow {}^{197}_{79}Au + {}^{2}_{1}X$$

Therefore, X must be a deuteron, $^{2}_{1}$H (or just d).

Study Break
Before you move on to the next section, give yourself a break to clear your head and let this all soak in. Go for a walk, listen to a song you love, grab a snack—don't burn yourself out!

Disintegration Energy

Nuclear reactions not only produce new nuclei and other subatomic particles, but also involve the absorption or emission of energy. Nuclear reactions must conserve total energy, so changes in mass are accompanied by changes in energy according to Einstein's equation $\Delta E = (\Delta m)c^2$.

A general nuclear reaction is written

$$A + B \rightarrow C + D + Q$$

where Q is the **disintegration energy**.

If Q is positive, the reaction is **exothermic** and the reaction can occur spontaneously; if Q is negative, the reaction is **endothermic** and the reaction cannot occur spontaneously. The energy Q is calculated as follows:

$$Q = [(m_A + m_B) - (m_C + m_D)]c^2$$

For spontaneous reactions—ones that liberate energy—most of the energy is revealed as kinetic energy of the least massive product nuclei.

Summary of Formulas

For the test, be sure you are familiar with the following concepts from this chapter.

- Nuclear physics

- The nuclear force

- Binding energy

- Radioactivity

- Alpha decay

- Beta decay

- β^- decay

- β^+ decay

- Electron capture

- Radioactive decay rates

- Nuclear reactions

- Disintegration energy

Survey of Natural Sciences (SNS)

Chapter 14
Biology

14.1 BIOLOGY OVERVIEW

The material in this section is not designed to be a comprehensive review, but rather is a set of outlines to help you guide your studying. Comprehensive Biology review for the OAT can be found in *Cracking the DAT*.

I. Biological Macromolecules
   A. Amino Acids and Proteins
      1. General structure of amino acids
      2. Isoelectric point
      3. Classification of amino acids (non-polar, polar, acidic, basic, sulfur containing)
      4. Protein structure (peptide bond, primary, secondary, tertiary, quaternary structures)
   B. Carbohydrates
      1. General structure of saccharides
      2. Monosaccharides (glucose, fructose, galactose)
      3. Disaccharides (maltose, sucrose, lactose)
      4. Polysaccharides (glycogen, starch, cellulose)
   C. Lipids and Steroids
      1. Hydrophobicity, saturated fats, unsaturated fats
      2. Triglycerides and phospholipids
      3. Steroids and cholesterol
   D. Nucleic Acids
      1. High-energy phosphate bonds
      2. Nucleotide structure
      3. DNA and RNA

Summary of Key Concepts:

- Amino acids (AAs) consist of a tetrahedral -carbon connected to an amino group, a carboxyl group, and a variable R group, which determines the AA's properties.

- The isoelectric point of an amino acid is the pH at which the net charge on the molecule is zero; this structure is referred to as the zwitterion.

- Electrophoresis separates mixtures of amino acids and is conducted at buffered pH. Positively charged AAs move to the "−" end of the gel, and negative AAs move to the "+" end.

- Proteins consist of amino acids linked by peptide bonds, or amide bonds, which have partial double bond characteristics, lack rotation, and are very stable.

- The secondary structure of proteins (-helices and -sheets) is formed through hydrogen bonding interactions between atoms in the backbone of the molecule.

- The most stable tertiary protein structure generally places polar AAs on the exterior and non-polar AAs on the interior of the protein. This minimizes interactions between nonpolar AAs and water, while optimizing interactions between side chains inside the protein.

- All animal amino acids are L-configuration and all animal sugars are D-configuration.

- Carbohydrates are chains of hydrated carbon atoms with the molecular formula $C_nH_{2n}O_n$.

- Sugars in solution exist in equilibrium between the straight chain form and either the furanose (five-atom) or pyranose (six-atom) cyclic forms.

- The anomeric forms of a sugar differ by the position of the OH group on the anomeric carbon; OH down = α, OH up = β.

- All monosaccharides and some disaccharides contain a free aldehyde, ketone, or hemiacetal group that allows them to act as reducing agents, and they are therefore called reducing sugars.

- The glycosidic linkage in a disaccharide is named based on which anomer is present for the sugar containing the acetal and the numbers of the carbons linked to the bridging O.

- Monosaccharides like glucose, fructose, and galactose are energy molecules for cells.

- Disaccharides include maltose, sucrose, and lactose.

- Polysaccharides are for either glucose storage or structure. Glycogen is a glucose storage molecule in animals, starch is glucose storage for plants, and cellulose is a plant structural molecule.

- Fats are hydrophobic molecules used for energy storage (triglycerides), membrane structure (phospholipids and cholesterol), or hormones (steroids).

- Saponification (or base mediated hydrolysis) of a triglyceride produces three equivalents of fatty acid carboxylates. These amphipathic molecules form micelles in solution.

- Cholesterol is a ring-shaped lipid that helps stabilize lipid bilayers. Steroid hormones are derived from cholesterol.

- The building blocks of nucleic acids (DNA and RNA) are nucleotides, which are comprised of a pentose sugar, a purine or pyrimidine base, and 2-3 phosphate units.

II. **Generalized Cellular Biology**
   A. **General cell structure**
   B. **Organelle structure and function**
      1. Nucleus
      2. Mitochondria
      3. Ribosomes
      4. Rough and Smooth ER
      5. Golgi apparatus
      6. Lysosomes
      7. Peroxisomes
   C. **Plasma Membrane Cytoskeleton, and Cell Junctions**
      1. Membrane structure
      2. Diffusion and osmosis
      3. Passive and active transport
      4. Endo- and exocytosis
      5. Cell surface receptors and G-proteins
   D. **Cytoskeleton and Cell Junctions**
      1. Microtubules, microfilaments, intermediate filaments
      2. Cilia and flagella
      3. Desmosomes, tight junctions, and gap junctions

Online Practice Tests
Remember to register your book online in order to gain access to your online practice tests.

E. **Cell Cycle and Mitosis**
   1. Interphase (G_1, S, and G_2)
   2. Mitosis (prophase, metaphase, anaphase, telophase)
F. **Prokaryotic Cells**
   1. General structure
   2. Transcription and translation
   3. Shape
   4. Cell membranes, cell walls, and Gram staining
   5. Flagella
   6. Temperature, nutrition, and growth media
   7. Oxygen use and tolerance
   8. Binary fission
   9. Conjugation
G. **Fungi**
   1. General structure
   2. Reproduction

Summary of Key Concepts:

- For the OAT, you should know the structures and functions of the following key eukaryotic organelles: nucleus, mitochondria, ribosomes, rough ER, smooth ER, Golgi apparatus, lysosomes, and peroxisomes.

- The rough ER is the site of translation of proteins to be either secreted from the cell, inserted into the membrane, or targeted to the lysosomes, ER, or Golgi apparatus.

- Signal sequences are specific amino acid sequences that direct proteins in translation to the rough ER and the secretory pathway (rough ER Golgi apparatus final location).

- Post-translational modification can occur in the rough ER or in the Golgi apparatus.

- All cellular membranes are composed of lipid bilayers with distinct hydrophobic and hydrophilic regions. The membranes act as selective barriers that regulate which molecules can cross.

- Molecules naturally want to move from regions of higher concentration to regions of lower concentration (with respect to that particular molecule). Diffusion is the movement of particles down their concentration gradient, and osmosis is the movement of water down *its* concentration gradient.

- Hydrophobic molecules (e.g., O_2, CO_2, and steroids) cross the membrane by simple diffusion, while hydrophilic, polar molecules (e.g., ions, glucose, and water) must cross the membrane with the help of a special membrane protein (a channel or a carrier). This is called facilitated diffusion.

- Active transport uses energy to move molecules against their concentration gradients (from low concentration areas to higher concentration areas). Primary active transport uses ATP directly, while secondary active transport relies on gradients previously established by a primary active transporter.

- The Na^+/K^+ ATPase is a primary active transporter that moves three Na^+ ions out of the cell for every two K^+ ions it moves into the cell. This helps establish the resting membrane potential of the cell, helps maintain osmotic balance in the cell, and sets up a Na^+ gradient that can be used for secondary active transport.

- G-proteins help transduce signals from extracellular ligands across the membrane. They change the level of cAMP or calcium (second messengers) in the cell, which changes the metabolic enzyme pathways active in the cell.

- Microtubules form centrioles, cilia, and eukaryotic flagella, while microfilaments participate in contractile activity.

- Tight junctions help form a seal between cells so that the flow of molecules across the entire cell layer is regulated. Desmosomes form general adhesions between cells. Gap junctions form connections between cells that allow the flow of cytoplasm from cell to cell.

- During the cell cycle, DNA replication occurs during the S-phase of interphase, and cell division occurs during mitosis (M-phase).

- Mitosis is comprised of four major phases (prophase, metaphase, anaphase, and telophase) and results in two daughter cells that are identical to each other and identical to the original parent cell.

III. **Biochemistry**
  A. **Thermodynamics and Kinetics**
    1. G
    2. Energy of Activation
    3. Reaction coordinate graph
    4. Reaction coupling
  B. **Enzymes**
    1. General structure: active site, allosteric site
    2. Regulation
    3. Kinetics
    4. Inhibition
  C. **Cellular Respiration**
    1. Oxidation and reduction
    2. Overview of cellular respiration (stages, locations, oxygen dependence)
    3. Glycolysis
    4. PDC
    5. Krebs cycle
    6. Electron transport chain and oxidative phosphorylation
    7. Fermentation
    8. Energy totals
    9. Other biochemical pathways (general overview)
  D. **Photosynthesis**
    1. Overview and location
    2. Light-dependent reactions
    3. Light-independent reactions

Summary of Key Concepts:

- A decrease in free energy (negative DDDG) means that a reaction is spontaneous, but not necessarily fast.

- The energy of activation of a reaction determines its rate; a high energy of activation means a slow rate of reaction, and a low energy of activation means a faster rate of reaction.

- Enzymes are biological catalysts which increase the rate of a reaction by lowering the activation energy.

- Unfavorable reactions in the cell are performed by coupling them to favorable reactions (such as ATP hydrolysis).

- Enzyme activity can be controlled via covalent modification, proteolytic cleavage, associations, or allosteric regulation.

- Competitive inhibitors bind at the active site of an enzyme, do not affect V_{max}, but increase K_m.

- Noncompetitive inhibitors bind at an allosteric site of an enzyme, decrease V_{max}, but do not change K_m.

- Cellular respiration is the oxidation of carbohydrates, reduction of electron carriers, and generation of ATP.

- Glycolysis occurs in the cytoplasm and generates two pyruvate molecules, two ATP, and two NADH per glucose.

- Under anaerobic conditions, the cell performs fermentation to regenerate NAD^+ so that glycolysis can continue.

- The pyruvate dehydrogenase complex (PDC) functions in the mitochondrial matrix, converts pyruvate into acetyl-CoA, and generates an NADH.

- The Krebs cycle in the mitochondrial matrix generates six NADH, two $FADH_2$, and two GTP per glucose.

- The electron transport chain in the inner mitochondrial membrane starts with the oxidation of the electron carriers NADH and $FADH_2$, and it ends with the reduction of oxygen and the generation of a proton gradient across the inner mitochondrial membrane.

- ATP synthase in the inner mitochondrial membrane uses the proton gradient to generate ATP (2.5 ATP per NADH from the mitochondrial matrix, 1.5 ATP per NADH from the cytoplasm, and 1.5 ATP per $FADH_2$).

- Both eukaryotes and prokaryotes perform cellular respiration, but prokaryotes use their plasma membrane for the electron transport chain and generate two more ATP per glucose than eukaryotes.

- There are several other metabolic pathways in the cell and many of them converge on the Krebs cycle.

- Photosynthesis is the process plants use to convert light to ATP. Although the summary equation is essentially the chemical reverse of respiration, the specific reactions are not just respiration in reverse.

- Photosynthesis occurs in two steps, the light-dependent reactions (which generate ATP and NADPH) and the light-independent reactions (which generate carbohydrates).

IV. Molecular Biology
  A. **DNA Structure and Function**
    1. Nucleotide structure
    2. Base pairing
    3. DNA packaging (prokaryotic vs. eukaryotic)
    4. The Central Dogma
    5. Mutations
  B. **Replication**
    1. Semiconservative
    2. Direction
    3. General process and enzymes
    4. Prokaryotic vs. eukaryotic
  C. **RNA and Transcription, and Translation**
    1. RNA vs. DNA
    2. Transcription general process and definitions (promoter, template strand, etc.)
    3. Prokaryotic transcription vs. eukaryotic transcription
  D. **Translation**
    1. tRNA
    2. Ribosomes
    3. General process

Summary of Key Concepts:

- DNA is the fundamental unit of inheritance in cells.

- DNA and RNA are polymers, made of nucleotide monomers. A nucleotide contains phosphate group(s), a sugar (either deoxyribose for DNA or ribose for RNA), and a nitrogenous base, either a purine (adenine or guanine) or a pyrimidine (thymine, cytosine, or uracil).

- Adenine always pairs with thymine via two hydrogen bonds, and cytosine always pairs with guanine via three hydrogen bonds.

- Uracil replaces thymine in RNA, and the ribose in RNA has an OH group on carbon 2.

- DNA is supercoiled in prokaryotes and packaged around histone proteins in eukaryotes.

- Point mutations are single nucleotide base pair substitutions.

- Point mutations are classified based on their effect on DNA (transition or transversion) or their effect on the amino acid sequence (missense, nonsense, or silent).

- Frameshift mutations are caused by insertions or deletions in the DNA base sequence that affect the reading frame of a gene. These are generally very serious mutations because they affect every amino acid codon from the point of the mutation on.

- DNA replication occurs in the S-phase of the cell cycle and is semiconservative in nature.

- Several enzymes are involved in DNA replication. Helicases unwind the parental DNA at the origin of replication. Primases synthesize an RNA primer. DNA polymerase synthesizes new DNA, proofreads, and replaces the RNA primer. DNA ligase attaches the Okazaki fragments in the lagging strand.

- Transcription is the first part of protein synthesis; it is the creation of an RNA transcript by an RNA polymerase that reads the DNA template. Translation is the second part of protein synthesis; it is the creation of a polypeptide chain by ribosomes that read the mRNA transcript.

- All nucleotide synthesis (replication of DNA or transcription of RNA) occurs 5' 3'.

- Key information about Prokaryotes (bacteria): theta replication, genome is a single circular piece of double-stranded DNA, three different DNA polymerases, one RNA polymerase, no mRNA processing, polycistronic mRNA, transcription and translation happen at the same time, smaller ribosomes (70S).

- Key info about Eukaryotes: replication bubbles, genome is several linear pieces of DNA, capping, tailing, and splicing of mRNA prior to translation, monocistronic mRNA, transcription in nucleus, translation in cytosol, larger ribosomes.

V. **Genetics**
   A. **Basic Definitions**
      1. Genes and alleles
      2. Genotype vs. phenotype
      3. Dominant vs. recessive
      4. Incomplete dominance and codominance
      5. Epistasis, pleiotropic genes, and penetrance
      6. Sex chromosomes
   B. **Meiosis**
      1. Meiosis I and meiosis II
      2. Nondisjunction
   C. **Mendelian Genetics**
      1. Law of Segregation
      2. Law of Independent Assortment
      3. Punnett squares
      4. Rules of probability
      5. Linkage and recombination frequency
   D. **Inheritance Patterns and Pedigrees**
      1. Common patterns
      2. Pedigree analysis
      3. Prokaryotic transcription vs. eukaryotic transcription
   E. **Population Genetics**
      1. Hardy-Weinberg Law and assumptions
      2. Hardy-Weinberg equations

Summary of Key Concepts:

- Organisms express phenotypes (physical characteristics) according to their genotypes (combinations of alleles).

- Classical dominance occurs when a phenotype or trait is determined by one gene with two alleles, and one allele is dominant (expressed) and the other is recessive (silent). There are several exceptions to classical dominance, including incomplete dominance, codominance, epistasis, pleiotropism, polygenism, and penetrance.

- Incomplete dominance occurs when two different alleles for a single trait result in a blended phenotype. Codominance occurs when two different alleles for a single trait are expressed simultaneously, but independently (no blending).

- Epistasis occurs when the expression of one gene depends on the expression of another.

- Pleiotropic genes affect many different aspects of the overall phenotype.

- Polygenic traits are affected by many different genes.

- Penetrance refers to the likelihood that a particular genotype will result in a given phenotype. Penetrance can be affected by several factors including age, environment, and lifestyle.

- From a single diploid precursor cell, meiosis generates four haploid cells (gametes) with a random mix of alleles. This is due to crossing over in prophase I, and separation of homologous chromosomes in anaphase I. Nondisjunction is a failure to separate the DNA properly during meiosis, and it can result in gametes with improper numbers of chromosomes.

- The Punnett square or the rules of probability can be used to determine the genotypes and phenotypes of offspring from given crosses, or the probability of having offspring with certain traits.

- The rule of multiplication states that the probability of A and B occurring is equal to the probability of A multiplied by the probability of B.

- The rule of addition states that the probability of A or B occurring is equal to the probability of A plus the probability of B, minus the probability of A and B together.

- Linkage occurs when two genes are close together on the same chromosome; it leads to alleles being inherited together (less recombination) instead of independently.

- Pedigrees can be used to analyze the patterns of inheritance of different traits. There are four primary modes of inheritance: autosomal recessive, autosomal dominant, Y-linked, and X-linked recessive.

- The Hardy-Weinberg Law can be used to study population genetics. It assumes classical dominance with only two alleles and unchanging allele frequencies. It is based on five assumptions: no mutation, no natural selection, no migration, large populations, and totally random mating.

- The Hardy-Weinberg equation for allele frequency is $p + q = 1$.

- The Hardy-Weinberg equation for genotype frequency is $p^2 + 2pq + q^2 = 1$.

VI. **Evolution, Diversity of Life, Ecology, and Animal Behavior**
    A. **Evolution and Speciation**
        1. Evolution by natural selection
        2. Fitness
        3. Modes of selection
        4. Species concept and speciation
    B. **The Diversity of Life**
        1. Taxonomy basics (binomial classification, taxonomic categories)
        2. General taxonomic characteristics of the main domains
        3. Specific taxonomic characteristics of:
            a) Domain Archaea
            b) Domain Bacteria
            c) Kingdom Protista
            d) Kingdom Fungi
            e) Kingdom Plantae
            f) Kingdom Animalia
    C. **The Origin of Life**
    D. **Ecology**
        1. Biomes
        2. Succession
        3. Population and community ecology
        4. Symbiotic relationships
    E. **Animal Behavior**
        1. Innate behavior
        2. Learned behavior

Summary of Key Concepts:

- Natural selection drives evolution by allowing individuals with random, beneficial mutations to survive and pass those beneficial mutations on to their offspring.

- Fitness refers to the ability of an organism to successfully reproduce and pass on its alleles to future generations, not just how well it is equipped for survival.

- Natural selection can occur in multiple forms, including:
  - Directional selection: a phenotype at one end of the bell-curve is selected for, eventually shifting the curve in that direction.
  - Divergent selection: phenotypes at both ends of the bell-curve are selected for, and the phenotype in the middle of the curve is lost, eventually splitting the population into two extremes.
  - Stabilizing selection: extreme phenotypes at the ends of the bell-curve are selected against, favoring the average phenotype.

- A species is a group of organisms that can reproduce sexually. Reproductive isolation keeps existing species separate. The creation of new species is called speciation.

- Homologous structures are the result of divergent evolution to form new species, and analogous structures are the result of convergent evolution, in which different species must meet similar environmental challenges.

- Taxonomy is the classification of organisms. The principal taxonomic categories are domain, kingdom, phylum, class, order, family, genus, and species. Each organism is given two names based on its genus and species, as specified by the binomial classification system developed by Carolus Linnaeus. Some examples are *Homo sapiens* and *Escherichia coli*.

- Domain Archaea is made up of unicellular prokaryotes that live in extreme conditions, while Domain Bacteria is made up of prokaryotes that live in more typical conditions. Both lack organelle and have single circular genomes. Domain Bacteria organisms also have a cell wall.

- Domain Eukarya is made up of four Kingdoms: Protista, Fungi, Plantae, and Animalia.

- Protists are typically single-celled organisms that are plant-like, animal-like, or fungus-like.

- Fungi are non-photosynthetic decomposers that acquire nutrition by absorption.

- Plants can be divided into non-vascular (mosses, liverworts, and hornworts) and vascular groups. The vascular plants can be further divided into seedless plants (like ferns and horse-tails) and seeded plants.

- Seeded plants can be divided into gymnosperms ("naked seed" plants, like conifers and cycads) and angiosperms ("flowering plants" like grass, orchids, sunflowers, and maple trees).

- Kingdom Animalia can be divided into many phyla, each with its own unique characteristics and subgroups.

- Biomes are large ecological communities with flora and fauna suited for certain climatic or geographic conditions. There are eight major terrestrial biomes (tropical forests, deserts, savanna, temperate deciduous forest, temperate grasslands, chaparral, taiga, and tundra) and two aquatic biomes (freshwater biome and marine biome).

- Ecological succession is the movement of a community through predictable stages. Primary succession is the colonization of barren ground by pioneer organisms (such as lichen and mosses) and proceeds until the stable climax community is reached.

- Populations can be affected by both density-dependent (increase in intensity with the size of the population) and density-independent (not related to population size) factors.

- Symbiotic relationships include commensalism (one member benefits and the other is unaffected), mutualism (both members benefit), and parasitism (one member benefits and the other is harmed).

- Producers are organisms capable of producing their own food (e.g., plants).

- Consumers are organisms that rely, directly or indirectly, on producers for nutrition (e.g., animals).

- Innate behaviors, such as fixed action patterns, are unlearned, preprogrammed behaviors that are genetically determined and present in all members of the species.

- Learned behaviors, such as habituation and conditioning, require interaction with the environment and the behavior develops as a result of individual experiences.

VII.   Anatomy and Physiology: Body Control and Communication
   A.   The Nervous System
       1.   Neuron structure
       2.   Resting potential and action potential
       3.   Myelin and saltatory conduction
       4.   Refractory periods
       5.   Synapses (electrical and chemical)
       6.   Divisions of the nervous system
       7.   CNS: anatomy and function
       8.   Sensory receptors
   B.   The Endocrine System
       1.   Hormone types and mechanism of action (peptide vs. steroid)
       2.   Regulation of the endocrine system
       3.   Major glands, hormones, and their effects
   C.   The Circulatory System
       1.   Components of the circulatory system
       2.   Heart anatomy (vessels, chambers, valves)
       3.   Cardiac cycle and heart sounds
       4.   Cardiac muscle cell structure
       5.   Cardiac action potentials: muscle and autorhythmic cells
       6.   Blood pressure
       7.   Components of blood
       8.   Blood typing
       9.   Gas transport
       10. Capillary exchange
       11. Lymphatic System
   D.   The Immune System
       1.   Innate immunity
       2.   Humoral immunity and B-cells
       3.   Cell-mediated immunity and T-cells

Summary of Key Concepts:

- The neuron is the basic structural and functional unit of the nervous system. It has several specialized structures that allow it to transmit action potentials.

- Neurons receive incoming information via dendrites. Signals are summed by the axon hillock, and if the signal is greater than the threshold, an action potential is initiated.

- The action potential is an all-or-none signal that includes depolarization (via voltage-gated sodium channels) and repolarization (via voltage-gated potassium channels); it begins and ends at the cell's resting potential of –70 mV.

- Since action potentials are all-or-none events, intensity is coded by the frequency of the action potential.

- Neurons communicate with other neurons, organs, and glands at synapses. Most synapses are chemical in nature; an action potential causes the release of a neurotransmitter into the synaptic cleft, and binding of the neurotransmitter to receptors on the postsynaptic cell triggers a change, either stimulatory or inhibitory, in that cell.

- The central nervous system includes the spinal cord and the brain; specialized areas control specific aspects of human behavior, movement, intelligence, emotion, and reflexes.

- The peripheral nervous system includes the somatic (voluntary) and autonomic (involuntary) subdivisions.

- The sympathetic branch of the autonomic system controls our fight-or-flight response; norepinephrine is the primary neurotransmitter of this system, and it is augmented by epinephrine from the adrenal medulla.

- The parasympathetic branch of the autonomic system controls our resting and digesting state; acetylcholine is the primary neurotransmitter of this system.

- Humans have several types of receptors (mechanoreceptors, chemoreceptors, nociceptors, thermoreceptors, electromagnetic receptors, and proprioceptors) that allow us to detect a variety of stimuli.

- The endocrine system controls our overall physiology and homeostasis by hormones that travel through the bloodstream. Hormones are released from endocrine glands, travel to distant target tissues via the blood, bind to receptors on target tissues, and exert effects on target cells.

- Peptide hormones are made from amino acids, bind to receptors on the cell surface, and typically affect target cells via second messenger pathways. Effects tend to be rapid and temporary.

- Steroid hormones are derived from cholesterol, bind to receptors in the cytoplasm or nucleus, and bind to DNA to alter transcription. Effects tend to occur more slowly and are more permanent.

- The circulatory and lymphatic systems transport materials (O_2, CO_2, nutrients, wastes, hormones, etc.) around the body. The lymphatic system helps to filter and return tissue fluid (lymph) to the circulatory system.

- Deoxygenated blood returning from the body enters the heart at the right atrium, and is pumped to the lungs by the right ventricle. The oxygenated blood returns to the heart at the left atrium, and it is pumped to the body by the left ventricle.

- AV valves (tricuspid on the right and bicuspid, or mitral, on the left) separate the atria and ventricles. Semilunar valves (pulmonary on the right and aortic on the left) separate the ventricles and the arteries.

- Veins always return blood to the heart. Most veins carry deoxygenated blood; an exception are the pulmonary veins, which return blood from the lungs to the heart.

- Arteries always carry blood away from the heart. Most arteries carry oxygenated blood; an exception are the pulmonary arteries, which carry blood from the heart to the lungs.

- The cardiac muscle cell action potential is prolonged by the opening of voltage-gated calcium channels. The influx of calcium causes a long plateau in the action potential.

- Cardiac muscle is a functional syncytium; cells are connected by intercalated disks, which contain gap junctions. The gap junctions are electrical synapses that easily allow the transmission of the action potential, and thus contraction, to spread from cell to cell.

- The SA node is the "pacemaker" of the heart. It has an unstable resting potential that rises until threshold is reached and an action potential is fired. This action potential (and subsequent contraction) is then transmitted throughout the heart.

- Systemic blood pressure is directly proportional to cardiac output (the volume of blood pumped per minute) and to peripheral resistance (the force opposing blood flow through the vessels).

- Cardiac output is directly proportional to stroke volume and heart rate, while peripheral resistance is inversely related to vessel diameter.

- Blood is approximately 55 percent plasma, 40 to 45 percent erythrocytes (red blood cells), and 1 percent leukocytes (white blood cells) and platelets.

- ABO and Rh antigens on the surface of erythrocytes determine blood type; type AB+ is the universal recipient and type O– is the universal donor.

- Oxygen is transported in the blood bound to hemoglobin, a protein in red blood cells. Carbon dioxide is transported in the blood primarily as bicarbonate ion; some also binds to hemoglobin.

- Innate immunity is nonspecific and includes things like the skin, lysozyme, stomach acid, phagocytes, and the complement system.

- Humoral immunity is the production of antibodies by B-cells that are highly specific for particular antigens (foreign molecules).

- Cell-mediated immunity is handled by T-cells. Killer (cytotoxic) T-cells destroy "self" cells that are displaying abnormal antigen on MHC I. Helper T-cells are activated by antigen displayed on MHC II, and secrete chemicals to help activate and stimulate the proliferation of killer T-cells and B-cells.

VIII. **Anatomy and Physiology: Nutrients and Waste**
    A. **The Respiratory System**
        1. Functions of the respiratory system
        2. The conduction zone
        3. The respiratory zone
        4. Ventilation and regulation of ventilation rate
    B. **The Digestive System**
        1. GI epithelium and muscle
        2. Exocrine secretion
        3. Myelin and saltatory conduction
        4. Mouth, pharynx, and esophagus
        5. Stomach
        6. Small and large intestines
        7. GI accessory organs: pancreas, liver, and gallbladder
        8. Vitamins
    C. **The Excretory System**
        1. Organs involved in excretion
        2. Kidney functions
        3. Urinary system anatomy
        4. Nephron structure and function
        5. Concentration and dilution
        6. Renal regulation of blood pressure and pH

Summary of Key Concepts:

- The primary functions of the respiratory system are gas exchange and pH regulation. pH regulation by the respiratory system is very fast.

- The organs of the respiratory system are divided into the conduction zone and the respiratory zone.

- The conduction zone is for ventilation only and includes the nose and nasal cavity, the pharynx, the larynx, the trachea, and the respiratory tree from the primary bronchi to the terminal bronchioles.

- The larynx is made entirely of cartilage, and it includes the epiglottis (which separates food and air) and the vocal cords (for sound production).

- The respiratory zone is for gas exchange and includes the respiratory bronchioles, the alveolar ducts, and the alveoli.

- Surfactant reduces the surface tension inside the alveoli and makes it easier to inflate them.

- Inspiration is an active process and requires the contraction of the diaphragm to expand the chest cavity. An increase in the size of the chest cavity (and lungs) reduces their pressure, and air flows in.

- Expiration is primarily a passive process; the diaphragm relaxes and lung elastic recoil helps return them to their resting state. Forced expiration requires the contraction of the abdominal muscles to forcibly reduce the size of the chest cavity. In either case, the reduction in the size of the chest cavity increases their pressure and pushes the air out.

- Ventilation rate is determined primarily by P_{CO_2} and the need to regulate pH, according to the following equilibrium: $CO_2 + H_2O \rightleftharpoons H_2CO_3 \rightleftharpoons H^+ \rightleftharpoons + HCO^-_3$. As CO_2 levels increase, pH falls, and ventilation rate increases (the reverse is also true).

- The digestive system organs are divided into two categories: the alimentary canal and the accessory organs. The alimentary canal is the long muscular tube consisting of the mouth, esophagus, stomach, small intestine, and large intestine. The accessory organs have a digestive role, but are not part of the tube. They include the salivary glands, the liver, the gallbladder, and the pancreas.

- The mouth breaks down food mechanically by chewing, and also begins starch digestion via salivary amylase.

- The stomach is primarily a storage tank for food. Mechanical digestion occurs through churning of the food, acid hydrolysis begins chemical digestion, and protein digestion is begun via pepsin.

- Almost all chemical digestion and nutrient absorption takes place in the small intestine. The large intestine primarily reabsorbs water and stores feces; no digestion takes place in the large intestine.

- The liver produces bile (secreted into the small intestine), which emulsifies fat to increase the efficiency of fat digestion. The gallbladder stores and concentrates bile.

- The pancreas secretes the majority of the digestive enzymes used in the small intestine, along with bicarbonate to help neutralize the acid entering the small intestine from the stomach. The pancreas is also a major endocrine organ, secreting insulin and glucagon to regulate blood glucose.

- The kidneys filter the blood to remove hydrophilic wastes. They also play a major role in homeostasis by regulating blood pressure, pH, ion balance, and water balance.

- Urine is produced by first filtering the blood, then by modifying the filtrate via reabsorption (moving substances from the filtrate to the blood) and secretion (moving substances from the blood to the filtrate), and finally by concentrating the filtrate to conserve body water.

- Filtration occurs at the glomerulus, most reabsorption and secretion occurs in the PCT, selective reabsorption and secretion occur in the DCT, and concentration occurs in the collecting duct.

- The Loop of Henle establishes a concentration gradient in the medulla; this gradient is critical to the reabsorption of water and the creation of a concentrated urine.

- ADH increases the water permeability of the collecting duct to allow reabsorption of water, and aldosterone increases Na^+ reabsorption at the distal tubule. Both hormones work together to help regulate blood pressure.

- When systemic blood pressure falls, the kidneys release renin. Renin is an enzyme that converts the blood protein angiotensinogen into angiotensin I, which is further converted to angiotensin II. Angiotensin II is a potent vasoconstrictor, and also increases the release of aldosterone; the ultimate goal is to increase blood pressure.

IX. **Anatomy and Physiology: Support and Structure**
    A. **The Muscular System**
        1. Joints
        2. Skeletal muscle structure
        3. Sliding filament theory
        4. Excitation-contraction coupling
        5. Neuromuscular junction (NMJ)
        6. Energy storage in muscle cells
        7. Cardiac and smooth muscle
    B. **The Skeletal System**
        1. Functions of the skeletal system
        2. Connective tissue
        3. Bone structure
        4. Cartilage, ligaments, and tendons
        5. Bone growth and remodeling
    C. **The Skin**
        1. Skin structure, layers, and tissue types
        2. Thermoregulation

Summary of Key Concepts:

- There are three types of muscle tissue: skeletal, cardiac, and smooth.

- Skeletal muscles are voluntary, striated, multinucleate, and attached to the bones. They are individually innervated.

- The group of skeletal muscle cells controlled by a single neuron is called a motor unit, and each muscle is made of several motor units. All the cells in a motor unit contract together; to increase the strength of a contraction, additional motor units are recruited.

- Skeletal muscles are bundled into fascicles of many myofibers (cells), which are composed of myofibrils (strings of sarcomeres).

- Actin and myosin are organized into sarcomeres, which are the contractile units of the skeletal muscle cell. The arrangement of actin and myosin produces a characteristic banding pattern (striations): A band, I band, A band, I band, etc. Overlap of actin and myosin during the sliding filament theory produces sarcomere shortening.

- The four steps of the sliding filament theory involve the binding of myosin to actin (cross-bridge formation), the pulling of actin toward the center of the sarcomere (power stroke), the release of actin (ATP binding), and resetting myosin to a high-energy conformation (ATP hydrolysis).

- Depolarization of the muscle cell triggers the release of calcium into the cytosol from the sarcoplasmic reticulum. Calcium binds to troponin, changing its shape, and subsequently changing the position of the tropomyosin to which the troponin is bound. This exposes the myosin binding sites on actin and allows contraction to occur. This is known as excitation-contraction coupling.

- Cardiac muscle is also striated, meaning that it, too, is organized into sarcomeres. Sliding filaments and excitation-contraction occur as in skeletal muscle. However, cardiac muscle is involuntary and autorhythmic. The cells are uninuclear and connected by gap junctions to form a functional syncytium.

- Cardiac muscle cells have an action potential that includes a long plateau phase. The plateau is the result of the opening of voltage-gated Ca^{2+} channels.

- Smooth muscle lacks striations and sarcomeres; however, calcium is still needed for smooth muscle cells to contract. They are involuntary.

- Bone is a dense connective tissue that functions primarily in body support and protection. Bones also play a role in mineral storage; resorption and deposition of bone is regulated by parathyroid hormone and calcitonin, respectively, to regulate blood calcium levels.

- Compact bone is organized into osteons, long cylinders of hard, dense bone. Compact bone forms the outer shell of all bones, and the shaft (diaphysis) of long bones.

- Spongy bone contains much more space than compact bone and is filled with red bone marrow; this is where blood cell formation takes place. Spongy bone forms the core of flat bones, and it is found at the ends (epiphyses) of long bones.

- There are three types of cartilage. Fibrous cartilage is strong and rigid, elastic cartilage is flexible, and hyaline cartilage is strong and slightly flexible.

- Ligaments connect bones to bones and tendons connect muscles to bones.

- The epiphyseal plate allows bone growth during childhood and adolescence, but closes at about age 18, preventing any further growth.

- Osteoblasts make bone, osteocytes are dormant and mature osteoblasts, and osteoclasts dissolve bone. These cells are stimulated or inhibited by the parathyroid hormone, calcitonin, and calcitriol (vitamin D).

- The skin is made of three main layers: the epidermis (epithelial tissue), the dermis (connective tissue), and the hypodermis (adipose tissue).

- The epidermis provides a barrier to infection and water loss.

- The dermis is where sweat glands, nerves, blood vessels, and sensory receptors are found.

- The hypodermis is a layer of fat for protection and insulation.

- Thermoregulation is primarily a function of the dermis. When temperatures rise, blood vessels in the dermis dilate to release heat, and sweat glands are activated. When temperature falls, blood vessels constrict to retain heat. Also, involuntary skeletal muscle contractions occur (shivering) to produce heat.

X. **Reproduction and Development**
   A. **The Male System**
      1. Anatomy
      2. Accessory glands
      3. Male sexual act
      4. Spermatogenesis
      5. Male and female reproductive development
      6. Androgens and estrogens
   B. **The Female System**
      1. Anatomy
      2. Female sexual act
      3. Oogenesis and ovulation
      4. The menstrual cycle
      5. Pregnancy and hormones
   C. **Development**
      1. Fertilization and cleavage
      2. Implantation and the placenta
      3. Gastrulation and neurulation
      4. Differentiation
      5. Birth and lactation
      6. Animal phylogeny and development
      7. Protostomes vs. deuterostomes

Summary of Key Concepts:

- The primary sex organs produce gametes and hormones. The testes are the male primary sex organ and the ovaries are the female primary sex organ.

- Male internal genitalia are formed from Wolffian ducts and female internal genitalia are formed from Müllerian ducts.

- Spermatogenesis takes place in the seminiferous tubules and results in four haploid sperm from a single spermatogonium. It begins at puberty and continues on a daily basis for the life of the male. FSH stimulates spermatogenesis and LH stimulates testosterone production.

- Sperm travel from the seminiferous tubules to the epididymis, then to the ductus deferens, then to the urethra. Semen is a supportive fluid for sperm, produced by the seminal vesicles, the prostate, and the bulbourethral glands.

- Oogenesis begins prenatally, producing primary oocytes. It occurs again on a monthly basis, beginning at puberty and ending at menopause; this produces one secondary oocyte (which is ovulated) and the first polar body. Oogenesis is only completed if the secondary oocyte is fertilized, in which case an ovum and the second polar body will be produced.

- FSH stimulates follicle development and estrogen secretion during the first half of the menstrual cycle. LH stimulates ovulation and the formation of the corpus luteum, as well as progesterone and estrogen secretion, during the second half of the menstrual cycle.

- Estrogen stimulates growth of the endometrium during the first half of the menstrual cycle; progesterone and estrogen maintain and enhance the endometrium during the second half of the menstrual cycle. If no fertilization takes place, estrogen and progesterone levels fall, and the endometrium is sloughed off.

- Arousal is mediated by the parasympathetic nervous system, while orgasm and resolution are mediated by the sympathetic nervous system.

- Fertilization takes place in the uterine tubes, and cleavage begins 24–36 hours later. The zygote becomes a morula, the morula becomes a blastula, and the blastula implants in the endometrium.

- The trophoblast becomes the placenta and the inner cell mass becomes the embryo.

- The first eight weeks of development are the embryonic stage, during which gastrulation (formation of the primary germ layers), neurulation (formation of the nervous system), and organogenesis occur.

- The fetal stage begins at the eighth week of development and ends at the birth of the baby.

- Labor is a positive feedback cycle triggered by mild (initially) uterine contractions that push the baby's head on the cervix. This stimulates the release of oxytocin, which causes a stronger uterine contraction, and a bigger stretch of the cervix. This positive feedback loop will continue until the birth of the baby.

- Prolactin stimulates milk production and oxytocin stimulates milk ejection in a baby-driven cycle.

- Animals with two primary germ layers are diploblastic and display radial symmetry (jellyfish and hydra). All other animals are triploblastic (have three primary germ layers) and display bilateral symmetry.

- Protostomes include annelids, mollusks, and arthropods. Their blastopore becomes their mouth, and they display spiral, determinate cleavage.

- Deuterostomes include echinoderms and chordates. Their blastopore becomes their anus, and they display radial, indeterminate cleavage.

14.2   BIOLOGY LAB TECHNIQUES

Why Do I Have To Know About Biology Lab Techniques?

Great question! We're glad you asked!

Since about 2012, the OAT has contained a handful of questions on biology lab techniques, mostly molecular biology and biotechnology protocols. These started with some straight forward questions on PCR, nucleotide content in DNA (Chargaff's rules), cDNA, electrophoresis, and plasmids. Over the last few years these questions have become trickier and have focused on things like cell fractionation, X-ray crystallography, mass spectrometry, and electron microscopy.

Because of this, you should be familiar with some common biology lab techniques. The tricky thing here is that there are so many biology techniques out there and the OAT appears to like asking questions about a wide range of protocols. The good news is that most tests contain fewer than three questions on biology lab techniques. Also, a basic understanding of molecular or cell biology helps with Process of Elimination (POE) on most questions. Finally, typical of the OAT, biology lab techniques questions tend to test *basic* information, and *not* advanced applications. You need to know a little bit about everything, but don't worry about an in-depth understanding.

The section below contains a summary of common biology lab techniques. Much of this you'll be familiar with from your undergraduate labs. If you're completely unfamiliar with a certain technique or concept, you may want to do some background reading or research. These topics represent a good cross section of the types of questions the OAT has tested in the past.

An Overview Of Biology Lab Techniques

Technique, Concept or Reagent	How it Works	Why It Is Useful
Polymerase Chain Reaction (PCR)	• Template DNA is replicated in a small tube • Uses a heat-stable DNA polymerase (Taq polymerase)	• Generate millions of copies of DNA • Especially useful when there is only a small amount of template DNA available
Centrifugation	• Liquid sample (or solution) is spun at high speeds in a tube	• Separates heavy/solid material from the liquid supernatant
Cell Lysis	• Detergent and buffer are added to cells, to break them open	• Releases macromolecules (such as DNA, RNA or proteins) from the cell so they can be used in experiments

Technique, Concept or Reagent	How it Works	Why It Is Useful
Cell Fractionation	• Lysed cell contents are centrifuged at varying speeds • Heavy components are isolated first • Light components are isolated last	• Isolates different cell components into different samples
Spectrophotometer	• Exposes macromolecules (such as DNA, RNA or protein) to UV light	• Quantifies the macromolecule, especially the concentration of the sample
Bradford Quantification	• Coomassie blue is added to lysate and control samples • Samples are analyzed via a spectrophotometer	• Quantifies proteins in a lysate sample
Gel Electrophoresis	• Macromolecules are added to a gel • Electric current is applied • Small molecules move quickly • Large molecules move slowly	• Separates a mixture of macromolecules in a gel by size and charge
Agarose Gels	• Solid gel used for gel electrophoresis	• Separating samples of RNA or DNA by size
Acrylamide Gels	• Solid gel used for gel electrophoresis	• Separating samples of proteins/lysates by size
Ethidium Bromide (EtBr)	• Intercalates between DNA bases • Fluoresces orange under UV light	• Allows nucleic acid samples to be visualized after gel electrophoresis
2D Gel Electrophoresis	• A gel with a pH gradient • Electric current is applied • Proteins separate in two dimensions into dots, based on their molecular mass and isoelectric point	• Separation of a complex mixture of proteins
Coomassie Blue	• A dye that can be added to lysate samples or acrylamide gels	• Allows visualization of protein or lysate samples
Radiograph	• An image of dark bands on an X-ray film • Produced by a pattern of radioactive decay	• Allows detection of radioactively labeled probes or molecules

Technique, Concept or Reagent	How it Works	Why It Is Useful
Southern Blot	• DNA samples are separated via electrophoresis • DNA is transferred to a membrane • Fragment of interest is detected via a complementary, radioactive probe • Probe is detected via a radiograph	• Allows you to detect a certain DNA fragment
Northern Blot	• RNA samples are separated via electrophoresis • RNA is transferred to a membrane • Fragment of interest is detected via a complementary, radioactive probe • Probe is detected via a radiograph	• Allows you to detect a certain RNA fragment
Western Blot	• Protein/lysate samples are denatured and reduced, then separated via electrophoresis • Proteins are transferred to a membrane • Protein of interest is detected via an antibody linked to an enzyme • Add the enzyme substrate to detect the antigen-antibody complex	• Allows you to detect and quantify a certain protein in a lysate sample
Eastern Blot	• Varying protocols	• Analyze post-translational modification of proteins
DNA Fingerprinting	• aka DNA profiling • See RFLP	• Unique DNA characteristics are used to identify individuals
Restriction Fragment Length Polymorphism (RFLP)	• Genomic DNA is digested with restriction enzymes and electrophoresed	• Unique banding pattern can be used to match and compare different DNA samples • Examples: forensics, paternity testing
Molecular Cloning	• Generating recombinant DNA	• Generate unique DNA sequences, not found in nature
Subcloning	• Move a particular DNA sequence between different vectors	• Easy and flexible manipulation of DNA in the lab
Genetic Engineering	• Manipulating an organism's genes via biotechnology	• Produce improved or novel organisms

Technique, Concept or Reagent	How it Works	Why It Is Useful
Restriction Enzymes	• Cut double-stranded DNA at specific sites	• Help move around DNA in molecular cloning • RFLP • Digest genomic DNA before starting a Southern blot
Plasmids	• Small, double-stranded, circular DNA molecules	• Study, manipulate, transfer and replicate small DNA fragments
Cloning Vector	• A plasmid, BAC, YAC or virus	• Transfer and replicate DNA
Selection	• Sensitive organisms die • Resistant organisms survive • Bacteria: often use antibiotics such as ampicillin, tetracycline, penicillin, or streptomycin • Can also use eukaryotic selection agents such as puromycin or neomycin	• Select for cells that have taken up a plasmid or carry a mutation of interest
Transformation	• Expose bacterial cells to heat or electric current	• Transfer plasmid DNA or a chromosome fragment into a bacterial host cell
Complementary DNA (cDNA)	• DNA made from single stranded RNA via reverse transcriptase	• Allows easy manipulation of eukaryotic genes (that contain introns) in the lab and bacterial cells • Study gene expression
cDNA Library	• Collection of cDNA molecules made from a certain cell, cloned into plasmids	• Study gene expression
gDNA Library	• Collection of gDNA fragments, cloned into plasmids	• Study genomic structure and function
Artificial Chromosomes	• Includes bacterial artificial chromosomes (BACs) and yeast artificial chromosomes (YACs) • Vectors for large DNA inserts	• Study, manipulate, transfer and replicate large DNA fragments
Tissue Culture	• Eukaryotic cells are grown *in vitro*, in a petri dish with liquid media	• Study, manipulate and replicate eukaryotic cells
Transfection	• Expose eukaryotic cells to chemicals, liposomes, or electric current	• Transfer plasmid DNA or a chromosome fragment into a eukaryotic host cell
Transduction	• Expose eukaryotic or bacterial cells to viruses carrying DNA	• Transfer DNA into a eukaryotic or bacterial host cell

Technique, Concept or Reagent	How it Works	Why It Is Useful
Reverse Transcription Polymerase Chain Reaction (RT-PCR)	• PCR performed on cDNA	• Detect gene expression by amplifying a certain mRNA template
Quantitative Polymerase Chain reaction (qPCR)	• aka real-time PCR • PCR where the product is detected and quantified	• Quantify presence and abundance of template DNA or cDNA
Enzyme-Linked Immuno-Sorbent Assay (ELISA)	• Serum or cells are exposed to antigen-antibody interactions in a microtiter well • Secondary antibody is enzyme-linked to detect a color change	• Test for the presence of an antibody or antigen
Radioimmunoassay (RIA)	• Similar to ELISA • Secondary antibody is radiolabelled instead of enzyme-linked	• Test for the presence of an antibody or antigen
Sanger Sequencing	• 4 PCR reactions with dideoxynucleotide triphosphates (ddNTPs), one per tube • Gel electrophoresis of the four samples side-by-side	• Sequence DNA
Comparative Genomics	• Many options	• Study genome structure and function across different species
Functional Genomics	• Many options	• Define gene function
Transcriptomics	• Many options	• Study gene expression and RNA molecules
Proteomics	• Many options	• Study proteins made by a cell (structure, modifications, functions, interactions)
Lipidomics	• Many options	• Study lipids made by a cell (structure, modifications, functions, interactions)
Metabolomics	• Many options	• Study metabolic processes and metabolites
Single Nucleotide Polymorphisms (SNPs)	• Single base-pair variations in the genome • Found at >0.01 frequency in the population	• Used to study human populations, migration, and evolution
Tandem Repeats	• Short sequences of nucleotides are repeated one right after the other, 3 to over 100 times • Includes microsatellites and minisatellites	• Important in some diseases (e.g., Huntington's disease) • STR Analysis

Technique, Concept or Reagent	How it Works	Why It Is Useful
Short Tandem Repeat (STR) Analysis	• Similar to RFLP • PCR amplify repetitive DNA • Southern blot	• Unique DNA pattern can be used to match different DNA samples
Exome Sequencing	• Sequence exons	• Smaller scale that whole-genome sequencing • Easier and more specific
Karyotyping	• Chromosomes are isolated, stained, and imaged	• Study genome structure
Fluorescence *In Situ* Hybridization (FISH)	• Fluorescent probes are used to detect specific sequences on isolated chromosomes • A type of staining	• Study genome structure
Comparative Genomics Hybridization (CGH)	• Isolate and label two samples of genomic DNA • Mix and apply to chip • Relative colors are measured	• Quantifies copy number variation (CNV) in genomic DNA, such as deletions or duplications
Microarrays	• A type of transcriptional profiling • Isolate and label two samples of RNA • Mix and apply to chip • Relative colors are measured	• Quantifies comparative gene expression
In Situ Hybridization (ISH)	• Similar to FISH • A type of staining • Use a probe to detect a DNA or RNA sequence in a tissue section on a microscope slide	• Analyze gene expression in a tissue sample
RNA-Seq	• RNA sequencing • aka whole transcriptome shotgun sequencing • A type of transcriptional profiling • Isolate RNAs, convert them to cDNA and sequence them	• Analyze gene expression and splicing
Edman Degradation	• Remove one amino acid at a time from a peptide chain • Identify it	• Determine amino acid sequence of a protein
X-ray Crystallography	• Purify the protein of interest • Crystallize it • Expose to X-rays • Record reflections (location and intensity) • Convert to atomic model via mathematical modeling	• Determine structure of rigid proteins

14.2

Technique, Concept or Reagent	How it Works	Why It Is Useful
Mass Spectrometry	• Ionize molecules • Shoot through a magnetic field of varying strength • Calculate a mass to charge ratio (m/z)	• Highly specific • Determine molecular weight or formula • Identify molecules • Determine protein structure
Nuclear Magnetic Resonance (NMR) Spectroscopy	• Purify protein of interest • Place in a magnetic field • Probe with radio waves	• Determine protein structure of rigid but small proteins
Light Microscope	• aka optical microscope • System of lenses and light	• Magnify small samples
Fluorescent Microscope	• A type of light/optical microscope • Illuminates a sample with varying and specific wavelengths of light	• Looking at fluorescent molecules under a microscope
Confocal Microscope	• A type of light/optical microscope • aka Confocal laser scanning microscopy (CLSM) • The microscope focuses a small beam of light (a laser) at one narrow depth level at a time	• Generates images with high optical resolution and contrast
Transmission Electron Microscope (TEM)	• Use a beam of accelerated electrons to illuminate a small sample	• Produce 2D images that have high magnification and great resolution
Scanning Electron Microscope (SEM)	• Use a beam of accelerated electrons to illuminate a small sample	• Produce 3D images that have high magnification and great resolution
Micrograph	• A photograph or digital image taken through a microscope	• Shows a magnified image of an object
Multiple Alignment	• DNA or protein sequences are aligned and compared	• Helps determine how sequences are similar or related
Protein Domains	• Conserved patterns in protein sequence and structure	• Helps determine how proteins are similar or related
GFP	• Green fluorescent protein • Fluorophore that emits green light	• Used to tag proteins and antibodies
RFP	• Red fluorescent protein • Fluorophore that emits red light	• Used to tag proteins and antibodies
CFP	• Cyan fluorescent protein • Fluorophore that emits cyan light	• Used to tag proteins and antibodies

Technique, Concept or Reagent	How it Works	Why It Is Useful
YFP	• Yellow fluorescent protein • Fluorophore that emits yellow light	• Used to tag proteins and antibodies
DAPI	• A blue fluorescent dye	• Used to dye the nuclei of cells
Immunohistochemistry (IHC)	• Similar to ISH • A type of staining • Use antibodies to detect protein expression in a tissue section on a microscope slide • Secondary antibody can be enzyme-linked or connected to a fluorophore	• Analyze protein expression in a tissue sample on a microscope slide
Serial Sections	• Sections of a paraffin block cut one right after the other • Stained by IHC • Images of tissue or cells are captured and stacked together	• Generate 3D images of stained tissues or cells
Z-Stacks	• Images obtained by optical sectioning	• Combined to generate 3D images of stained tissues or cells
Optical Sectioning	• One section is stained via IHC • A confocal microscope is used to take a series of images (Z-stacks) at different depths • Images of tissue or cells are stacked together	• Generate 3D images of stained tissues or cells
Tissue Microarray (TMA)	• A type of staining • Several tissue samples are preserved together in one paraffin block • Section is cut and stained via IHC	• Analyze protein expression in many tissue samples on one microscope slide
Flow Cytometry	• Individual cells are stained via antibodies linked to fluorophores • Cells are passed through a laser beam of light • Data is collected and graphed for each individual cell	• Analyze protein/antigen expression for a collection of cells • Several proteins can be analyzed for each cell • Information on cell size is also collected
Fluorescence-Activated Cell Sorting (FACS)	• Cell sorting that follows flow cytometry	• Cells are sorted into populations based on antigen/protein expression

14.2

Technique, Concept or Reagent	How it Works	Why It Is Useful
Mass Cytometry	• aka Cytometry by time of flight (CyTOF) • Similar to flow cytometry but antigens are labeled with heavy metal ion tags instead of an antibody linked to a fluorophore • Antigens are identified via mass spectrometry	• Identification of up to 100 different molecules per cell being analyzed by flow cytometry
RNA Interference (RNAi)	• Use microRNA (miRNA) or small interfering RNA (siRNA) • Both these RNAs bind mRNA • Double-stranded RNA is degraded	• Decrease gene expression
Morpholino	• Synthetic DNA molecules • Bind and sterically block RNA	• Decrease gene expression
Knock-In	• Gene of interest is over-expressed by incorporating it into the genome with a strong promoter • Can go into its own locus (endogenous) or elsewhere	• A way to increase expression of the protein of interest
In Vitro Mutagenesis	• A gene is cloned, specifically mutated, then returned to a cell	• A way to study the effect of a certain mutation
Immunoprecipitation (IP)	• Lysate is collected • Add an antibody specific to your protein of interest • Isolate the antibody via a heavy bead or a magnet	• Isolate your protein of interest and all its binding partners • Binding partners can be identified via western blot or mass spec
Yeast Two-Hybrid (Y2H)	• Fuse your protein of interest to the DNA-binding domain (BD) of a transcription factor via cloning • Fuse a potential binding partner (or many) to the activation domain (AD) of a transcription factor via cloning • Add both to the same cell that has a reporter gene downstream of the promoter for the transcription factor	• If the reporter gene is transcribed: bait and prey proteins must interact • If the reporter gene is not made: they do not • Therefore, used to determine if proteins interact with each other

Technique, Concept or Reagent	How it Works	Why It Is Useful
Fluorescence Resonance Energy Transfer (FRET)	• Similar to Y2H, but use fluorophores instead of transcription factor domains and a reporter gene • Fuse your protein of interest to one fluorophore • Fuse a potential binding partner to a different fluorophore • Add both to the same cell • Expose the cell to the light for the first fluorophore using a fluorescent microscope	• If the color emitted matches the fluorophore on your protein of interest, the two proteins do not interact • If the color matches the other fluorophore, the two proteins must interact (energy was transferred between fluorophores because they are close together) • Therefore, used to determine if proteins interact with each other
Solid-Phase Synthesis	• Used for peptides and nucleic acids • Molecules are bound on a solid bead and synthesized step-by-step in a reactant solution	• Biomolecule synthesis
Solid-Phase Peptide Synthesis (SPPS)	• Amino acids are connected C-terminus to N-terminus on a bead • Reactive groups are protected to control the reaction	• Peptide synthesis in the opposite direction as *in vivo*
Totipotent Stem Cells	• Zygote • Morula • Can become any cell in the trophoblast	• Most undifferentiated cells
Pluripotent Stem Cells	• Inner cell mass cells (aka embryonic stem cells, ESC) • Can become any cell in the adult organism	• Isolated and used for stem cell work in the lab • Many possible uses in regenerative medicine • Can be genetically altered to generate transgenic animal models • Use of human ESCs is controversial because they're isolated from IVF blastocysts
Multipotent Stem Cells	• Ectoderm, mesoderm, endoderm and adult stem cells • Can become a subset of cells in the adult	• Lineage and tissue specific stem cells
Stem Cell Therapy	• Manipulate embryonic stem cells in the lab	• Use stem cells to treat diseases such as blood and immune system genetic disorders, many cancers, spinal cord injuries, Parkinson's disease, juvenile diabetes, burns, and blindness

Technique, Concept or Reagent	How it Works	Why It Is Useful
Induced Pluripotent Stem Cells	• Isolate adult somatic cells • Express a subset of genes • Induce the cells back to a pluripotent state	• Their use is still being determined • These cells act like ESC in some ways but not in other ways • Patient-specific drug screens
Reproductive Cloning	• Isolate a nucleus from a donor somatic (adult) cell • Transfer it into an egg with no nucleus • The egg develops into an animal	• Making an animal genetically identical to another
Cloned Animal	• Made via reproductive cloning	• Genetically identical to another animal • Example: Dolly the sheep
Transgenic Plants	• Genetically altered plant	• Increase the use/productivity of plants • Make plants more robust or efficient
Transgenic Animals	• Genetically altered animals	• Model human diseases • Optimize food production (e.g., milk)
Genetically Modified Foods (GMF)	• Food produced from organisms that have had their DNA altered	• Increase nutritional value • Decrease food rot and waste • Increase shelf-life • Decrease pesticide use • Decrease contamination and pollution
Recombinant Treatments	• Therapies and pharmaceuticals synthesized via genetic engineering	• Better vaccines • Insulin production • Synthesis of molecules and proteins needed to treat disease

Chapter 15
General Chemistry

15.1 GENERAL CHEMISTRY OVERVIEW

The material in the OAT Chemistry section is not designed to be a comprehensive review, but rather is a set of outlines to help you guide your studying. Comprehensive Chemistry review for the OAT can be found in *Cracking the DAT*.

I. **Chemistry Basics**
   A. **Metric Units**
   B. **Molarity**
   C. **Density**
   D. **Assessing Molecular Composition**
      1. Molecular Formulas
      2. Molecular Weight
      3. The Mole
      4. Empirical Formula Calculations
      5. Percent Composition by Mass
   E. **Chemical Equations and Stoichiometry**
      1. Chemical equations
      2. The Limiting Reagent
      3. Stoichiometric Relationships in Balanced Reactions
   F. **Oxidation States**

Summary of Key Concepts:

- In chemistry, concentration of solutions is commonly expressed in molarity

- Molarity (M) = moles of solute per liter of solution. This is usually stated as $C = n/V$

- Density is a measure of the mass per volume for a given material.

- Density (ρ) = mass (kg)/volume (m^3).

- Water has a density of 1 g/cm^3 or 1000 kg/m^3.

- A molecular formula provides information about the atomic makeup of a compound, including the identity and the number of atoms.

- The molecular weight (MW) of a compound is the sum of the atomic weights of all the atoms.

- One mole of any substance contains 6.02×10^{23} molecules (Avogadro's number).

- Number of moles of a compound = mass (g)/molecular weight. This is usually stated as $n = m/M$.

- An empirical formula shows the lowest whole-number ratio of the elements that constitute a compound. For example, the molecular formula of glucose is $C_6H_{12}O_6$, but the empirical formula is CH_2O.

- Chemical equations represent chemical reactions.

- Limiting reagents are reactants depleted first in a chemical reaction, thereby determining the amount of product produced.

- An oxidation state is a positive or negative number assigned to an element based on its degree of oxidation. Be familiar with the rules for assigning oxidation states.

II. **Atomic Structure**
   A. **Elements and the Periodic Table**
   B. **The Atom**
      1. Subatomic Particles
      2. Isotopes
      3. Atomic Weight
      4. Ions
   C. **Electron Quantum Numbers**
      1. First Quantum Number
      2. Second Quantum Number
      3. Third Quantum Number
      4. Fourth Quantum Number
   D. **Electron Configurations**
      1. Blocks in the Periodic Table
      2. Anomalous Electron Configurations
      3. Electron Configurations of Ions
      4. Diamagnetic and Paramagnetic Atoms
      5. Excited State and Ground State
   E. **Atomic Structure**
      1. Absorption and Emission Spectra
      2. Bohr Model of the Atom
   F. **Nuclear Structure**
      1. Stability and Radioactivity
      2. Alpha Decay
      3. Beta Decay (β^- and β^+)
      4. Electron Capture
      5. Gamma Decay
      6. Half Life
      7. Nuclear Binding Energy

Summary of Key Concepts:

- The periodic table is organized into blocks based on the architecture of electron orbitals. Therefore, valence electron configurations can be determined based on an element's location in the table.

- The nucleus contains protons and neutrons. Their sum corresponds to the atomic mass (A).

- The number of protons corresponds to the atomic number (Z).

- Each electron in an atom has a distinct set of four quantum numbers (Pauli Exclusion Principle). These numbers describe the energy of the electron and what kind of orbital it resides within.

- The four quantum numbers describe the shell (n), subshell (l), orbital (m_l), and spin (m_s) of an electron.

- In their ground state, electrons occupy the lowest energy orbitals available (Aufbau Principle), and occupy subshell orbitals singly before pairing (Hund's Rule).

- The *d* subshell is always backfilled: for an atom in the *d* block of period *n*, the *d* subshell will have a principle quantum number of *n* – 1.

- A half filled (d^5) or filled (d^{10}) *d* subshell is exceptionally stable.

- Transition metals ionize from their valence *s* subshell before their *d* subshell.

- Electrons exist in discrete energy levels within an atom. Emission spectra are obtained from energy emitted as excited electrons fall from one level to another.

- An overabundance of either protons or neutrons can result in unstable nuclei, which decay via the emission of various particles.

- For nuclear decay reactions, the sum of all mass and atomic numbers in the products must equal the same sum of these numbers in the reactants.

- The rate of nuclear decay is governed by a species' half-life.

III. **Periodic Trends and Bonding**
   A. **Groups of the Periodic Table**
   B. **Periodic Trends**
      1. Shielding
      2. Atomic Radius and Ionic Radius
      3. Ionization Energy
      4. Electron Affinity
      5. Electronegativity
      6. Acidity
   C. **Covalent Bonding**
      1. Lewis Dot Structures
      2. Covalent Bonding
      3. Formal Charge
      4. Resonance
      5. Polar Covalent Bonding
      6. Coordinate Covalent Bonds
      7. VSEPR Theory and Hybridization
   D. **Ionic Bonding**
   E. **Types of Solids**
      1. Ionic Solids
      2. Network Solids
      3. Metallic Solids
      4. Molecular Solids
   F. **Intermolecular Forces**
      1. Ion-dipole Forces
      2. Dipole-dipole Forces
      3. London-dispersion Forces
      4. Hydrogen Bonding

Summary of Key Concepts:

- Atoms and ions are most stable when they have an octet of electrons in their outer shell.

- The apparent magnitude an electron feels due to its position and the quantity of electrons between it and the nucleus is called the Effective Nuclear Charge (Z_{eff}), and will have a quantity less than or equal to the Z of an atom.

- Atomic radius increases to the left and down the periodic table; for charged species, cations < neutral atom < anions for a given element; for isoelectronic ions, the species with more protons (larger Z_{eff}) will have the smaller radius.

- Ionization energy, electron affinity, and electronegativity increase up and to the right on the periodic table, while acidity increases to the right and down the periodic table.

- The relative electronegativities of common atoms in decreasing order are F>O>N>Cl>Br>I>S>C~H.

- The best Lewis dot or resonance structures have 1) octets around all atoms, 2) minimized formal charge, and 3) negative charges on more electronegative elements.

- Ionic bonds form between elements with large differences in electronegativity (metals + nonmetals), and the strength of that bond depends on Coulomb's Law; larger charges and smaller ions make the strongest ionic bonds.

- Covalent bonds form between elements with similar electronegativities (two nonmetals).

- Coordinate covalent bonds form between a Lewis base (e^- pair donor) and a Lewis acid (e^- pair acceptor); electrons are shared.

- Nonpolar bonding means equal electron sharing; polar bonding means unequal electron sharing, and electron density is higher around the more electronegative element.

- VSEPR theory predicts the shape of molecules; angles between electron groups around the central atom are maximized for greatest stability.

- If bond dipoles are symmetrically oriented in a molecule, the molecule as a whole is nonpolar; if the dipoles are asymmetrical, the molecule will be polar.

- The hybridization of an atom is dependent on the number of electron groups on the atom (e.g., two e^- groups = sp, three e^-~groups = sp^2...six e^-~groups = sp^3d^2).

- Nonpolar molecules have London dispersion forces and polar molecules have dipole forces.

- Hydrogen bonding occurs between hydrogen attached to F, O, or N and lone electron pairs of F, O, or N.

- Hydrogen bonding is a very strong type of dipole forces

- Intermolecular forces are cohesive, and the relative strengths of these forces determine the physical properties (melting and boiling points, solubility, vapor pressure, etc.) of a compound.

IV. Phases
   A. Phase Transitions
      1. Heats of Phase Changes
      2. Calorimetry
      3. Phase Transition Diagrams
   B. Phase Diagrams
      1. Triple Point and Critical Point
      2. Difference between Diagram of Water and Carbon Dioxide

Summary of Key Concepts:

- Changes in pressure and/or temperature of a substance can induce changes in phase.

- The three important phases are (in order of increasing entropy and increasing internal energy / kinetic energy) solid, liquid, and gas.

- Specific heat (c) is an intrinsic property that defines how resistant a substance is to temperature change.

- The change in temperature associated with the input or extraction of heat when phase is unchanged is given by $q = mc\Delta T$, where c is the specific heat of a substance and m is the amount (either mass or moles, depending on c).

- Heat capacity (C) is given by $C = mc$, where m is the mass of the sample. Heat capacity is a proportionality constant that defines how much heat is required to change the temperature of a sample by 1°C.

- A substance cannot simultaneously undergo a phase change and a temperature change.

- The heat associated with a phase change is given by $q = n\Delta H_{phase\ change}$, where n is the number of moles of substance (or mass if ΔH is given in energy/weight).

- Lines on a phase diagram correspond to equilibria between phases and phase transitions. The intersection of all three lines on a phase diagram is known as the triple point, and it represents equilibrium between all three phases.

- The phase diagram of water is unique in that its solid/liquid equilibrium line has a negative slope. This results in ice melting under increased pressure, and the density of ice being less than that of liquid water. Most substances (such as carbon dioxide) exhibit a positive solid/liquid equilibrium line because pressure favors the more dense phase (which almost always is the solid phase; water is the exception).

V.   Gases
  A.   Gases and the Kinetic-Molecular Theory
  B.   Units of Volume, Temperature, and Pressure and STP Conditions
  C.   The Ideal Gas Law
  D.   P-V-T Gas Laws
       1.   Charles' Law
       2.   Boyle's Law
       3.   Avogadro's Law
  E.   Dalton's Law of Partial Pressures
  F.   Graham's Law of Effusion
  G.   Real Gases and Deviations from Ideality

Summary of Key Concepts:

- The Ideal Gas Law states that $PV = nRT$.

- Standard temperature and pressure (STP) conditions are at 1 atm and 273 K.

- Molecules of an ideal gas take up no volume and experience no intermolecular forces.

- Real gases approach ideal behavior under most conditions, but deviate most from ideal behavior under conditions of high pressure and low temperature.

- Dalton's Law of Partial Pressures states that the total pressure inside a container is equal to the sum of the partial pressures of each constituent gas. The partial pressure of a gas divided by the total pressure of all gases is equal to its mole fraction within the gaseous mixture.

- Temperature is a measure of the average kinetic energy of molecules within a sample.

- Graham's Law of Effusion states that the rate of effusion of a gas is inversely proportional to its molecular weight. In other words, lighter gases effuse more quickly than heavier gases.

VI.   Solutions
  A.   Dissolution and Solubility
       1.   Concentration Measurements
       2.   Electrolytes
       3.   Solubility Rules
  B.   Colligative Properties
       1.   Vapor-pressure Depression
       2.   Boiling Point Elevation
       3.   Freezing Point Depression
       4.   Osmotic Pressure

Summary of Key Concepts:

- Concentration is generally given in either molarity (mol solute/L solution, M) or molality (mol solute/kg solvent, m). Molality is independent of temperature, while molarity is not.

- Electrolytes are free ions in solution produced by dissociation of ionic substances.

- The van't Hoff (or ionizability) factor, i, tell us how many ions one unit of a substance will produce in solution.

- All Group I, ammonium, nitrate, perchlorate, and acetate salts are completely soluble. All silver, lead, and mercury salts are insoluble, except when they are paired with nitrate, perchlorate, or acetate.

- The solubility of solids in liquids increases with increasing temperature, and of gases in liquids decreases with increasing temperature and increases with increasing pressure.

- Colligative properties depend on the number of particles in solution. Colligative properties include vapor pressure depression, boiling point elevation, freezing point depression, and osmotic pressure.

- In the context of OAT questions, the colligative strength of a substance can usually be determined based on its van't Hoff factor (i).

- As the concentration of solute increases in solution, the vapor pressure of the solution (relative to the pure solvent) will decrease according to the equation:
$$P_{vap\ (soln)} = X_{solvent}\ P^\circ_{vap\ (pure\ solvent)}.$$

- Increases in solute concentration and the van't Hoff factor correlate with decreases in solution freezing point or increases in solution boiling point.

- Increases in concentration, van't Hoff factor, and temperature correlate with increased osmotic pressure (Π) according to the equation: $\Pi = MRTi$.

VII. **Kinetics**
- A. **Reaction Mechanisms**
  - 1. Transition States and Intermediates
  - 2. Rate-Determining Step
- B. **Reaction Rates**
  - 1. Activation Energy
  - 2. Catalysts
  - 3. Rate Constant and Rate Laws

Summary of Key Concepts:

- Kinetics is the study of how quickly a reaction occurs, but it does not determine *whether or not* a reaction will occur.

- All rates are experimentally determined by measuring a change in the concentration of a reactant or product compared to a change in time (often given in M/s).

- Molecules must collide in order to react, and the frequency and energy of these collisions determines how fast the reaction occurs.

- Increasing the concentration of reactants *often* increases the reaction rate due to an increased number of collisions.

- Increasing the temperature of a reaction *always* increases the reaction rate since molecules move faster and collide more frequently; the energy of collisions also increases.

- Activation energy (E_a) is the minimum amount of energy required to start a reaction and proceed to the formation of products.

- Catalysts lower E_a, thereby increasing the reaction rate, and are not consumed in the reaction.

- Transition states are at energy maxima, while intermediates are at local energy minima along a reaction coordinate.

- A reaction mechanism must agree with experimental data, and suggests a possible pathway by which reactants and intermediates might collide in order for a chemical reaction to occur.

- The sum of all elementary steps of a mechanism will add to give the overall chemical reaction.

- The slow step of the mechanism is the rate limiting step, and it determines the rate of the overall reaction.

- A rate law can only be determined from experimental data or if given a mechanism, and it has the general form: Rate = k [reactants]^x, where x is the order of the reaction with respect to the given reactant, and k is the rate constant.

- The overall order of a reaction is the sum of all exponents in the rate law.

- The value of the rate constant, k, depends on temperature and activation energy, and its units will vary depending on the reaction order.

- Coefficients of the reactants in the rate limiting step of a mechanism can be used to determine the order of a reaction in the rate law; coefficients from the overall reaction alone CANNOT be used to find the order of a reaction.

VIII. **Equilibrium**
   A. **Equilibrium Definitions and Constants**
   B. **Reaction Quotient**
   C. **Le Châtelier's Principle**
       1. Adding Reagents
       2. Removing Reagents
       3. Effects of Changes in Pressure and Volume
       4. Effects of Changes in Temperature
       5. Addition of Inert or Non-Reactive Reagents
       6. Addition of Catalysts
   D. **Solubility Product Constant**
       1. Molar Solubility Calculations
       2. Ion Product Calculations
       3. Common Ion Effect

Summary of Key Concepts:

- The equilibrium constant dictates the relative ratios of products to reactants when a system is at equilibrium.

- For $aA + bB \rightarrow cC + dD$: $K_{eq} = ([C]^c[D]^d)/([A]^a[B]^b)$

- Pure solids and liquids are not included in the equilibrium constant.

- If $K > 1$, products are favored. If $K < 1$, reactants are favored.

- The reaction quotient, Q, is a ratio of products and reactants with the same math as K, but used when the reaction isn't at equilibrium. If $Q < K$, the reaction will proceed in the forward reaction; if $Q > K$, the reaction will proceed in the reverse direction until equilibrium is achieved.

- The only factor that changes the equilibrium constant is temperature.

- Changing the concentrations of the products or reactants of a reaction at equilibrium will force the system to shift according to Le Châtelier's principle.

- Increasing the temperature of a system at equilibrium favors the products in an endothermic reaction and the reactants in an exothermic reaction. Decreasing the temperature will have the opposite effect on both types of reactions.

- In a gaseous reaction, increasing the pressure by decreasing the volume favors the side of the reaction with fewer moles of gas. Decreasing the pressure has the opposite effect.

- The degree to which a salt dissolves in water is given by its solubility product constant (K_{sp}).

IX. Acids and Bases
   A. Definitions
      1. Arrhenius Acids and Bases
      2. Brønsted-Lowry Acids and Bases
      3. Lewis Acids and Bases
      4. Conjugate Acids and Bases
   B. Strengths of Acids and Bases
      1. Strong and Weak Acids
      2. Strong and Weak Bases
      3. Relative Strength of Conjugate Acid-Base Pairs
      4. Relationship Between K_a and K_b and Strength
      5. Amphoteric Substances
   C. Autoionization of Water and pH
      1. Autoionization of Water
      2. pH scale
      3. Relationship between pH and pOH
   D. pH Calculations
      1. Strong Acid and Base Solutions
      2. Weak Acid and Base Solutions
   E. Neutralization Reactions
   F. Hydrolysis of Salts
   G. Buffer Solutions
   H. Indicators
   I. Acid-Base Titrations

Summary of Key Concepts:

- Acids are proton donors and electron acceptors; bases are proton acceptors and electron donors.

- Strong acids completely dissociate in water ($K_a > 1$). You should memorize the list of strong acids and bases.

- The higher the K_a (lower the pK_a), the stronger the acid. The higher the K_b (lower the pK_b), the stronger the base.

- For any conjugate acid and base pair, $K_a K_b = K_w$. Therefore, it follows that the stronger the acid, the weaker its conjugate acid. Conjugates of strong acids and bases have no acid/base properties in water.

- Amphoteric substances may act as either acids or bases.

- Water is amphoteric, and autoionizes into OH^- and H_3O^+. The equilibrium constant for the autoionization of water is $K_w = [OH^-][H_3O^+]$. At 25°C, $K_w = 1 \times 10^{-14}$.

- pH = $-\log[H_3O^+]$. For a concentration of H_3O^+ given in a 10^{-x} M notation, simply take the negative exponent to find the pH. The same is true for the relationship between $[OH^-]$ and pOH, K_a and pK_a, and K_b and pK_b.

- At 25°C, pK_a + pK_b = 14.

- If a salt is dissolved in water and the cation is a stronger acid than water, the resulting solution will have a pH < 7. If the anion is a base stronger than water, the resulting solution will have a pH > 7.

- Buffers resist pH change upon the addition of a small amount of strong acid or base. A higher concentration of buffer resists pH change better than a lower concentration of buffer (i.e., the solution has a higher buffering capacity).

- A buffer consists of approximately equal molar amounts of a weak acid and its conjugate base, and it maintains a pH close to its pK_a.

- The Henderson-Hasselbalch equation can be used to determine the pH of a buffer solution.

- Indicators are weak acids that change color upon conversion to their conjugate base.

- In a titration, the equivalence point is the point at which all of the original acid or base has been neutralized.

- When a strong acid is titrated against a weak base, the pH at the equivalence point is < 7. When a strong base is titrated against a weak acid, the pH at the equivalence point is > 7. When a strong base is titrated against a strong acid, the pH at the equivalence point is = 7.

- At the half equivalence point of a titration of a weak plus a strong acid or base, the solution has equal concentrations of acid and conjugate base, and pH = pK_a.

Summary of Key Concepts:

- Energy flow into a system has a positive sign. Energy flow out of a system has a negative sign.

- The First Law of Thermodynamics states that energy cannot be created or destroyed. Based on this, $\Delta E = q + w$.

- For an adiabatic process, $q = 0$.

- An isobaric process occurs at constant P, isothermal at constant T, and isochoric at constant V.

- The Second Law of Thermodynamics states that all processes tend toward maximum disorder, or entropy (S).

- Enthalpy (H) is a measure of the heat energy.

- Breaking bonds requires energy ($+\Delta H$), while forming bonds releases energy ($-\Delta H$).

- Standard state conditions are 1 atm and 298 K, 1 M concentrations. Standard state conditions are denoted by a superscript "O."

- An endothermic reaction has a $\Delta H > 0$. An exothermic reaction has a $\Delta H < 0$.

- $\Delta H_{reaction} = H_{products} - H_{reactants}$. This equation can also be applied to ΔG and ΔS.

- ΔG, the Gibbs free energy, is the amount of energy in a reaction available to do chemical work.

- For a reaction under any set of conditions, $\Delta G = \Delta H - T\Delta S$.

- If $\Delta G < 0$, the reaction is spontaneous in the forward direction. If $\Delta G > 0$, the reaction is nonspontaneous in the forward direction. If $\Delta G = 0$, the reaction is at equilibrium.

- For a reaction at equilibrium under standard state conditions, $\Delta G° = -RT\ln K_{eq}$.

- For a reaction under nonequilibrium conditions, ΔG can be calculated using $\Delta G = \Delta G° + RT\ln Q$.

XI. Electrochemistry
     A. Oxidation-Reduction Reactions
     B. Galvanic Cells
     C. Standard Reduction Potentials
     D. Electrolytic Cells

Summary of Key Concepts:

- Oxidation is electron loss; reduction is electron gain (remember "OIL RIG").

- A species that is oxidized is a reducing agent, and a species that is reduced is an oxidizing agent.

- In all electrochemical cells, oxidation occurs at the anode and reduction occurs at the cathode.

- Electrons always flow from the anode to the cathode.

- Salt bridge anions always migrate toward the anode, and cations always migrate toward the cathode.

- The free energy of an electrochemical cell can be calculated from its potential based on $\Delta G = -nFE$.

- A galvanic cell spontaneously generates electrical power ($-\Delta G$, $+E$).

- An electrolytic cell consists of nonspontaneous reactions and requires an external electrical power source ($+\Delta G$, $-E$).

- In a galvanic cell, electrons spontaneously flow from the negative (–) terminal to the positive (+) terminal. Therefore, it follows that in a galvanic cell the anode is negatively charged (–) and the cathode is positively charged (+).

- In an electrolytic cell, electrons are forced from the positive (+) terminal to the negative (–) terminal, and therefore the anode is positively charged (+) and the cathode is negatively charged (–).

- Standard reduction and potentials are intrinsic values and therefore should not be multiplied by molar coefficients in balanced half reactions.

- For a given reduction potential, the reverse reaction, or oxidation potential, has the same magnitude of E but the opposite sign.

XII. LAB TECHNIQUES
  A. Calorimetry
  B. Electrolysis
  C. Splint tests
  D. Density calculations
  E. Laboratory equipment
  F. Precision and accuracy

Summary of Key Concepts:

- Calorimetry is the process of measuring the amount of heat exchange in a reaction or a sample using a calorimeter.

- The method of using electrical current to drive a non-spontaneous reaction is known as electrolysis.

- Splint tests are used to determine the combustibility or presence of a certain gas.
  - In a sample containing hydrogen or oxygen, a splint would burn.
  - In a sample containing nitrogen or carbon dioxide, a burning splint would be extinguished.

- The volume of an object is equal to the volume of water displaced when the object is submerged in water. Once the volume of the object is known, its density can be easily determined by the following equation: $\rho = m/V$.

- Be familiar with the following laboratory equipment, including their uses and limitations: buret, pipette, Erlenmeyer flask, volumetric flask, graduated cylinder, beaker, crucible.

- The strength of data depends on two parameters: precision and accuracy.

  - Precision refers to how close data points are to one another
  - Accuracy refers to how close data points are to the true value.

Chapter 16
Organic Chemistry

16.1 ORGANIC CHEMISTRY OVERVIEW

The material in the OAT Organic Chemistry section is not designed to be a comprehensive review, but rather is a set of outlines to help you guide your studying. Comprehensive Organic Chemistry review for the OAT can be found in *Cracking the DAT.*

I. Organic Chemistry Basics
    A. Basic Nomenclature and Functional Groups
        1. Common Functional Groups
        2. Line Structures
        3. Nomenclature of Alkanes
        4. Nomenclature of Haloalkanes
        5. Nomenclature of Alcohols

Summary of Key Concepts:

- Hydrocarbons are named according to the longest continuous chain of carbon atoms.

- A number of common functional groups are common to organic structures, and nomenclature is modified to reflect the number and position of functional groups.

- Line structures involve connection of non-hydrogen atoms and labeling of heteroatoms with the number of lines reflecting the number of bonds between atoms.

- Haloalkanes are named according to the position of the halogen substituent and are described according to a prefix for each atom (e.g., fluoro-).

- Alcohols are named by position and the suffix "-ol" is added to the end of the name of compound to reflect the hydroxyl group.

II. **Structure and Bonding**
   A. **Bonding and Hybridization**
      1. Hybridization
      2. Sigma (σ) Bonds
      3. Pi (π) Bonds
   B. **Structure**
      1. Degrees of Unsaturation
      2. Bond Length and Bond Dissociation Energy
      3. Constitutional Isomers
      4. Conformational Isomers
      5. Stereoisomers and Chirality
      6. Enantiomers
      7. Diastereomers
      8. Optical Activity
      9. Meso Compounds
     10. Geometric Isomers
   C. **Physical Properties of Hydrocarbons**
      1. Melting and Boiling Points
      2. Solubility
      3. Carbocations, Alkyl Radicals, and Carbanions
      4. Inductive Effects
      5. Resonance Stabilization
      6. Acidity
      7. Ring Strain

Summary of Key Concepts:

- Sigma (σ) bonds generally form through the end-on-end overlap of hybrid orbitals; pi (π) bonds form through the side-to-side overlap of unhybridized p orbitals.

- Saturated compounds have the general formula C_nH_{2n+2}; unsaturated molecules contain rings or π bonds.

- Compounds with the same molecular formula are known as *isomers*; structural, or constitutional isomers differ by the connectivity of atoms in the molecule.

- Conformational isomers differ by rotation around an σ bond.

- Stereoisomers have the same atom connectivity but different spatial orientation of atoms.

- Chiral molecules have chiral centers (carbon with four different substituents), are not superimposable on their mirror image, and rotate plane-polarized light.

- Enantiomers are non-superimposable mirror images and have opposite absolute configuration at all chiral centers.

- Enantiomers rotate plane-polarized light an equal magnitude, but in opposite direction, therefore a 50:50 mixture of enantiomers, or a racemic mixture, is not optically active.

- Diastereomers are stereoisomers that are not mirror images; they differ in absolute configuration for at least one, but not all carbons.

- Epimers are diastereomers that differ in absolute configuration at only one stereocenter.

- Geometric isomers are diastereomers that are *cis/trans* (or *Z/E*) pairs on a ring or double bond. When highest priority groups are on the same side of a ring or bond the molecule is *cis* (or *Z*); when they're on opposite sides, the compound is *trans* (or *E*).

- Meso compounds are achiral molecules with chiral centers and an internal mirror plane.

- As the substitution of carbocations and radicals increases, so does their stability due to the inductive effect; carbanions are more stable when they are less substituted.

- Resonance stabilization results from the ability of π electrons or charge to move and delocalize through a system of conjugated π bonds or unhybridized p orbitals.

III. **Substitution and Elimination Reactions**
  A. **Free Radical Halogenation**
    1. Initiation
    2. Propagation
    3. Termination
    4. Inhibition of Free Radical Halogenation
    5. Stereochemistry
    6. Stability of Radicals
    7. Selectivity
  B. **Nucleophilic Substitutions**
    1. Nucleophiles and Electrophiles
    2. S_N2 Reactions
    3. S_N1 Reactions
    4. Substitution Reactions of Ethers and Amines
  C. **Elimination Reactions**
    1. E1 Reactions
    2. E2 Reactions
  D. **Properties of Alcohols**
    1. Hydrogen Bonding
    2. Acidity
  E. **Formation of Alkyl Halides**
    1. Reactions of Alcohols with Phosphorus Halides
    2. Reactions of Alcohols with Thionyl Chloride

Summary of Key Concepts:

- Radical brominations are regioselective for tertiary bromides, while chlorinations yield mixtures of substitution products.

- All free radical halogenations are non-stereoselective, giving racemic mixtures of products when one new stereocenter is formed.

- Radical selectivity = product distribution/# of identical hydrogens.

- Nucleophiles are Lewis bases and are electron rich, while electrophiles are Lewis acids and are electron deficient.

- Nucleophiles are stronger when negatively charged, less electronegative, or larger in size.

- Leaving groups are more likely to leave as their stability in solution increases (uncharged and/ or larger groups are usually better LGs).

- More substituted substrates and protic solvents favor S_N1 over S_N2.

- Carbocation intermediates formed in either S_N1 or E1 reactions will rearrange if possible to form a more stable carbocation.

- Second order reactions (S_N2 or E2) require specific spatial orientations of the reacting species (S_N2 = backside attack of Nuc-; E2 = antiperiplanar conformation of H and LG).

- First order reactions (S_N1 or E1) do not depend on the concentration of the Nuc- or base.

- Eliminations break two σ bonds and form one π bond.

- Non-nucleophilic bases and heat favor eliminations over substitutions, and strong bases favor E2 over E1.

- Zaitsev's rule favors the formation of the more substituted bond in elimination reactions (E2 reactions must use small bases), and *trans* double bonds are favored over *cis*.

IV.   **Electrophilic Addition Reactions**
   A.   **Markovnikov Additions**
      1.   Electrophilic Additions and the Pi bond
      2.   H-X Addition Across a Bond
      3.   Acid-catalyzed Hydration of Alkenes
      4.   Oxymercuration-demercuration Reactions
   B.   **Anti-markovnikov Additions**
      1.   Hydroboration
      2.   HBr Addition in the Presence of Peroxides
   C.   **Other Electrophilic Additions**
      1.   Addition of Halogens to a π Bond
      2.   Epoxide Formation and Hydrolysis
      3.   Oxidation of π Bonds with Dilute $KMnO_4$
      4.   Hydrogenation of Alkenes and Alkynes
      5.   Ozonolysis
   D.   **Aromatic Compounds**
      1.   Hückel Numbers and Aromaticity
      2.   Electrophilic Aromatic Substitution

Summary of Key Concepts:

- The loosely held electrons in C=C π bonds can act as nucleophiles in addition reactions, which replace one π bond with two σ bonds.

- When p electrons attack electrophiles, the resulting carbocation will be on the more substituted carbon and yield the Markovnikov (more substituted) product.

- Addition reactions that put the new, non-hydrogen group on the less substituted carbon are termed anti-Markovnikov additions.

- Anti-addition puts two new substituents on opposite sides of the planar double bond, while syn-addition puts two new substituents on the same side of the planar double bond.

- Addition reactions are usually not stereospecific since the alkene is planar. Electrophiles will add with equal frequency to both faces of the bond, giving mixtures of enantiomers.

- Double bonds are split by ozonolysis, yielding two carbonyl-bearing compounds.

- Alkenes and alkynes can be hydrogenated by use of H_2 and metal catalysts.

- Aromatic compounds are cyclic, planar, conjugated (all sp^2 hybridized atoms), have $4^{n+2\pi}$ electrons, and are exceptionally stable.

- Under the influence of very strong electrophiles, aromatic electrons can be nucleophilic, resulting in aromatic substitution.

- Substituents that add electron density to a benzene ring are activating for substitution chemistry, and they favor reaction at *ortho* and *para* positions.

- Substituents that withdraw electron density from benzene are ring deactivating, and all but the halogens favor substitution at *meta* positions.

V.   **Nucleophilic Addition and Cycloaddition Reactions**
  A.   **Aldehydes and Ketones**
    1.   Addition of Oxidizing Agent to Primary and Secondary Alcohols
    2.   Acidity and Enolization
    3.   Keto-enol Tautomerism
  B.   **Nucleophilic Addition Reactions**
    1.   Addition of Reducing Agent to Ketones and Aldehydes
    2.   Organometallic Reagents
    3.   Wittig Reaction
    4.   Acetals and Hemiacetals
    5.   Imine Formation
    6.   Aldol Condensation
    7.   Conjugate Addition to α,β-Unsaturated Carbonyl Compounds
  C.   **Carboxylic Acids**
    1.   Acidity and Hydrogen Bonding
    2.   Inductive Effects on Carboxylic Acid Acidity
    3.   Decarboxylation Reactions of β-Keto Acids
    4.   Carboxylic Acid Derivatives
    5.   Esterification Reactions
  D.   **Cycloaddition Reactions**

Summary of Key Concepts:

- The C=O bond is very polarized due to the high electronegativity of oxygen, resulting in the carbon of the carbonyl group being electrophilic.

- Protons α to a carbonyl are acidic and can be removed by a strong base to yield a nucleophilic carbanion, or enolate.

- Keto-enol tautomerism is the rapid equilibration of the more stable keto form of a carbonyl and the less stable enol form where the α-proton shifts to the carbonyl oxygen.

- Nucleophilic additions involve the attack of a nucleophile on the carbon of an aldehyde or ketone; these reactions break one π bond to form two σ bonds.

- Hydride reduction, a type of nucleophilic addition, can convert ketones or aldehydes into alcohols; alcohols can be converted back to carbonyl compounds using oxidizing agents.

- An aldol condensation is a C—C bond forming reaction where the carbonyl carbon of one molecule is the electrophile, while the a-carbon of another carbonyl is the nucleophile.

- α,β-Unsaturated carbonyl compounds are electrophilic at the β-carbon and undergo Michael, or conjugate addition reactions.

- Acidity of carboxylic acids results from the resonance stability of the carboxylate anion.

- Electron withdrawing groups increase the acidity of carboxylic acids by stabilizing the negative charge of the carboxylate anion via the inductive effect.

- The reactivity of carboxylic acid derivatives decreases as follows: acid halide > acid anhydride > ester > amide.

- Nucleophilic addition to the carbonyl carbon in a carboxylic acid derivative is usually followed by elimination due to the presence of a good electronegative leaving group.

VI.   **Laboratory Techniques and Spectroscopy**
   A.   **Separations**
      1.   Extractions
      2.   Crystallization and Precipitation
      3.   Thin-layer (TLC) and Flash Chromatography
      4.   Gas Chromatography
      5.   Distillations
   B.   **Spectroscopy**
      1.   Infrared (IR) Spectroscopy
      2.   UV/Vis Spectroscopy
      3.   Proton (^{1}H) Nuclear Magnetic Resonance (NMR) Spectroscopy
      4.   Carbon (^{13}C) NMR

Summary of Key Concepts:

- Organic compounds are separated via extraction based on their differing solubility in polar (aqueous) or nonpolar (organic) solvents.

- Organic acids (COOHs and PhOHs) and bases (amines) can undergo acid-base reactions to generate ions, which preferentially dissolve in the aqueous layer during an extraction.

- Thin layer chromatography (TLC) separates molecules based on polarity; the more polar compound travels the least distance up the plate and has the lowest R_f value.

- Distillation and gas chromatography separate compounds based on boiling point.

- IR spectroscopy identifies the functional groups present in molecules.

- The most common IR resonances tested on the DAT are the C=O bond (~1700 cm^{-1}), the C=C bond (~1650 cm^{-1}), and the O–H bond (~3600 cm^{-1}).

Study Break

Before you move on to the next section, give yourself a break to clear your head and let this all soak in. Go for a walk, listen to a song you love, grab a snack— don't burn yourself out!

- The number of resonances in a ^{1}H NMR spectrum indicates the number of non-equivalent hydrogens present in a molecule.

- The number of Hs each signal represents is determined by the integration of the peak.

- Protons that are more deshielded (near electronegative groups) will be further downfield (at higher ppm), and protons that are more shielded (near electron donating groups) will be more upfield (at lower ppm).

- Splitting in a ^{1}H NMR spectrum occurs when one H has non-equivalent protons located on an adjacent atom (signal will be split into $n + 1$ lines; n = # of nonequivalent adjacent hydrogens).

- The number of resonances in a ^{13}C NMR spectrum indicates the number of non-equivalent carbons present in a molecule.

Reading Comprehension Test (RCT)

Chapter 17
Overview of the RCT

17.1 INTRODUCTION

The Reading Comprehension Test (RCT) on the OAT contains 50 questions that you must answer in 60 minutes. There are 3 passages, each of which has between 10 and 20 questions associated with it. Each passage has about 1500 words, and between 7 and 20 paragraphs. The questions are not in any particular order (for example, they are not arranged in the order that they appear in the passage, chronologically). The passages are extremely dense with information, usually (but not always!) about a science or health-related topic. Additionally, most students find that they do not have time to complete the section comfortably and must rush, at least to some extent, to complete the section in the allotted time.

No Outside Knowledge

One aspect of the RCT that is peculiar is that it does not test your knowledge of any particular subject area. While the Survey of Natural Sciences, for example, is supposed to test your knowledge of biology, general chemistry, and organic chemistry, the RCT is supposed to test your ability to "read, comprehend, and analyze...basic scientific information," according to ADA. What this means, in practical terms, is that everything that you need to know is in the passage. If the passage says it, it's true. If the passage doesn't say it, you can't use it as the basis for an answer. Don't bring in specialized knowledge from outside the passage for answering questions. (ADA, in their characteristic manner, puts this in the following fashion: "Prior understanding of the science topics is not a prerequisite to answering the test items.")

Also, while most passages are about topics that are at least somewhat related to a typical science undergraduate curriculum and thus might discuss information that you are already familiar with, don't worry if a passage is about a topic that you know less about. Even if the passage is about, say, pianos, all of the information that you need is in the passage. You don't have to be a consummate musician or professional piano tuner in order to answer RCT questions about a piano.

Self-Evaluation

So how do you study for a test that doesn't test your knowledge of something? Obviously, you can't approach studying for RCT the way that you approach studying for the SNS, physics, or QRT. You have to become familiar with the basic structure of the test, the common question types, and the essentials of eliminating answers. Then you have to practice. And practice. And practice. But simply doing lots of passages will not, in itself, help you, at least not much. You also have to review your work carefully. If you miss a question (or spend too long on a question), you have to figure out why, and how you can avoid doing so in the future when you see a similar question.

Often, when students are studying for the RCT, if they miss a question, they will say to themselves (once they've checked the answer and seen where it comes from in the passage), "Oh, well, all I have to do next time is just read a little more carefully." And then, the next time, when they miss more questions, they will make the same comment to themselves: "I'll just read more carefully next time." This continues, over and over.

This is not a specific enough plan for improvement. Formulating a better plan for improvement depends on figuring out where in the process things went wrong. Perhaps the comment should go something like this: "I only read the first few words of this answer before making up my mind that it was right, choosing it, and moving on, but the entire second half of the answer was wrong. What I will do in the future is read answer choices all the way to the end before making up my mind, and I will focus more closely on the way answer choices end, and not just how they begin, in order not to make the same sort of mistake."

Notice that this is still, in essence, "reading more carefully." However, it is specific enough that the student can probably do this, whereas "reading more carefully" is so vague that it is hard to accomplish. Be specific with your self-evaluation!

17.2 CORE STRATEGIES

Basic Approach for the RCT

For comprehensibility, we will split the strategies for the RCT into two parts, and we will start with the broadest, section strategy. The following is the **Basic Approach for the RCT** as a whole:

Step 1: Choose an order for the passages.
The passages are not of uniform difficulty, and, as discussed earlier, most students do not find that they can finish the entire test comfortably (and lose points by rushing too much). Thus, it is recommended that you do the passages in an order that you choose, rather than the order that is presented in the test. You can usually tell how hard a passage is going to be by reading the title and first sentence or two and glancing at the questions.

Thus, take about a minute at the beginning of the section to read the titles and first few sentences of each passage. To get from one passage to the next, you must press "Next" through all of the questions; as you are doing this, take a quick glance at each question, just to note whether it looks like a common question or a rare question type (discussed later). Based on this, quickly determine an order in which to work the passages.

Step 2: Work the passages in that order.
Begin with the first passage that you have chosen to do, and work it according to the Basic Approach for Passages given below. Then move to the second passage. If you have time, continue to the third passage.

Step 3: Inspect the section.
When the 5-minute warning pops up, consider where you are in the section. Unless you are completely certain that you will finish all questions in the time allotted, now is a good time to use the Review screen to check what remains unanswered and enter your guessing letter for those questions. Then return to where you were in the section and continue to work.

Basic Approach for Passages

Stepping down a level in scope, here is the **Basic Approach for Passages**:

Step 1: Skim read, and map the passage.

On the RCT, the passages are extremely long, and there are a great many questions about each one, with a fairly restrictive time limit. Thus, if you spent a great deal of time reading each passage before you got to the questions, you would not have anywhere near enough time to work the questions. However, the passages are also extremely thick with information, and it's certainly not possible to remember all the details from a quick read. Thus, you must read the passage relatively quickly and focus on main points and locating information, not on the mess of details. Ideally, this step takes no more than 3–4 minutes (closer to 3 minutes if you intend to finish 2.5–3 passages, close to 4 minutes if you intend to finish 2–2.5 passages).

As you are doing this, use your noteboard. For each paragraph, write the number of the paragraph and a word or two (no more than two) on the topic of the paragraph. Your goal is to summarize what the paragraph is about. Generating this **passage map** will tell you quickly what information is where. There is a good reason for doing this: the answer is usually straightforward if you are looking at the relevant portion of the passage. However, none of the questions contain line or paragraph references, and they are not in any useful order. Thus, the primary goal of an initial reading of the passage is to read quickly and create a map that can guide you through the questions.

You will also have the option of highlighting the passage (anything from a single word to a full paragraph) and these yellow highlights will be retained as you navigate around the RCT section. You can use highlighted words or phrases to generate a passage map, but be critical in what you highlight. Again, your goal is to generate a table of contents for each paragraph, or a map of what is where.

Step 2: Work the questions.

Proceed through the questions more or less in order, skipping questions if they look confusing or time-consuming or if you have no idea where in the passage to look for the answer. (Come back to these questions before you move on to the next passage.) For each question, read it carefully to make sure that you understand what it's asking. Remember that you can highlight key words in the question stem if this will help you keep track of what the question is asking. Next, refer back to the relevant part of the passage and figure out what the answer will have to say or do, and come back to the answer choices. Now it is time for POE.

In the RCT, if there are five answers, knowing that four answers are wrong is a good way to find the correct answer, especially on harder questions. Furthermore, while several of the answers may superficially look tempting, all but one will be flawed, so looking for the right answer is less reliable than finding four wrong answers. Process Of Elimination (POE) is a crucial element of your strategy. Doing POE in your head is slow and likely to cause problems, so be sure to use the strike out function available on the computer (right click). Eliminate answers until only one remains, and choose the last answer standing (after reading it to make sure it makes sense).

When you are doing POE on challenging questions, use the **Two Pass Technique:** the first time you are going through the answer choices, eliminate the worst options. Keep anything you're not sure about, tempting answer choices, options that look good, and keep anything you don't understand. You can probably work relatively quickly on your first pass. When you're down to two or three tempting answer choices, go back and do a second pass: slow down, pay attention and read carefully. You can use a **comparison strategy** to find the best answer. Compare the remaining choices to the passage, the question stem, and each other. One of these comparisons will help you see that one answer choice is the best one there and the others have something wrong with them.

There are several common patterns for wrong answer choices. Watch for these as you're doing POE on your practice passages. Spend some time thinking about which ones from the list below you find particularly tempting:

- Not supported: when an answer choice contains information that was not in the passage, goes beyond the passage, or requires background information.
- Not relevant: when an answer choice contains irrelevant information from the passage. These answer choices sometimes contain statements from the wrong part of the passage, or common words from the passage. Remember, just because a statement is true and from the passage, doesn't mean it actually answers the question
- Wrong scope or tone: when an answer choice is too specific or too general to answer the questions, or is too extreme. Look out for words like only, solely, no, none, all, always, never, every, must, etc.
- Partially correct: when an answer is partially correct, it can be really tempting. However, be sure you read answers choices through to the end. If they're partially wrong, they're all wrong and you should strike that option out.
- Contradicts the passage: sometimes an answer option will contradict something in the passage, meaning it is not the correct answer. Read answer choices carefully: adding one small word (such as "no" or "not") or slightly modifying a word (such as changing "typical" to "atypical") can mean a statement says the exact opposite of what it did before.
- Wrong direction or opposite: be careful not to pick a true statement on a false question, or vice versa. Also be careful when you're doing POE on least, most, not, and except question stems. Highlighting these key words in the question stem may help you keep track of what the question is asking.

Be aware that the primary skill that the RCT is testing is **scanning**. Scanning is a particular type of reading that involves searching for a key word or phrase. For example, if a question asks about John Hunter, and John Hunter appeared only in one part of the passage, then the most reliable way to answer that question is to find "John Hunter" in the passage. If you have no idea where to look, you have to scan across the entire passage until you find the name. In this case, "John Hunter" is a **lead word**, a word or phrase that leads you to the appropriate part of the passage. In general, your passage map should allow you to confine your scanning to a small portion of the passage, which will help you save time.

17.3

17.3 WORKING QUESTIONS

Question Strategy

First, let's review fundamental question strategy and discuss in further detail some of the crucial aspects.

In working each question, you should:

1. Read the question carefully and make sure that you understand what it's asking.
2. Refer back to the relevant part of the passage and figure out what the answer will have to say/do.
3. Eliminate answers until only one remains.

Sometimes students struggle with reading the question carefully after having just read the passage so quickly. However, while you do not need every last detail of the passage on an initial reading, you do need to notice every word of a question, because if it is phrased in a slightly peculiar way, there is probably a reason. Thus, you must change gears when you reach the questions.

The second step is vital to a degree that is hard to overstate. The person who wrote the questions for the passage that you're reading was looking right at a particular part of the passage when he or she wrote the question and the right and wrong answers. At the time, it was clear to him or her what the answer was, based on looking at this part of the passage. In order for it to be clear to you which answers are right and which are wrong, you should be looking at the same part of the passage. Thus, *find it!* Determine lead words in the question stem, try to locate the relevant area of the passage from your notes, and then scan for those lead words in the passage.

Also, by the time you are done reading the relevant portion of the passage—which usually involves not only the sentence or two that contain the words of interest, but also the context, which often extends a sentence or two before and a sentence or two after the bit that was referenced, so you should probably just re-read the entire paragraph mentioned in the question—you should have a reasonably good idea what the answer needs to be. At first, you should practice answering questions in your own words (or, when the answer should be exactly what the passage says, in the passage's own words) to work on this. Over time, it will probably become so automatic that you do not need to work on it consciously anymore.

Finally, even if one answer looks superficially tempting, you must not simply choose that answer and move on without at least glancing at the rest of the answers. Likewise, if two answers look tempting, don't just guess between them without forming a solid reason to eliminate one and choose the other. This test is constructed such that many of the answers look vaguely similar to a right answer, but only one will have no flaws that make it wrong. POE is fundamental, perhaps more fundamental than any other single strategy on the RCT.

Retrieval

By far, the most common type of question on the RCT is the **Retrieval** question, which asks something to the effect of, "What did the passage say about [x]?" The next most common is the **Inference** question, which asks, "What did the passage suggest about [x]?" (Inference questions may also use the words "imply" or "infer.") On either type of question, the right answer can consist of either the **exact words** of the passage about that subject or **a close paraphrase** of the passage, although the former is more common on Retrieval questions and the latter more common on Inference questions. To illustrate, consider the following excerpt (from a much longer passage) and example question about this portion:

The platypus was first reported to Europeans in 1798 by Vice-Admiral John Hunter, a British naval officer and second governor of New South Wales, Australia. In 1797, he watched a local Australian observe a platypus for over an hour and then kill it with a spear. After this, he sent a remarkably accurate description back to Britain. In 1799, George Shaw gave the platypus its scientific name, *Platypus anatinus* (which was changed later to *Ornithorhynchus anatinus*), and in 1800, Thomas Bewick, a British wood engraver, circulated an image of the strange creature.

At first, many thought it was an elaborate hoax...

1. Who gave the platypus the name *Platypus anatinus*?

    A. John Hunter
    B. Thomas Bewick
    C. George Shaw
    D. A local Australian

Notice that this question asks for something that the passage outright says, so we expect the exact words of the passage to be the right answer. According to the middle of the excerpt, "George Shaw gave the platypus its scientific name, *Platypus anatinus*," so the answer must be George Shaw. That eliminates everything but (C). Many of the questions on the RCT will be this straightforward.

Inference

However, some questions on the RCT will require a little more matching of meaning, rather than matching words. Consider the following example:

Among venomous mammals, most bite in order to deliver their venom into victims. This is the method employed by venomous shrews, solenodons, and moles. The slow loris can also deliver a toxin via a bite, although its status as "venomous" is not without controversy. The platypus, however, attacks with spurs on its legs to deliver its cocktail of poisons. The venom can kill smaller animals, and while it is not strong enough to be deadly to humans, it can cause extreme pain. In contrast to the bites of certain snakes and spiders, platypus stings do not cause necrosis...

2. Which of the following does the passage suggest about venomous mammals?

A. The bite of a venomous shrew causes extreme pain.
B. Some people dispute that the slow loris is venomous.
C. The platypus is more poisonous than other mammals.
D. The platypus uses its poison to kill prey during hunting.
E. A single poison is responsible for the effects of the platypus's sting.

In this case, because the question is more open-ended, it is hard to predict what the answer will be. The passage indicates many things about venomous mammals. Use POE. Eliminate (A), because it garbles two parts of the passage: According to the second-to-last sentence, the bite of a platypus causes extreme pain, but no explicit connections is made between that effect and the effect of the bite of a venomous shrew (in the second sentence). Choice (B) matches the third sentence adequately, so leave it alone for the moment. Eliminate (C), because no comparison of degree of poison was made in the passage, so to say that the platypus is "more poisonous" is not justified. Eliminate (D), because no reference was made to hunting or any related behavior, so no such conclusion can be drawn (in fact, the platypus actually uses the spurs for self-defense). Eliminate (E), because the passage describes the venom as a "cocktail" of poisons in the fourth sentence, which means that there is more than one. Thus, the answer must be (B).

Notice that B is not particularly a logical leap away from the passage. The passage says about the slow loris that "its status as 'venomous' is not without controversy," and this answer says that some people dispute this. These are close paraphrases, even if they are not the same exact words. Bear in mind that the *meaning* is the most important thing, not the words. Many of the wrong answers repeat some of the words of the passage, but only one will mean the same thing as what the passage said.

It is particularly important to note that the right answer to this question is not much of a leap from the passage since the word "suggest" might make you think that you have license to make stuff up. Maybe the passage doesn't *say* that the platypus is more poisonous than other mammals, but doesn't it *suggest* it? Or maybe the passage doesn't say that the bite of a venomous shrew causes extreme pain, but doesn't it *suggest* it? The answer is no. If the passage doesn't say it, it doesn't say it. The same is true of words such as "imply" and "infer," as well.

Think of it this way: this is a standardized test. They can't make things up. If you decided that their question was fraudulent and unfair and sued them, they would have to be able to stand in court before a judge and defend their question, and they know it. They don't write questions for which their only defense would be, "But Your Honor, doesn't (B) just *feel* cosmically right?" They write questions for which their defense would be, "Your Honor, if you read the third sentence of the paragraph, you will clearly see that (B) is supported more than any of the others." They would be able to rattle off specific reasons that the rest of the answers are wrong (such as "more poisonous" in (C)). You should hold yourself to the same standard: You must be able to point to the part of the passage that supports the answer you are about to choose, and, equally, find the wrong parts of the answers that you are eliminating.

Because you need to find something directly stated in the passage, answering retrieval questions will be doable once you've found your strategy and have had lots of practice. Inference questions are usually more challenging and take a bit more time.

You will also see open-ended questions on the OAT. These questions ask things like "Which of the following is true based on information in the passage?" They give you no information on where to go in the passage, and often the answer choices are from different parts of the passage. Because of this, these questions require POE and take time. You may want to mark these questions and come back to them later, once you've worked with the passage a little more.

17.4 OTHER QUESTION TYPES

While the overwhelming majority (generally more than 80%) of questions on the RCT are of the Retrieval or Inference variety, there are some other questions that are asked with some frequency, and these deserve a close look here. Bear in mind that the most common of these are the New Information and Two Parts questions, of which you are likely to see a few on any given RCT. The others may or may not show up at all, but they are here for completeness.

New Information

Sometimes a question will provide new information in the question stem and ask you a question about the new information, informed by what is already in the passage. This is a **New Information** question. In general, you must first determine how the information relates to the passage, and then you can use POE aggressively. Consider the following example:

Among venomous mammals, most bite in order to deliver their venom into victims. This is the method employed by venomous shrews, solenodons, and moles. The slow loris can also deliver a toxin via a bite, although its status as "venomous" is not without controversy. The platypus, however, attacks with spurs on its legs to deliver its cocktail of poisons. The venom can kill smaller animals, and while it is not strong enough to be deadly to humans, it can cause extreme pain. In contrast to the bites of certain snakes and spiders, platypus stings do not cause necrosis…

3. The New Guinean quoll is a very small mammal. Which of the following can be concluded about it on the basis of the information in the passage?

A. It is not venomous.
B. It sometimes bites humans.
C. Its habitat overlaps with that of the platypus.
D. It is closely related to the platypus.
E. It could be killed by a platypus sting.

Notice that the first sentence provides the new information: the New Guinean quoll is a very small mammal. Now, find anything relevant in the passage. It is tempting just to latch onto the word "mammal" and read the first few sentences of the passage. However, this might be misleading. The word "small" may also be important, which relates to the portion, "The venom can kill smaller animals." Bear this in mind as you eliminate answers.

While (A) may be tempting (and true by outside knowledge), it goes beyond what the passage says. The passage lists certain poisonous mammals but never says that these are the only ones. Thus, based on the information given, the quoll could be poisonous. Eliminate (A). Also, eliminate (B), because this is never mentioned anywhere; even the biting animals in the passage are not described as biting humans in particular. Eliminate (C), because this part of the passage does not give enough information to determine the habitat of the platypus. (Strictly speaking, if the earlier excerpt were from the same part of the passage, we could determine that the habitat of the platypus includes Australia, and the name "New Guinean" implies that the habitat of this type of quoll includes New Guinea. These are near each other but not necessarily overlapping, so the answer is still wrong.) Eliminate (D), because no biological or evolutionary relationship was described in the passage or question. At this point, hopefully it's (E), because everything else is gone, and indeed it is: the passage indicated that the platypus's venom could kill small animals, and the question stem indicates that the New Guinean quoll is a small mammal. Thus, the quoll could be killed by a platypus sting.

In general, the right answer will do what this right answer does, namely, relate the passage and the new information in the question stem accurately. If the answer does not come from the passage or is not relevant to the new information in the question stem, it is likely wrong.

Two Parts

A **Two Parts** question usually provides a statement and a reason (though it can occasionally provide two separate statements) and asks both whether they are true and whether they are related. Begin with the first consideration: Are they true or not? Once you have decided that, you can continue determining whether they are related. Consider the following example:

At first, many thought it was an elaborate hoax, because of its exotic appearance and characteristics. Like a duck, the platypus has a long, flat, broad bill. Also like a duck, it has webbed feet, and when on land, it must walk on its knuckles to avoid damaging the webbing. Onlookers observe that when it walks, it looks more like a reptile, since its feet are lateral to its body instead of underneath. Like a beaver, it has a paddle-shaped tail. Its body, however, is shaped like an otter's body. As a result, when a skin of a dead platypus was shipped back to Britain as one of the first pieces of evidence that such animals existed, the first to see it speculated that it had been sewn together by a taxidermist. However, they soon found out that this animal was genuine, and its other odd abilities included laying eggs and manufacturing poison.

Among venomous mammals…

4. British experts still living in Europe were skeptical that early specimens of the platypus were genuine because it walks like a reptile, not like most mammals.

    A. Both the statement and the reason are true, and they are related.
    B. Both the statement and the reason are true, but they are unrelated.
    C. The statement is true, but the reason is not true.
    D. The statement is not true, but the reason is true.
    E. Neither the statement nor the reason is true.

First, determine whether the first part (the statement) is true. It definitely is, because the first sentence of the excerpt says so, and the last two sentences of the paragraph confirm it. Thus, you can eliminate (D) and (E), since these say that the statement is not true. Next, check whether the second part (the reason) is true. It is true, too, since the fourth sentence of the excerpt indicates this. Thus, eliminate (C), because it says that the reason is not true. Now, you must decide whether the two statements are related. The passage indicates that the British in Europe were inspecting the "skin of a dead platypus" and suspected that it had been "sewn together by a taxidermist." Thus, they had to have been looking at the bizarre features of the body, such as the duck bill and feet, the beaver tail, and the otter body. More specifically, it was a skin, not a live animal, so they could not see it walk. (The passage specifically notes that "[o]nlookers" are the ones who observe its strange gait, which does not include experts speculatively reconstructing the appearance of the body in motion from a skin. Granted, some scientists have tried to infer how animals walked from their dead remains, such as fossils, but we have no evidence that happened here.) Thus, its method of walking could not have been fuel for their skepticism. Eliminate (A), and the answer must be (B).

Notice, by the way, that if either of the statements had been false, you could have eliminated both (A) and (B) and would not have had to determine whether the statements were related. This is the reason to determine the statements' truth first and their relationship later. Indeed, some Two Parts questions do not even ask whether the statements are related.

Tone/Attitude

Occasionally, a **Tone/Attitude** question will ask about the author's, well, tone or attitude. The author's tone or attitude will be revealed in the author's word choice. Words that indicate positive or negative value judgments or indicate agreement or disagreement are tone words, and such words will help you answer these questions. Consider the following example:

Recent research has located these peculiar features within the genome of the platypus. Because the evolution of monotremes, including the platypus and the echidna, split from that of all other mammals before the development of many non-reptilian features, such as viviparity, many unusual characteristics of the platypus come from genetic similarities to reptiles. This promising research has opened up the possibility of deeper understanding both of the platypus itself, which has always been difficult to study due to the animal's shy and reclusive nature, and of its relation to other animals…

5. The author's attitude toward recent research on the platypus can best be described as

A. Cynical
B. Shy
C. Confused
D. Optimistic
E. Apathetic

The question asks for the author's attitude toward the recent research, so search the passage for tone words. Until the last sentence of the excerpt, not much tone is indicated, but the final sentence describes the research as "promising" and points out that it "has opened up the possibility of deeper understanding" that "has always been difficult" to achieve. These are all good things, so the passage is generally positive towards the research and believes that it can do good things in the future. Next, evaluate answers.

Eliminate (A), which means skeptical of others' motives or the value of something, so it is completely off the mark. While (B) is a word that is used in the passage, it is used of the platypus, not of the author, so it is also wrong. Choice (C) may be how you feel after reading some particularly dense RCT passages, but it is almost never how authors feel about their subjects (if they were confused, they would figure out what they're talking about before writing about it), so not only is it wrong here, but it is also probably never going to be the right answer on any question. Choice (D) is fine, so leave it. Choice (E) means not caring or lacking interest, so it, too, is almost certainly never going to be the right answer to any question about the attitude of the author (authors care about their subjects, even if no one else does). Thus, (D) is the best answer.

Notice that this question asks about something that might not seem very concrete ("attitude"), but the answer must still be based on the words in the passage. Even a question about tone or attitude is not an excuse to make stuff up. The answer is in the passage, no matter how buried in a mass of details. It has to be there, somewhere, and your task is to find it.

Insertion

Very rarely, you may be asked to insert something into some portion of the passage, usually a final sentence. This is an **Insertion** question, and your goal is to be as close to what the passage has already said as possible. The right answer will be as redundant with the rest of the passage as it can be; it will not take the passage in a crazy, new direction or contradict information already presented in the passage. You are trying to summarize and support what has already been said. Consider the following example:

...This promising research has opened up the possibility of deeper understanding both of the platypus itself, which has always been difficult to study due to the animal's shy and reclusive nature, and of its relation to other animals.

One result that has arisen in the past few years from such research is the discovery that platypus sex determination in some way resembles the system in birds. In any mammal, including the platypus, the homogametic sex is female, with two X chromosomes, and the heterogametic sex is male, with an X and a Y. In birds, the homogametic sex is male, with two Z chromosomes, and the heterogametic sex is female, with a Z and a W. However, the platypus's X chromosome shows remarkable homology with a bird's Z chromosome, suggesting that the differences between the sex chromosomes in other mammals, such as humans, and those in birds evolved later than was previously thought, after the split between monotremes and other mammals.

Other genetic studies have yielded similarly remarkable results, and experiments continue with remarkable speed.

6. Which of the following sentences would be best to insert at the end of the passage?

   A. The confusion that early biologists had regarding the platypus also inspired the title of *Kant and the Platypus*, a book regarding how humans perceive the things around us.

   B. It is also remarkable that when threatened, the platypus can also emit low growls as well as use its leg stinger.

   C. However, such experiments should be considered with skepticism, given the ongoing uncertainty whether the platypus is in fact a hoax.

   D. Although we have come a long way from the early British explorers who doubted the platypus's authenticity, research continues into this odd but fascinating creature.

The passage concludes with paragraphs regarding the research into the platypus's genes, so the correct answer will likely relate to platypus gene research. The rest of the passage, as we've seen up to this point, had to do with how strange and exotic the platypus is and how this utterly flummoxed the first Europeans to encounter it, so there is a pretty good chance that this, too, will show up in the right answer. Given this, evaluate the answers.

Eliminate (A), because while this relates somewhat to the beginning of the passage about the early biologists, this is a complete non sequitur from the end of the passage. It has nothing to do with the genetic research and instead brings up problems of perception. Eliminate (B), even though it is probably not wise to argue with a growling platypus, because this sentence's only connection with the end of the passage is the fact that this is "remarkable" (which is a tenuous connection at best). Eliminate (C), because it contradicts much of the rest of the passage. There is no "ongoing uncertainty whether the platypus is in fact a hoax" anymore; this was a problem in the early history of the study of the platypus, not now. The answer is (D) because this relates both to the beginning of the passage about the confusion of the British explorers and to the end of the passage about the genetic research.

In general, on Insertion questions, relevance is the most crucial issue. Is the sentence still on topic, or does it veer off in a strange new direction? Does it match the sorts of things that were said before, or does it seem to contradict them? Keep to the central points of the passage and the point of view that the author has already expressed. In this way, even if the right answer says something that is not exactly what the passage has already said, your answer will still be based on the text of the passage, which it must be in order to be right. This is not an exercise in creative writing; it's a Reading Comprehension Test.

Miscellaneous

From time to time, the RCT will ask questions that are not easy to categorize, because they differ from each other. Make sure to read these **Miscellaneous** questions carefully, because they may ask strange things that differ in some ways from the above. Always bear in mind that the right answer must be based on the text of the passage, and it will generally agree in tone and main point with what the author has already said. Consider the following example:

Few animals have caused the sheer amount of confusion and consternation that the platypus has. Even the name itself is strange. Although the casual layperson might expect the plural of "platypus" to be "platypi," in the same way that the plural of "cactus" is "cacti," this turns out to be incorrect. The word "cactus" is derived from the Greek cactos, which in Greek has a plural of cactoi that in Latin becomes cacti and is retained in English. The word "platypus," on the other hand, is derived from a Greek compound platypos that in Greek has a plural of platypodes. Thus, in English, we might count "one platypus," "two platypodes." However, this is so strange that English speakers sometimes discard this notion and use the English plural "platypuses" rather than the Greek. The fact that we can hardly even speak about the platypus without confusion is no surprise when one considers the unique history and biology of the animal, which is equally baffling.

The platypus was first reported to Europeans in 1798...

7. The author mentions the plural of the word "platypus" most likely in order to

A. lament the inconsistencies of the English language.
B. correct a common misunderstanding.
C. present himself as a linguistic expert.
D. argue in favor of the English plural "platypuses."
E. illustrate a confounding subject of study.

17.4

This question asks about the author's purpose in mentioning the plural. The passage introduces the topic by mentioning how much "confusion and consternation" there has been around the platypus, and it concludes by mentioning, "the unique history and biology of the animal...is equally baffling." Thus, the point that the passage makes about the plural is that it is confusing and strange in exactly the same way as the animal is. Now eliminate answers.

Eliminate (A), because it misses the essential point of this example. The point that the author makes is not about language, but about biology. The platypus's name is just one example of how strange it is. Eliminate (B), because it also is about language, not biology. The author's point is not just that the plural of "platypus" is not "platypi"; his point is that the confusion surrounding this is much like the confusion about the nature of the animal itself. Eliminate (C), because this, too, focuses excessively on linguistics, and besides, one does not have to be a linguistics expert to know one's etymology. Eliminate (D), because the author never does this anywhere. The answer is (E), because the discussion of the plural shows one example of how strange the platypus is, which is what (E) brings up.

Miscellaneous questions in particular and rare question types in general tend to be testing higher-level comprehension than straight Retrieval and Inference questions. Where a Retrieval question typically asks you to fetch the exact wording of the passage and an Inference question typically asks you to fetch the meaning of a particular sentence, Miscellaneous questions often depend on understanding the author's point. This is still not a huge leap from the passage. Focus on synthesizing or summarizing what you've read and what you know about the passage. Answering these questions near the end of the questions for this passage can be helpful. Finally, don't panic: these questions are rare and you may not see even one on the test that you take.

Here are some additional types of Miscellaneous questions:

- **Meaning in Context:** asks about the meaning of a word or phrase in the context of the passage. Go back to the passage and read a few lines above and a few lines below the term you're being asked about. Predict what it means or why it is there, and focus on use in the passage instead of on general definitions.

- **Purpose:** asks about the purpose of the passage, a paragraph, an example, a phrase, or a word. Find it in the passage, predict the answer (in general terms), and do POE with the answer choices. Ask yourself "why is that there?".

- **Main Point:** asks for the author's thesis, conclusion or main point. Focus on the big picture of the passage and POE. The best answer will address the whole passage, but focusing on the first and last paragraph may help. Ask yourself why the author wrote the passage. What are they trying to convince you of?

17.5   PACE IN RCT

Difficulty Level of Questions

You must remember that all questions are worth 1 point, no matter how long you spend working on them! Many questions in the RCT will be doable: you will be able to work quickly and confidently. You will use your passage map to find the content you need in the passage and you will be able to quickly find the right answer and move on. These questions are good to do right away (these are your "now" questions), because they boost your confidence and allow you to gain familiarity with the passage. They often have clear question stems and short answer options.

Some retrieval questions will take more time: sometimes the question stems gives you clear information on where to go, but the answer choices are longer and you need to carefully read each one and do POE. In other questions, the question stem gives you no information on where to go, so the answer is hard to find. Once you find it in the passage however, you can answer the question really quickly. You should also slow down when working on inference questions, and remember to stay within the scope of the passage. The questions we're talking about here are your "later" questions. Mark them on your first pass through the passage and come back to them when you're done with the "now" questions.

Finally, some questions on the RCT are going to be just plain hard. They will take you a long time to answer or maybe you never feel completely confident about the answer you end up picking. These questions are often open-ended or application questions, include content from all over the passage, and require effective POE skills. These time-wasting questions are good candidates for "never" questions. Get used to recognizing these so you save them for last, or skip them completely.

No matter what, make sure you've answered all the questions for a given passage before you move on to another passage.

Skipping Questions in RCT

Some test takers don't have time to answer every RCT question, and that is okay. Many students aim to complete 2 and a half passages with high accuracy, instead of rushing through all three passages and making silly mistakes. Another option is aiming to get through all three passages but skipping a couple (the hardest) questions on each. Either way, make sure you're working at a pace on test day that ensures you're getting questions you're working on correct. To do this, find and do the "now" questions on your first pass, and "later" questions on your second pass. Identify and skip the "never" questions and answer them using your Letter of the Day. Note, that you must skip the hardest questions; don't spend any time on these questions, just select your Letter of the Day and move on.

READING COMPREHENSION DRILL

PASSAGE 1: KOMODO DRAGON

1. The Komodo dragon, also known as the Komodo monitor, is the largest living reptile species in the world. Like the famed Galapagos tortoise, the largest living tortoise species in the world, the Komodo dragon has two competing (but non-exclusive) explanations for its great size. One is island gigantism. According to this explanation, mainland lizards are kept from growing larger by predators. Larger lizards are more visible and are eaten. On an island with few existing large predators, however, no such evolutionary pressure to stay small exists. On the contrary, a larger lizard can eat larger prey that otherwise would have no predators. Thus, islands that lack large predators will evolve them, possibly from animals that are not normally large elsewhere.

2. The other explanation is relict survival. There were many large animals among the Australasian megafauna of the Pleistocene, most of which went extinct about 40,000 years ago. The Komodo dragon evolved alongside other giant monitor lizards, such as *Varanus priscus,* which may have been 7 or 8 meters long. However, lizards were not the only giant animals of the era and region. *Bullockornis planei,* the so-called "Demon Duck of Doom," was a duck or duck-like animal that stood approximately 2.5 meters tall. *Diprotodon* was a genus of marsupial related to the wombat or koala but of the size and appearance of a rhinoceros or hippopotamus. *Meiolania* was a turtle half again as large as the Galapagos tortoise. *Procoptodon* was a giant kangaroo that likely stood over 2 meters tall. Unlike the preceding animals, a few Australiasian megafauna survived to the present day. The goanna and the saltwater crocodile are two enormous reptile species that, like the Komodo dragon, are still alive. The emu, the red kangaroo, and the Australian Giant Cuttlefish are all extant species of very large animals in the Australian region.

3. Most living megafauna are endangered or threatened. There are perhaps 5,000 Komodo dragons living on Komodo and other nearby islands, though their numbers may be jeopardized by a lack of breeding females. The Indonesian islands that are home to the dragons are very near the equator, so they remain warm year-round, which is essential to the health of the dragons' eggs. Although the dragons are excellent swimmers, they do not often move from one island to another.

4. The dragons are obviously physically striking. They can grow as long as 3 meters and 136 kilograms, though their average length is approximately 2.5 meters and somewhat under 100 kilograms, and they live approximately 30 years in the wild. Half of their length is taken up by tail, and the other half is body. When prey ascends a tree to escape, young dragons can clamber up after it, while older dragons can stand on their hind legs and balance with their tails to reach the prey. Dragon skin is usually grayish brown, tough, and scaly, though sometimes it is a dirt-colored red.

5. Each individual has approximately 60 teeth that grow up to 2.5 centimeters in length, which are effective in tearing flesh. Komodo dragon teeth are viciously serrated, like those of a flesh-eating shark, such as the great white. Unlike humans, who have a baby set of teeth and an adult set of teeth, Komodo dragons lose their teeth continuously throughout their life. Whenever their teeth are worn down or dulled, they are replaced with new teeth in order to keep their ripping and tearing capacity. Dragons also have sharp claws, which they use to rend prey.

6. Komodo dragons do not rely exclusively on the damage their teeth and claws can do in order to kill prey. Their saliva, which is usually reddish from the dragon's own blood, contains an incredible variety of virulent pathogens. They have what appear to be venom glands, although it is not clear whether venom plays a role in bites. A bite from a dragon is usually followed by severe infection. Humans experience swelling followed by shooting pains; most other animals likely experience similar symptoms. The dragon follows its bitten victim until the infection renders it completely helpless, usually within 24 hours, and then the dragon feeds. As a result, while the dragon is capable of brief, rapid sprints, it usually employs these to achieve an initial bite, not to finish off prey. The dragon has a flexible head and jaws, and when an animal is sufficiently weakened, a dragon can place it between its jaws and slam it into a tree so as to force it down the dragon's throat.

7. The dragon can track prey even if the prey runs a long distance away, because the dragon has an acute sense of smell. The dragon primarily uses a vomeronasal organ, rather than its nostrils. It sticks out its long, forked tongue, swinging its head from side to side, and then retracts the tongue and touches it to the back of its mouth; thereby it can detect smells even at a great distance. Its other senses are not very sharp: It can hear, but only at a limited range of frequencies, and it can see, but it is thought not to see well when light is limited, such as at night.

8. Komodo dragons usually feed on carrion, and they can smell dead or dying prey at distances of several kilometers. However, when prey that is already dying is not available, they will attack prey with teeth and claws. They eat a wide variety of different animals, regularly including deer and other mammals, but also sometimes birds, other reptiles, and insects. Humans tend to make them skittish and likely to retreat, which makes them more difficult to study, but a few dragons are not afraid and will eat humans. They also will dig up shallow graves. They swallow most prey whole, regurgitating hair, teeth, and horns in mucus. They cannot digest bones either, but these are generally excreted. Dragons have slow metabolisms, so they can subsist on as few as a dozen meals per year when necessary. They can speed digestion by lying in the sun.

9.   The dragons may be monogamous, which is rare among reptiles. Mating season typically begins shortly before the Southern Hemisphere's winter and continues to its end. Eggs are laid in September and hatch in the following April. Clutches contain around 20 eggs. Dragons struggle their way out of the eggs with the aid of egg teeth, which drop out soon after hatching. Newly hatched dragons are quite vulnerable to predators and even to cannibalistic adult dragons; one survey suggests that young dragons represent as much as 10% of a typical adult dragon's diet. As a result, young dragons spend much of their time in trees. They also spread out from their hatching place. This may be to reduce competition when they become adults or to reduce the possibility of inbreeding. Other than for reproduction, dragons are normally solitary.

10.   Female dragons are capable of parthenogenesis in addition to normal sexual reproduction. Females produce several cells in meiosis that can become egg cells. Usually all but one of these is reabsorbed, but occasionally one will act like a sperm and fertilize an egg. The result is not a clone of the mother, since her genes are shuffled in the process. Consider the analogous situation with a hypothetical human parthenogenesis. If a brown-eyed mother were heterozygous with a blue-eye gene, then she could create two cells that each had brown-eye genes, two cells that had blue-eye genes, or one cell of each. Only the third possibility would produce a child with the same eye color genes as the mother.

11.   One obvious difference between Komodo dragon mother and child is that parthenogenically produced dragon offspring are all male. This is a consequence of the WZ system of sex determination in reptiles: Unlike the XY system, in which the heterozygous XY is male and the homozygous XX is female, in the WZ system, the homozygous ZZ is male and the heterozygous WZ is female (and the WW is unviable, just as a YY is unviable among humans). In parthenogenesis, when the egg is fertilized, it duplicates its sex-determining chromosome. Thus, a WZ mother produces either unviable WW or male ZZ offspring. Nonetheless, even though the child is not a clone, parthenogenesis may threaten genetic diversity.

12.   The first Western expedition to retrieve Komodo dragons was undertaken in 1926. Sightings of dragons had been reported at least since 1912, but no one had been able to retrieve physical evidence of the dragons' existence. William Douglas Burden, an American from the wealthy Vanderbilt family and a representative of the American Museum of National History, led a group to Komodo and took two live dragons back to the New York Zoo. He published a sensationalist book about his adventures in the following year, describing several near brushes with deadly dragons and the difficulties of keeping the dragons captured once they were initially trapped. More than once, a dragon appeared to be restrained but escaped. Burden's exciting stories inspired further scientific investigations into the Komodo dragon as soon as the following year, as well as significant popular curiosity. They also were among the inspirations for the 1933 movie, *King Kong.* While the dragon has been known to science for a century, investigations are ongoing, and surprisingly little is known about this provocative and fascinating species.

1. According to the passage, which of the following is a reason Komodo dragons are difficult to study in the wild?

    A. They spend most of their time camouflaged in treetops.
    B. They are aggressive toward humans and require extensive safety precautions.
    C. They are hard to distinguish from other gigantic island reptiles.
    D. Humans make them skittish and likely to hide or act defensively.
    E. They are nearly extinct in the wild.

2. Which of the following can be inferred about the goanna?

    A. It went extinct about 40,000 years ago.
    B. It is a large reptile still found in Australia and surroundings.
    C. It can reproduce parthenogenically.
    D. It was the so-called "Demon Duck of Doom."
    E. It lives approximately 30 years in the wild.

3. In which of the following years did William Douglas Burden publish a book about his expedition to Komodo?

    A. 1912
    B. 1926
    C. 1927
    D. 1933

4. Komodo dragons inhabit

    A. only Komodo Island.
    B. only Komodo and other nearby islands.
    C. only Australia.
    D. only mainland Southeast Asia and Indonesian islands.
    E. southeast Asia, Indonesian islands, and Australia.

5. A Komodo dragon egg was refrigerated on its way from Komodo to the United States. Which of the following is most likely to be true about the dragon that hatches from this egg?

    A. It is unhealthy.
    B. It is small.
    C. It is immature.
    D. It is strong.
    E. It is particularly vicious.

6. According to the passage, approximately how long does a Komodo dragon egg take to hatch?

    A. 1 month
    B. 4 months
    C. 7 months
    D. 9 months
    E. 12 months

7. How long is an average Komodo dragon's tail?

    A. 0.5 m
    B. 1 m
    C. 1.25 m
    D. 1.5 m
    E. 2 m

8. Each of the following is part of a typical Komodo dragon's diet except:

    A. deer.
    B. birds.
    C. young Komodo dragons.
    D. other reptiles.
    E. humans.

9. If a human father could create a fertilized egg from a pair of sperm in the way that a Komodo dragon mother can create a fertilized egg parthenogenically from a pair of unfertilized eggs, which of the following would be true of the fertilized eggs he would produce by himself?

    A. All males
    B. All females
    C. All unviable
    D. A mixture of males and unviable
    E. A mixture of females and unviable

10. According to the passage, Komodo dragon saliva includes

    I. dragon blood.
    II. deadly pathogens.
    III. mucus.

    A. I only
    B. II only
    C. I and II only
    D. II and III only
    E. I, II, and III

11. The author's attitude toward the two theories of the Komodo dragon's size is best described as

   A. disinterested.
   B. enthusiastic.
   C. cynical.
   D. apathetic.
   E. sardonic.

12. Of the following, the Komodo dragon would have the most difficulty seeing a

   A. fast-moving deer in a bright jungle.
   B. slow-moving pig in mud.
   C. young Komodo dragon in a tree.
   D. baby goat with no scent developed yet.
   E. horse galloping at night.

13. The author describes hypothetical human parthenogenesis primarily in order to

   A. explain how human children can differ from their parents.
   B. discuss eye color genetics in humans.
   C. begin a digression away from the subject of the passage.
   D. illustrate how a parthenogenic child is not a clone with a comparison.
   E. show how an egg can act like a sperm.

14. Where are young Komodo dragons most likely to be found?

   A. In trees, dispersed from their hatching site
   B. In their mother's nest
   C. Following other dragons to feed on the carrion they leave behind
   D. Lying in the sun
   E. Hunting in groups

15. Which of the following can be inferred about the great white shark?

   A. They eat swimming Komodo dragons.
   B. They inhabit the waters around Indonesia.
   C. They compete with Komodo dragons to eat birds.
   D. They have viciously serrated teeth.
   E. It is a relict survival of the Australasian megafauna of the Pleistocene.

16. Which of the following best describes the author's attitude toward William Douglas Burden and his stories?

   A. Reverential
   B. Approving
   C. Skeptical
   D. Populist
   E. Anxious

17. What color are Komodo dragons?

   A. Grayish brown or dirt-colored red
   B. Green or greenish yellow
   C. Gray or grayish green
   D. Blood red or crimson
   E. Bone white or pitch black

PASSAGE 2: FISSION YEAST AND CELL CYCLE

1. The eukaryotic cell cycle and its control mechanisms are highly conserved through evolution. The cell cycle is divided into 5 main phases: G_1, S, G_2, M and the optional G_0 phase. S (synthesis) phase is when the cell actively replicates its genome. M phase includes mitosis and cytokinesis. Mitosis is the partitioning of cellular components (genes, organelles, etc.) into two halves. Cytokinesis is the physical process of cell division. Between M phase and S phase, there are two "gap" phases, G_1 and G_2. The gap phases plus S phase together form the part of the cell cycle between divisions, known as interphase.

2. Most cells spend most of their time in interphase, growing and busily metabolizing and synthesizing materials. During the gap phases, cells actively make proteins (via transcription and translation), perform metabolic functions (such as cell respiration and the pentose phosphate pathway), grow, and make organelles. In G_1, the cell prepares for the S phase; in G_2, the cell prepares for mitosis.

3. Non-cycling cells exit the cell cycle during G_1. These non-dividing or non-proliferative cells can either enter senescence or quiescence. Entering senescence is an irreversible process. Cells in this state remain metabolically active but cannot divide. In contrast, entering quiescence is reversible. These cells stay alive and metabolically active, but take a "time-out" from the cell cycle. Finally, in multicellular organisms, cells may exit the cell cycle to undergo apoptosis (cell-regulated cell death) or differentiation. Differentiation is when a cell becomes more specialized in structure and function.

4. The most vital checkpoint pathways function at the G_1/S transition and the G_2/M transition. Once a cell leaves G_1, it has committed to finishing the cell cycle. Once a cell leaves G_2, it must stop growing and complete mitosis. Since both of these are big decisions for a cell to make, these transitions are tightly regulated.

5. The fission yeast *Schizosaccharomyces pombe* is a model organism commonly used to study the cell cycle and checkpoint pathways. Fission yeast are non-pathogenic, and use many of the same general biochemical pathways that mammals do. For example, they perform translation using a 40S/60S ribosome and use the same transcriptional machinery as most other eukaryotes. Fission yeast are also easy to culture in the laboratory; they can be grown on agar plates or in liquid culture, and they have a relatively short doubling time. Like all fungi, *S. pombe* have a chitin cell wall.

6. The nuclear genome of fission yeast has been completely sequenced. The *S. pombe* genome contains 12.5 megabases of DNA, divided into 3 chromosomes. There are a little over 5000 protein-coding genes and the average length of a gene is 1,400 base pairs. Approximately 400 replication origins have been found and current predictions state that 94% of the genome is transcribed, although there is extensive variation in different life stages and growth conditions. The mitochondrial genome of *S. pombe* has also been sequenced; it is 20 kilobases in length and codes for 11 genes.

7. The fission yeast cell cycle is characterized by relatively short G_1 and S phases and a long G_2 phase that typically takes up to 70% of the cell cycle. Cell cycle progression is controlled by cyclin-dependent kinases (CDKs) and their cyclin binding partners. Protein levels of the cyclins rise and fall with the cell cycle due to periodic transcription and regulated protein degradation. Fission yeast have only one CDK, called Cdc2, which can bind to one of 7 different cyclin partners, depending on the cell cycle phase. Cdc13 is the only cyclin that controls the G_2/M transition; activation of the Cdc2-Cdc13 complex triggers the cell to enter the M-phase.

8. Cdc2 is expressed throughout the cell cycle, but the activity levels change with the cell cycle phase. For example, Cdc2 activity is low in G_1, moderate in S-phase and G_2, and high during mitosis. The activity of Cdc2 is regulated by cyclin binding and via phosphorylation; Cdc2 can be phosphorylated on its fifteenth amino acid, which is a tyrosine (Y15).

9. Entry into mitosis is mediated by a complex network of proteins. First, Cdc13 protein levels start to rise through G_2. Cdc13 associates with Cdc2 and this complex is moved to the nucleus. One of two kinases (either Mik1 or Wee1) phosphorylate Y15 on Cdc2 and keep it inactive. Once proper cellular checkpoints have been passed, the cell is ready to proceed to M-phase: Wee1 and Mik1 are inactivated, and Cdc25 is transported to the nucleus by a transporter protein called Sal3. Cdc25 is a phosphatase and has the opposite function as Wee1 and Mik1. Many of the cellular checkpoint pathways function to control Wee1 and Cdc25 and this is how they regulate progression through the cell cycle. Once dephosphorylated on Y15, Cdc2 is active and phosphorylates many proteins in the cell to cause entry into mitosis.

10. Cdc25 activity is controlled partially through its subcellular location. Cdc25 is localized in the cytoplasm during G_1, S and part of G_2. It has been shown that Cdc25 is bound to the 14-3-3 protein Rad24 during interphase, which may anchor the mitosis-promoting protein in the cytoplasm and away from Cdc2. This association requires phosphorylation of Cdc25, although the kinase that accomplishes this is currently unknown. Cdc25 accumulates in the nucleus throughout G_2 and this nuclear transport is facilitated by the importin-β protein, Sal3. Once in the nucleus, Cdc25 dephosphorylates tyrosine 15 of Cdc2, which activates the Cdc2-Cdc13 complex and triggers the cell into mitosis.

11. Cdc25 is exported from the nucleus late in M-phase although it does not contain an identified nuclear export signal (NES). Cdc25 is likely phosphorylated, although the kinase machinery that accomplishes this has not been identified. Phosphorylation of Cdc25 leads to the association of the 14-3-3 proteins, Rad24 and Rad25, in either homodimer or heterodimer (Rad24-Rad25) configurations. 14-3-3 proteins initially bind Cdc25 in the nucleus and then mediate the cytoplasmic localization of Cdc25 in two ways. The dimer blocks the nuclear localization signal (NLS) on Cdc25, therefore causing it to remain in the cytoplasm. Rad24 also contains a NES between residues 219 and 234, which facilitates the association of the exportin Crm1. Crm1 is a highly conserved export protein, which transports Cdc25 to the cytoplasm via the standard export mechanism.

12. In addition to a change in subcellular localization, Cdc25 protein levels also decrease at the end of mitosis, and this is mediated by proteolysis. Cdc25 is dephosphorylated by Clp1 late in mitosis. This functions to destabilize and deactivate Cdc25, which is then degraded by the anaphase-promoting complex (APC) ubiquitin ligase.

13. When the cell has undergone DNA damage, or if DNA replication is incomplete, progression through mitosis would be disastrous. Therefore, the cell uses a complex checkpoint system to ensure that the genome is duplicated and intact before G2/M progression is allowed. Several complexes are involved in recognizing DNA damage. First, Rad3 is activated in response to the damage and associates with damaged chromatin. Rad3 forms a complex with and phosphorylates Rad26. Next, the 911 complex (Rad9-Rad1-Hus1) is recruited to the site of damage. Both Rad9 and Hus1 are phosphorylated by Rad3. The 911 complex is loaded onto the DNA by a third complex, the checkpoint loading complex (CLC), consisting of 5 proteins: Rad17, Rfc2, Rfc3, Rfc4 and Rfc5. Finally, after Rad3-Rad26 and the 911 complex are bound to the damaged DNA, Chk1 and its two helper proteins Crb2 and Cut5/Rad4 are recruited. These proteins are responsible for propagating the signal that DNA is damaged.

14. The effector kinase Chk1 is phosphorylated and possibly activated by Rad3. Chk1 phosphorylates and activates Wee1, causes accumulation of the tyrosine kinase Mik1, and causes extensive phosphorylation of Cdc25 in the N-terminal regulatory domain, thereby inactivating the phosphatase. Overall, the actions of Chk1 function to limit mitotic entry.

15. Cds1 is another checkpoint effector protein in the DNA damage and replication checkpoint system. Its activation requires much the same machinery as Chk1, including Rad3-Rad26, the 911 complex and the checkpoint loading complex. Cds1 functions to pass the checkpoint signal to replication machinery but also phosphorylates Cdc25, inhibiting phosphatase activity and mitotic progression. It has been shown that Cdc25 can be phosphorylated up to 12 times by Chk1 and Cds1. These responses, including inhibition of Cdc25, allow the cell time to repair DNA damage and complete genomic replication.

16. Fission yeast cells can be exposed to a wide variety of stresses, including osmotic and oxidative stresses, heat shock and exposure to toxic chemicals in the environment. Stress can be sensed in a variety of ways and the signal is fed into a MAP kinase pathway which results in phosphorylation of a protein called Spc1. Activated Spc1 translocates to the nucleus and activates the transcription factors Atf1 and Pap1 via phosphorylation. This causes the transcription of stress response genes and allows the cell to cope with the current environment. One of the genes that undergoes transcriptional activation during osmotic stress is Srk1. This protein is also phosphorylated by Spc1. Srk1 is important for cell cycle progression because it phosphorylates Cdc25 on many residues in the N-terminal region between amino acids 56 and 375, similar to Chk1 and Cds1 during the DNA checkpoint. This change in phosphorylation state stabilizes Cdc25, but causes cytoplasmic retention via Rad24 binding. This inhibits Cdc25 phosphatase activity and mitotic progression in times of cellular stress, but leaves Cdc25 protein levels high in order to reinitiate cell cycle progression under more favorable conditions.

1. The fission yeast genome contains:

    A. 4 diploid chromosomes.
    B. Approximately 5000 protein-coding genes.
    C. 20 kilobases of DNA.
    D. 1400 replication origins.
    E. 94 genes that are about 1400 base pairs in length.

2. A fission yeast mutant is isolated in the lab and examined under the microscope. The cells are much smaller than wild type control cells. This mutant most likely has a:

    A. mutation in the promoter of Wee1 that causes decreased transcription.
    B. an activating mutation in Wee1.
    C. silent mutation in Cdc13.
    D. mutation in the promoter of Sal3 that causes transcription silencing.
    E. nonsense mutation in Cdc25.

3. Cells that over-express Sal3 are:

    A. larger than wild type cells and spend more time in G_2.
    B. smaller than wild type cells and spend more time in G_2.
    C. larger than wild type cells and spend less time in G_2.
    D. smaller than wild type cells and spend less time in G_2.

4. Which of the following proteins is expressed throughout the cell cycle?

    A. Cdc13
    B. Cdc2
    C. Rfc4
    D. Chk1
    E. Cds1

5. Which of the following are determinants of the G_2/M checkpoint?

    A. Ensure that genomic replication is complete, and that DNA is stable
    B. Take inventory of nucleotide levels
    C. Check that mutations in DNA have been appropriately repaired
    D. Ensure that genomic replication is complete, DNA is stable, and mutations have been repaired
    E. Take inventory of nucleotide levels and check the quality of DNA replication.

6. Which of the following is the function of Wee1?

    A. Phosphorylates Mik1 on Cdc25
    B. Phosphorylates Cdc25 on Mik1
    C. Phosphorylates Cdc2 on Y15
    D. Transports Sal3 to the nucleus
    E. To oppose the function of Mik1

7. Fission yeast have evolved strategies to deal with each of the following except:

    A. Apoptosis
    B. Heat shock
    C. Osmotic stress
    D. Oxidative stress
    E. Exposure to toxins

8. A phosphatase is:

    A. An enzyme that reverses the action of a kinase and removes phosphate groups
    B. An enzyme that adds phosphate groups to molecules, using ATP as the phosphate source
    C. An enzyme that removes phosphate groups from only proteins
    D. A protein that increases the activation energy barrier to a reaction, increasing the rate
    E. An enzyme that has the same function as a kinase

9. The 911 complex:

    A. contains the proteins Rad9, Rad1 and Hus1.
    B. is active in the M phase.
    C. binds RNA.
    D. destabilizes Crb2, Cut5 and Rad4.
    E. phosphorylates Chk1.

10. The regulation of CDKs includes:

    A. post-translational modification and allosteric regulation.
    B. allosteric regulation and proteolytic cleavage.
    C. proteolytic cleavage and protein associations.
    D. protein associations and post-translational modification.

11. *S. pombe* cells have:

    A. a cell wall made of peptidoglycan and a 70S ribosome.

    B. a cell wall made of chitin and an 80S ribosome.

    C. a cell wall made of cellulose and either a 70S or an 80S ribosome.

    D. no cell wall and an 80S ribosome.

    E. no cell wall and a 70S ribosome.

12. A pharmaceutical company is trying to develop drugs to treat onychomycosis, fungal infections of the nails. Which one of the following would be their best drug to pursue?

    A. A drug that promotes and increases chitin synthesis

    B. A drug that inhibits redox reactions in the electron transport chain

    C. A drug that decreases production of ergosterol, a plasma membrane component

    D. A drug that limits associations between the 40S and 60S ribosome

    E. A drug that inhibits the ability of eukaryotic RNA polymerase to bind its promoter

13. What is meant by the term "time-out," as it was used in paragraph 3?

    A. A time for rest or recreation

    B. Time away from one's usual work or studies

    C. A cancellation or cessation that automatically occurs

    D. A break or pause in activity

    E. A recovery period

14. An area of future work could be to determine:

    A. the protein that imports Cdc25 into the nucleus.

    B. the kinase that phosphorylates Cdc25 before is associates with Rad24.

    C. if Cdc25 has a nuclear export signal.

    D. whether Rad24 and Rad25 form homodimers or heterodimers.

    E. if Cdc25 is localized in the nucleus or the cytosol.

15. Sal3 is an importin protein that brings Cdc25 into the nucleus. Crm1 is an exportin which binds Cdc25.

    A. Both statements above are true.

    B. Both statements above are false.

    C. The first statement is true and the second is false.

    D. The first statement is false and the second is true.

16. The checkpoint loading complex includes each of the following except:

    A. Rfc2

    B. Rad17

    C. Rfc3

    D. Rad1

    E. Rfc5

17. Recognizing DNA damage in fission yeast involves each of the following except:

    A. Chk1, Crb2 and Cut5/Rad4 send the signal that DNA is damaged.

    B. Rad3 is activated and associates with chromatin.

    C. the 911 complex is recruited to the site of DNA damage.

    D. Rad26 forms a complex with Rad3 and phosphorylates it.

    E. the checkpoint loading complex loads the 911 complex onto damaged DNA.

18. Which of the following is supported by the passage?

    A. Spc1 and Srk1 help the cell deal with oxidative stress.

    B. Cdc2 dephosphorylates Cdc25 on Y15.

    C. Cdc25 can be degraded via ubiquitination.

    D. Fission yeast have one cyclin protein and 7 different CDKs.

    E. Cdc25 binds Rad13 (a 14-3-3 protein) during mitosis.

19. Both senescence and quiescence involve exiting the cell cycle during interphase. Fission yeast can undergo differentiation in some cases.

    A. Both statements above are true.

    B. Both statements above are false.

    C. The first statement is true and the second is false.

    D. The first statement is false and the second is true.

20. Each of the following has kinase activity except:

    A. Cdc2

    B. Crm1

    C. Mik1 and Wee1

    D. Rad3

    E. Cds1 and Chk1

PASSAGE 3: AFFINITY CHROMATOLOGY

1. Chromatography is a laboratory technique for the separation of a mixture. The mixture is dissolved in a fluid called the mobile phase, which carries it through a structure holding the stationary phase. The various constituents of the mixture travel at different speeds, causing them to separate. The separation is based on differential partitioning between the mobile and stationary phases. Subtle differences in a compound's partition coefficient result in differential retention on the stationary phase and thus affect the separation.

2. The chromatography experiments performed today are based on work done in the first five decades of the 20th century. Chromatography was first employed in Russia by the Italian-born scientist Mikhail Tsvet in 1900. He continued to work with chromatography in the first decade of the 20th century, primarily for the separation of plant pigments such as chlorophyll, carotenes, and xanthophylls. Since these components have different colors (green, orange, and yellow, respectively) they gave the technique its name.

3. New types of chromatography were developed during the 1930s and 1940s, and made the technique more versatile. Chromatography techniques developed substantially as a result of the work of Archer John Porter Martin and Richard Laurence Millington Synge during the 1940s and 1950s, for which they won the 1952 Nobel Prize in Chemistry. They established the principles and basic techniques of partition chromatography, and their work encouraged the rapid development of several chromatographic methods: paper chromatography, gas chromatography, and what would become known as high-performance liquid chromatography. Since then, the technology has advanced rapidly. Researchers found that the main principles of Tsvet's chromatography could be applied in many different ways, resulting in the different varieties of chromatography used in laboratories today. Advances are continually improving the technical performance of chromatography, allowing the separation of increasingly similar molecules.

4. Affinity chromatography is used to separate biochemical mixtures, and is based on highly specific interactions between macromolecules. Affinity chromatography is most commonly used to purify proteins and uses many of the same principles as other chromatography techniques: you start with a heterogeneous mixture of molecules (such as cell lysate, growth media or blood). To isolate a protein of interest, you can either use an antibody or tag the protein with an affinity tag. The target molecule is trapped on a stationary phase due to specific binding, and the stationary phase is washed to increase purity. The target protein is then released (or eluted) off the solid phase, in a highly purified state.

5. Antibodies are highly specific and can be used to purify a protein of interest. Many high quality antibodies are commercially available. To isolate a protein of interest from a lysate sample, an antibody specific for the protein is added to the mixture. Next, antigen-antibody complexes need to be isolated. This is done using a Protein A-, Protein G- or Protein L-linked solid. These three proteins are isolated from microbes and are useful because they bind mammalian immunoglobulins (or antibodies). Each can be covalently linked to a solid support, such as agarose beads, magnetic beads, or polyacrylamide resin. The idea then is that complexes form in solution, which are made of the protein of interest bound to an antibody; this antibody is bound to Protein A/G/L, which is attached to a solid bead or resin.

6. Large-scale or small-scale purifications are possible. In large scale work, the stationary phase is a column packed with solid resin. The sample is poured through the column and slowly drips out the other end. The antigen-antibody complex is retained in the column due to interactions between the antibody and Protein A/G/L attached to the solid phase. Finally, the protein of interest is eluted off the solid phase; it leaves the column and is collected at the end of the experiment.

7. In smaller scale experiments, the solid phase can be added to a small tube of sample and mixed to allow interaction with the components of the mixture. The sample is then centrifuged (spun at high speeds) and the heavy solid resin settles to the bottom of the tube. The liquid (or supernatant) is removed, since the protein of interest is bound to the solid resin.

8. Magnetic beads can also be used as the solid phase. Here, beads are isolated from solution by putting the tube in a magnet. The magnetic beads (bound to the protein of interest) go the sides of the tube, and the liquid is dumped out. The magnetic beads are left in the tube and are released from the tube walls when the tube is removed from the magnet.

9. Not all proteins of interest have a commercial antibody available. In this case, researchers can either generate "home-made" antibodies, or can use an affinity tag. Antibodies are typically produced in laboratory animals; making an antibody is tedious and technically challenging. It also requires optimization, since it's characteristics (binding affinity, optimal concentrations, titer values) aren't known. Instead of going through this, many labs work with affinity tagged proteins. Here, a small molecular tag is added to the N-terminus or the C-terminus of the protein. Many proteins can be tagged on either end, but only one end works well on other proteins. For example, if the C-terminus of a protein codes for the catalytic domain, and the N-terminus of the protein is mostly structural, it would be better to tag the N-terminus. A good understanding of protein domains and function can help in deciding where to tag a protein. This also depends on the size of the tag being added. Large tags often affect the structure or function of the

protein of interest if they're added to a suboptimal region, whereas small tags usually have no effect on either end of the protein.

10. Adding a tag is done using recombinant technology. DNA sequences coding for affinity tags are well known, and these can be cloned into a plasmid with the gene of interest. If a eukaryotic gene is being cloned, a cDNA version of the gene is usually used to ensure the fragment is shorter and more manageable. The cloned plasmid can then be transformed into bacteria. Large cultures of the bacteria can be produced to replicate either the plasmid, the protein itself or both. The purified plasmid could also be transfected into eukaryotic cells.

11. There are many commonly used affinity tags. His tags are made of 6-10 histidine amino acids, and can bind ions such as nickel, zinc, copper, and cobalt. Generally, nickel-based resins have higher binding capacity, while cobalt-based resins offer the highest purity. His tags easily bind these metals in solutions containing 20 mM imidazole and a high pH. The bound proteins are eluted by adding imidazole up to 150-300 mM, or by lowering the pH. At low pH (~6 for cobalt and ~4 for nickel), histidine becomes protonated and is competed off the metal ion.

12. GST (glutathione-S-transferase) tags are 220 amino acids in length, and bind to glutathione-coupled beads. Glutathione is a tripeptide (Glu-Cys-Gly) and the substrate for GST. After washing, the purified GST-tagged protein can be eluted from the column by adding free reduced glutathione. This competitively displaces GST from the glutathione beads, and allows the protein of interest to emerge from the affinity column.

13. TAP (tandem affinity purification) tags have three components: protein A, a tobacco etch virus (TEV) protease cleavage site, and a calmodulin-binding peptide (CBP). They are 172 amino acids in length and about 20 kDa in size. First, TAP-tagged proteins are isolated by affinity chromatography on an IgG matrix (which binds protein A). Next, a TEV protease is added and cleaves the TEV site. This releases the protein of interest (still with a CBP tag) to solution. Next, the protein is incubated with calmodulin-coated beads in the presence of calcium. The CBP binds the beads and the protein of interest is isolated again. Because this system uses two purification steps, it leads to a highly purified protein product.

14. Some additional smaller tags are often used, and can usually be added to either terminus of a peptide. The HA tag is a 9 amino acid fragment from an influenza virus surface glycoprotein, and a FLAG tag is a synthetic octapeptide. Because they are so short, these tags rarely interfere with protein function, and antibodies for these tags are commercially available.

15. A typical affinity chromatography experiment with an HA tag would look like this: First the gene of interest is cloned into an expression plasmid, with either an N-terminal or C-terminal HA tag. The cloned plasmid is transferred into bacteria and grown on an agar plate containing a selection agent. Individual colonies of bacteria are selected and screened for the correct plasmid. A successful sample is grown into a large culture of cells (usually about 4 L of growth media). Cells are collected via centrifugation and lysed to release cellular lysate. Next, an anti-HA antibody is added to the lysate, and incubated at 4°C for an hour, mixing. Next, Protein A-linked-agarose beads are added to the mixture, and incubated at 4°C for an hour, mixing. The mixture is transferred to a centrifuge, and spun at high speeds to collect the agarose beads at the bottom of the tube. The liquid layer (or supernatant) is removed and discarded; the solid mass at the bottom of the tube contains complexes of Protein of Interest – HA – Anti-HA Antibody – Protein A – Agarose. The complex is washed several times to increase the purity of the final product, and then finally eluted off the agarose beads to obtain the purified protein of interest.

1. In a typical affinity chromatography experiment, what is the volume of a standard large culture of bacterial cells?

    A. 1 mL
    B. 500 mL
    C. 1 L
    D. 4 L
    E. 10 L

2. Which of the following matches the author's use of the term 'versatile' in the passage?

    A. Unable to be adapted to many different functions or activities
    B. Able to be used in other fields, such as physics or inorganic chemistry
    C. Useful for many separation processes
    D. Unchangeable, or constant
    E. Reliant on new technology

3. The catalytic subunit of phosphatidylinositol 3-kinase is a 110 kDa protein with the catalytic domain at the C-terminus. If a technologist wanted to tag this peptide with an HA tag, the best experimental plan would be to add the HA tag:

    A. to the N-terminus of the peptide.
    B. to the middle of the peptide.
    C. to the C-terminus of the peptide.
    D. to either the N- or C-terminus.
    E. anywhere in the protein.

4. Protein G binds antibodies made in mammalian organisms. Solid resins are used in both small scale and large scale purifications.

    A. Both statements above are supported by the passage.
    B. Neither statement is supported by the passage.
    C. The first statement is supported by the passage but the second is not.
    D. The second statement is supported by the passage but the first is not.

5. The passage mentions each of the following reagents except:

    A. Protein A-agarose beads.
    B. Protein G-magnetic beads.
    C. Protein L-polyacrylamide resin.
    D. Imidazole.
    E. Iron-based resin.

6. Glutathione is:

    A. a Glu-Cys-Gly tripeptide.
    B. 172 amino acids in length.
    C. a synthetic octapeptide.
    D. isolated from influenza virus.
    E. a magnetic bead.

7. What is a supernatant?

    A. A solid pellet formed after centrifugation
    B. The liquid layer formed after centrifugation
    C. A heterogeneous solution before centrifugation
    D. The tube used for centrifugation
    E. The machine used for centrifugation

8. Each of the following is part of the TAP tag protocol except:

    A. TEV protease cleavage.
    B. CBP binds calmodulin in the presence of calcium.
    C. Matrix functionalized with IgG binds protein A.
    D. Protein of interest is released with a CBP tag.
    E. Elution at low pH conditions.

9. The catalytic subunit of phosphatidylinositol 3-kinase is a 110 kDa protein with the catalytic domain at the C-terminus. If a technologist wanted to tag this peptide with an GST tag, the best experimental plan would be to add the GST tag:

    A. to the N-terminus of the peptide.
    B. to the middle of the peptide.
    C. to the C-terminus of the peptide.
    D. to either the N- or C-terminus.
    E. anywhere in the protein.

10. What is the smallest affinity tag discussed in the passage?

    A. FLAG
    B. GST
    C. HA
    D. His
    E. TAP

11. Each of the following techniques is mentioned in the passage except:

    A. Centrifugation.
    B. Electrophoresis.
    C. Lysis.
    D. Transfection.
    E. Transformation.

12. Which of the following is supported by the passage?

    A. The development of chromatography happened between 1900 and 1950.
    B. TAP tags are purified using a three-step tandem strategy.
    C. TEV protease cleaves a TEV site in a GST tag.
    D. HA is an octapeptide and FLAG is from an influenza virus surface glycoprotein.
    E. Chromatograph is so named because Martin and Synge initially used it to study plant pigments.

13. Which of the following correctly pairs an affinity tag with its elution conditions?

    A. His—20 mM imidazole and high pH
    B. TAP—IgG matrix
    C. GST—reduced glutathione
    D. TAP—calmodulin-coated beads
    E. His—cobalt-based resin

14. Mikhail Tsvet used chromatography to study:

    A. plant pigments.
    B. chlorophyll.
    C. carotenes.
    D. fucoxanthin.
    E. more than one of the above.

15. Who advanced chromatography in the 1950s?

    A. Mikhail Tsvet and James Watson
    B. Archer Martin and Richard Synge
    C. Richard Synge and Mikhail Tsvet
    D. Mikhail Tsvet and Archer Martin
    E. James Watson and Francis Crick

16. What is the largest affinity tag discussed in the passage?

    A. FLAG
    B. GST
    C. HA
    D. His
    E. TAP

17. Home-made antibodies must be optimized because which of the following is not known?

    A. The animal it was made in
    B. Its structure
    C. Its expiration date
    D. Its titer values
    E. Whether it is primarily IgG or IgM

18. Each of the following can be used as the solid phase in affinity chromatography except:

    A. agarose beads.
    B. immunoglobulins.
    C. magnetic beads.
    D. polyacrylamide resin.

19. Martin and Synge contributed to development of each of the following chromatography methods except:

    A. filtration chromatography.
    B. gas chromatography.
    C. high-performance liquid chromatography.
    D. paper chromatography.
    E. partition chromatography.

20. TAP-tagged proteins are eluted using:

    A. TEV protease and calcium.
    B. TEV protease and a calcium chelator.
    C. magnetic beads and a magnet.
    D. 20 mM imidazole and a high pH.
    E. 200 mM imidazole and a low pH.

PASSAGE 4: PRACTICAL APPLICATIONS OF DNA TECHNOLOGY

1.   Techniques in molecular biology and genetic engineering have been widely used for decades. Whole genomes have been sequenced. DNA technology has been applied to practical uses, such as forensics and paternity testing. Many useful transgenic organisms have been developed; these are organisms that carry a foreign gene that has been deliberately inserted into the genome. While these animals have many amazing applications, it is important to be aware of ethical considerations that come with both biotechnology and genetically engineered organisms.

2.   Recombinant bacteria are commonly used by pharmaceutical companies in drug production. Insulin to treat diabetes, clotting factors to treat hemophilia, growth hormone to treat dwarfism, interferon to treat viral infections, tumor necrosis factor to treat some cancers and prourokinase or tissue plasminogen activator (TPA) to treat heart attacks have all been produced in laboratory bacteria. To do this, an expression plasmid is made that contains a promoter and the gene of interest. The plasmid is transformed into competent bacteria and large cultures of the bacteria are grown in selective media. To harvest the drug of interest, the bacteria are either harvested and lysed (if the drug is produced inside the bacterial cell), or the growth media is collected, and the drug is purified from solution (if the bacteria have been modified so that the drug is transcribed and translated, then secreted from the bacterial cell). Genetically modified yeast have also been used to produce pharmaceuticals. Many plants have also been genetically modified to produce biopharmaceuticals. For example, transgenic carrot cells have been made to produce an enzyme to treat Gaucher's disease, a lysosomal storage disease. Algae, mosses and tobacco cells have also been genetically engineered to produce possible treatments. It's important to note that genetically modifying plant species requires different genetic tools than modifying bacteria or animals. The Ti plasmid from a strain of soil bacteria is the mostly commonly used tool to genetically alter plants.

3.   Genetic engineering and biotechnology have also been important in the development of vaccines. Here, the gene for a surface protein from a harmful pathogen can be cloned into a harmless virus, which is then used as a vaccine against the pathogenic microbe. This vaccine can be safely administered, since the body will recognize the surface protein as foreign (and will therefore mount an immune response), but will not be infected by the actual pathogen. Without the ability to cut and paste segments of DNA from one source to another (using restriction enzymes, PCR and plasmids), development of these vaccines would not be possible.

4.   Novel vaccine delivery systems are also being developed. For example, one group has developed transgenic potato plants that express proteins from the cholera bacterium. Ingestion of these potatoes causes production of anti-cholera antibodies, meaning the potato is effectively acting like a cholera vaccine. Although not yet widely available, this could offer a major benefit to impoverished areas, where people must travel long distances to medical clinics to receive vaccination shots.

5.   Genetically modified organisms are also useful in food processing and production. For example, the gene for chymosin has been cloned into both prokaryotic and eukaryotic expression plasmids, and bacteria or yeast containing these plasmids produce large amounts of the enzyme chymosin. This enzyme is then purified and used to clot milk in cheese production. Transgenic cows are being generated to produce milk that has the same characteristics as human breast milk. Additional transgenic animals are being made to produce useful substances (such as goats that excrete silk proteins in their milk, or pigs that produce omega-3 fatty acids).

6.   Both bacteria and plants (such as algae, corn and poplars) have been genetically modified for use in biofuel production. Biofuel is derived from living organisms and contains energy from geologically recent carbon fixation. Bioethanol (made from carbohydrates via fermentation) and biodiesel (made from animal and plant fats) are common example of biofuel.

7.   DNA technology has had a great impact on the science of agriculture. Scientists have been able to transfer genes to plants in order to optimize crop yield. For example, some plants express a transgenic enzyme that is harmful to pests, which decreases the need for pesticide use. Others express enzymes making them resistant to diseases or herbicides.

8.   Transgenic plants that are capable of nitrogen fixation are also in production. Most plants need large amounts of nitrate, which is produced from atmospheric nitrogen (a process call nitrogen fixation) by bacteria. Some plants, such as legumes, can fix their own nitrogen. Scientists have identified genes involved in this process and are working on developing transgenic corn and rice strains that are capable of nitrogen fixation. Success in this project would mean a decrease in global fertilizer use, which could have a beneficial impact in the environment.

9.   Genetically modified crops are common; food has been modified to increase shelf life and nutritional value. For example, tomatoes have been altered to stay firm during ripening. This means green tomatoes can be picked and transported to grocery shelves without going soft. Golden rice, which contains beta-carotene, has been developed to combat vitamin A deficiency. New rice strains with higher iron content are also being developed.

10.   DNA technology has also been applied to agriculture biotechnology in the form of animal husbandry. DNA fingerprinting has been applied to certain endangered animals (such as the Puerto Rican parrot, orangutans and some species of African livestock). This allows scientists to identify individual animals, verify their pedigree and ancestors, and track both

desirable and undesirable traits. Animals can be registered, and mating pairs can be tracked to make sure the population maintains enough variation to be viable, and that deleterious traits are not passed on to offspring. This is especially important for species that have a small population. These biotechnology-based breeding programs have also been applied to common agriculture livestock species such as cattle and horses.

11. Transgenic organisms are being engineered to express genes that will help cope with some environmental problems. For example, genetically engineered bacteria have been made to help with sewage treatment, and to degrade harmful compounds. Some bacteria have been made to extract heavy metals from the environment. These metals are then incorporated into different compounds what can be isolated and used to extract the metal. This means bacteria could play a role in the future of both cleaning up toxic mining waste, and also in the actual mining process itself. Phosphorus water pollution promotes algae growth. Genetically modified pigs, which produce the enzyme phytase in their saliva, are able to break down indigestible phosphorus. These pigs may help reduce water pollution, as their manure contains about half the amount of phosphorus as normal pigs. Genetically modified zebrafish are also being used in environmental biotechnology. For example, transgenic fish have been developed to detect aquatic pollution.

12. Gene therapy is when a genetic disorder is treated by introducing a gene into a cell. This is often to correct or supplement a defective gene. Gene therapy uses genetically modified viruses (such as retroviruses, adenoviruses or lentiviruses) to deliver genes to somatic human cells. Ideally, the targeted gene will be incorporated into the genome of the cell, but this doesn't always occur. This means treatment efficacy can gradually decrease over time, and repeated treatments may be necessary. Because the targeted cells are somatic, the treatment will only affect the individual patient and will not be passed to later generations. Gene therapy-based treatments for sickle cell anemia, Parkinson's disease, cystic fibrosis, cancer, HIV, diabetes, muscular dystrophy and heart disease are currently being developed. While the theory behind this technology is not new, it has been difficult to optimize gene therapy in practice. Because of this, gene therapy is not in widespread practice, but shows promise as a future treatment. Gene therapy of the germ line is also possible in theory, but because of ethical controversy, has not been well developed. There are some problems associated with gene therapy. Because a foreign particle is being introduced, there is a chance the immune system will respond, and this can reduce treatment efficacy. Current gene therapies are limited to one or two genes, while many disorders are caused by many genes. Finally, there is a small chance of tumor development if the therapy DNA integrates into the genome incorrectly.

13. Biotechnology has also been crucial in developing DNA-based tests. RFLP and STR analysis can be used in forensics (to compare crime scene samples to suspects for example). DNA tests can also establish relationships between people, or to study the evolutionary relationship between two species. Genetic testing is another application of these tests. Genetic testing can be done before birth (to look for diseases like hemophilia, cystic fibrosis, and Duchenne muscular dystrophy) or after birth (to test for mutations that may lead to increased disease risk). For example, mutations in BRCA1 and BRCA2 are hereditary and are associated with a very high risk of developing ovarian and/or breast cancer. The test for BRCA mutation carriers is a simple DNA test, where DNA from blood or saliva is extracted and checked for cancer-associated mutations.

1. Which of the following is not a correct pairing of disease and treatment?

   A. Clotting factors and hemophilia
   B. Growth hormone and dwarfism
   C. Interferon and viral infections
   D. Tissue plasminogen activator and heart attack
   E. Tumor necrosis factor and stroke

2. Gene therapy treatments are being developed to treat each of the following except:

   A. cystic fibrosis.
   B. hemophilia.
   C. muscular dystrophy.
   D. Parkinson's disease.
   E. sickle cell anemia.

3. What plasmid is commonly used to genetically alter plants?

   A. BRCA
   B. RFLP
   C. STR
   D. TI
   E. TPA

4. Which plants can fix their own nitrogen?

   A. Carrots
   B. Corn
   C. Legumes
   D. Rice
   E. Tomatoes

5. Which of the following is supported by the passage?

   A. Biofuel is derived from living organisms and contains energy from geologically ancient carbon fixation.
   B. Chymosin can be produced in prokaryotes or eukaryotes in the lab.
   C. Bioethanol is made from animal and plant fats.
   D. Corn and rice strains that are capable of nitrogen fixation would increase global fertilizer use.
   E. Biodiesel is made from carbohydrates via fermentation.

6. Transgenic potatoes that may be an effective cholera vaccine are in production. Transgenic goats are being studied in the hopes that they will produce milk very similar to human breast milk.

   A. Both statements above are supported by the passage.
   B. Neither statement is supported by the passage.
   C. The first statement is supported by the passage but the second is not.
   D. The second statement is supported by the passage but the first is not.

7. Which of the following is used to treat vitamin A deficiency?

   A. Golden rice
   B. Chymosin
   C. Prourokinase
   D. Transgenic potato plants that express proteins from the cholera bacterium
   E. Nitrogen-fixing corn

8. The author would agree with which of the following statements?

   A. Advances in biotechnology are plentiful and exciting, but ethical issues should be considered.
   B. The use of recombinant bacteria is promising in food processing, but not drug production.
   C. Transgenic organisms can be used to increase the nutritional value of foodstuffs, but not their shelf life.
   D. The public should beware of genetically modified foods, since they cannot be completely sure if they are safe.
   E. Only unicellular organisms such as bacteria and yeast should be used in genetic engineering.

9. Gene therapy uses each of the following except:

   A. adenoviruses.
   B. cytomegalovirus.
   C. lentiviruses.
   D. retroviruses.

10. It is most likely that the author wrote the passage in order to:

    A. compare and contrast several different topics.
    B. educate, using a narrative writing style and many examples.
    C. advocate the expanding use of biotechnology in creating genetically modified foods.
    D. correct a misconception about the role of genetic engineering in society.
    E. defend the use of cloning and transgenic animals in medical research.

11. Genetic testing can be used to detect each of the following except:

    A. BRCA1 and BRCA2 mutations.
    B. cystic fibrosis.
    C. Duchenne muscular dystrophy.
    D. hemophilia.
    E. sickle cell anemia.

12. If a paragraph were to be added to the end of the passage, it would mostly likely contain:

    A. a warning about the dangers of genetic engineering.
    B. examples of some drugs that have been produced in bacteria and can be used to treat human conditions.
    C. some information on how ethical considerations affect the DNA technology field.
    D. a rebuttal to the first paragraph, where the author circles back to the downsides of DNA technology.
    E. information on how DNA technology can be used to develop more and better vaccines.

13. The author discusses a novel vaccine option for which of the following?

    A. Cholera
    B. HIV
    C. Cancer
    D. Papillomavirus
    E. Hemophilia

14. Genetically modified pigs can produce which of the following in the saliva?

    A. Chymosin
    B. Nitrogen
    C. Phosphorus
    D. Phytase
    E. Prourokinase

15. Which of the following endangered animals is mentioned in the passage?

    A. Puerto Rican parrot and orangutan
    B. Red parrot and the great gorilla
    C. Orangutan and African lion
    D. Puerto Rican parrot and African lion
    E. Wooly mammoth and African cattle

16. How can genetically engineered bacteria help minimize or solve environmental problems?

    A. They can extract heavy metals from the environment, and thus contribute to mining practices.
    B. They can break down indigestible phosphorus, thus reducing water pollution.
    C. They are used in sewage treatment, to degrade harmful compounds.
    D. They can detect pollution in aquatic biomes.
    E. More than one of the above.

PASSAGE 5: NOTCH CELL SIGNALING

1. Mammals are eukaryotic organisms, and use cell signaling events to communicate. Effective communication governs basic cell activities and coordinates all cell actions. Cells in multicellular organisms need to perceive and correctly respond to their environment. Being able to do this well is the basis of development, tissue repair, and immunity, as well as normal tissue homeostasis. Errors in signaling events can cause illness and diseases such as cancer, autoimmunity, and diabetes. By understanding cell signaling, diseases may be treated more effectively, and human health will therefore improve.

2. The Notch signaling system is a commonly studied eukaryotic signaling pathway. It consists of three different types of proteins: receptors, ligands that bind to the receptors, and modifying enzymes. While this basic setup seems straightforward, in an actual organism it is anything but! There are many options for the three components of the Notch system, and they interact in very complex ways. Scientists have spent decades trying to understand how the Notch system signals in vertebrates.

3. In 1914 through 1919, several papers were published on gene linkage in the fruit fly *Drosophila melanogaster*. Specifically, a wing phenotype was described, where the flies had notches in their edges of their wings. This was found to be associated with loss of one copy of a gene, which was subsequently named Notch. This was one of the first genetic variations observed in *Drosophila melanogaster*. Soon after, it was discovered that when both copies of the Notch locus were lost, the flies died before birth and during embryonic development (a phenomenon known as embryonic lethality). This phenotype brought the Notch locus to prominence. In fact, this finding was very important because it was the first time mutations were linked to embryonic development. Before this finding, it was unclear whether the action of genes was linked with embryonic development. Several years later, the Notch locus was cloned (in the late 1970s and early 1980s). This work demonstrated that Notch was a large protein that passed through the plasma membrane, and suggested that Notch may function in cell interactions.

4. There are four types of Notch receptors in vertebrates, coded by the genes Notch1, Notch2, Notch3 and Notch4. Each receptor has an intracellular domain (inside the cell), a transmembrane domain (going across the plasma membrane) and an extracellular ligand-binding domain (outside the cell). The Notch receptor proteins are made in the secretory protein pathway (through the rough endoplasmic reticulum, the Golgi apparatus and secretory vesicles). While going through this pathway, Notch receptors are cleaved close to the transmembrane domain. This turns the Notch polypeptide into two separate molecules, but they remain closely associated together via non-covalent associations. This first cleavage event is called "S1" and is performed by a furin-like convertase enzyme. It is an important step in generating a functional Notch receptor on the surface of the cell.

5. There are five Notch ligands which are part of the Delta or Jagged families of proteins. Notch ligands bind the Notch receptors. The ligands' names are: Delta1, Delta3, Delta4, Jagged1 and Jagged2. These ligands are also transmembrane proteins. Typically, the extracellular domain of a Delta or Jagged ligand protein on one cell binds to a Notch receptor on a neighboring cell. This initiates another two cleavage reactions on the Notch receptor: after ligand binding, an ADAM metalloprotease TACE enzyme cleaves the Notch receptor 12 amino acids outside of the plasma membrane. This cleavage event is called "S2". Finally, γ-secretase (a presenilin containing multi-subunit protease) cleaves the C-terminus of the transmembrane domain on the Notch receptor. This releases an intracellular domain, which goes to nucleus. This final cleavage event is called "S3."

6. Once the Notch intracellular domain is translocated to the nucleus, it associates with two proteins that can bind DNA. The first is called suppressor of hairless, or Su(H), and is a DNA-binding effector. The second is a nuclear protein called MAM (or mastermind). The complex of Notch, Su(H) and MAM is essential for triggering the transcription of target genes. For example, the transcription of basic helix–loop–helix (bHLH) proteins changes in response to Notch signaling.

7. There is one final aspect to Notch signaling: both the receptor and ligand proteins can be modified by a class of sugar transferase enzymes called Fringes. There are three enzymes in the Fringe family, and they are named Lunatic, Manic and Radical. These enzymes glycosylate the Notch receptors and their ligands, controlling receptor specificity for ligands.

8. Notch signaling controls many aspects of development, including development of the central nervous system (CNS). The CNS includes two organs in humans: the brain and the spinal chord. It is protected by the skull and spine (respectively) and floats in cerebrospinal fluid. The nervous system is made of neurons, as well as support cells called glial cells. Glial cells are specialized, non-neuronal cells that typically provide structural and metabolic support to neutrons. Glia maintain a resting membrane potential but do not generate action potentials. There are several kinds of glial cells. First, Schwann cells are found in the peripheral nervous system (PNS) and form the myelin sheath. This structure increases the speed of action potential conductance along an axon. In other words, myelin insulates neurons. Oligodendrocytes have the same function but are found in the CNS. Astrocytes are also found in the CNS. They guide neural development, and regulate synaptic communication via regulation of neurotransmitter levels. Astrocytes are also part of the blood-brain barrier. Next, microglia are found in the CNS and they are important

because they remove dead cells and debris from the tissue. Finally, ependymal cells in the CNS produce and circulate cerebrospinal fluid. These five glial cell types are less well known than neurons, but none-the-less, play very important physiological roles in the nervous system.

9.   From a developmental point of view, the CNS starts as a neural stem cell, which has the ability to differentiate into two types of progenitor cells. Neuronal progenitor cells differentiate into only mature neurons. Neurons are the functional unit of the CNS and are responsible for information processing and signal relay. Neural stem cells can also differentiate into glial progenitor cells, which can produce two types of mature glial cells: astrocytes and oligodendrocytes.

10.   It has recently been found that Notch signaling inhibits the development of neuronal progenitor cells into neurons and also inhibits the development of glial progenitor cells into oligodendrocytes. However, Notch signaling promotes astrocyte differentiation. This complex relationship was defined using mice that either over-express certain Notch signaling proteins (knock-in mice), or lack certain Notch signaling proteins (knock-out mice).

11.   While Notch signaling was initially studied for its critical role in development, more recent work has shown that it also has complex and tissue-dependent roles in cancer and other diseases. Activation of the Notch signaling pathway can be either oncogenic (tumor-promoting) or cause tumor suppression. Deregulation of the Notch signaling pathway has been implicated in many types of cancerFor example, oncogenic Notch signaling was first found in T-cell acute lymphoblastic leukemia (T-ALL). Many T-ALLs have point mutations in a Notch gene that causes ligand-independent cleavage and increased stability of the intracellular domain. This leads to Notch pathway activation. In addition, preliminary work on mammary gland development suggests that Notch signaling is associated with cell growth and proliferation. High levels of Notch ligand and receptor expression are positively correlated with breast tumor aggressiveness. It has therefore been concluded that elevated Notch signaling is also oncogenic in the breast. While Notch1 mutations are oncogenic in T-ALL and breast cancer, it is tumor suppressive in prostate cancer cells, where it up-regulates PTEN expression. Elucidating roles for Notch in other cancers has been difficult: the effect of active Notch signaling seems to depend on the tissue, cell type, niche and timing.

1. Where are furin-like convertase enzymes expressed in the cell?

    A. Extracellular
    B. Plasma membrane
    C. Secretory pathway
    D. Nucleus
    E. Mitochondria

2. Which of the following are post-translational modifications of the Notch receptor?

    A. Glycosylation only
    B. Phosphorylation only
    C. Proteolytic cleavage only
    D. Glycosylation and phosphorylation
    E. Glycosylation and proteolytic cleavage

3. The blood-brain barrier is formed at least in part by:

    A. astrocytes.
    B. ependymal cells.
    C. microglia.
    D. oligodendrocytes.
    E. Schwann cells.

4. The author would most likely agree with which of the following statements?

    A. The Notch signaling pathway is the most complex signaling pathway found so far.
    B. The roles of genetics in development was not well understood in the early 20th century.
    C. The roles of Notch signaling in development and disease are now well understood.
    D. The Notch singling pathway is a straight-forward system with only a few components.
    E. While interesting to some, the Notch signaling pathway is over-studied and not important.

5. The author discusses the role of Notch singling in each of the following except:

    A. insect development.
    B. mammary gland development.
    C. musculoskeletal development.
    D. nervous system development.
    E. wing phenotypes.

6. How many Notch ligands are there?

    A. 1
    B. 2
    C. 3
    D. 4
    E. 5

7. A knock-out mouse that does not express a certain Notch receptor in the CNS would most likely have:

    A. fewer neurons and fewer oligodendrocytes than a wildtype mouse.
    B. fewer astrocytes than a wildtype mouse.
    C. fewer neurons and fewer astrocytes than a wildtype mouse.
    D. more neurons and fewer oligodendrocytes than a wildtype mouse.
    E. no change in the development of CNS cells.

8. What is the function of Fringe proteins?

    A. Receptors
    B. Ligands
    C. Modifying enzymes
    D. Transcription factors
    E. Secretory pathway

9. A mouse that over-expresses Jagged in the CNS would most likely have:

    A. fewer neurons and fewer oligodendrocytes than a wildtype mouse.
    B. more neurons and more astrocytes than a wildtype mouse.
    C. fewer neurons and fewer astrocytes than a wildtype mouse.
    D. more astrocytes and more oligodendrocytes than a wildtype mouse.
    E. no change in the development of CNS cells.

10. Which proteins have transmembrane domains?

    A. Notch receptor and ligands
    B. Notch receptors and Fringe proteins
    C. Notch ligands and Fringe proteins
    D. Only Notch receptors
    E. Only Notch ligands

11. Oligodendrocytes have the same function as:

    A. astrocytes.
    B. ependymal cells.
    C. microglia.
    D. neurons.
    E. Schwann cells.

12. The function of γ-secretase is to:

    A. bind Notch receptors.
    B. cleave Notch receptors in S2.
    C. cleave Notch receptors in S3.
    D. act at a Notch ligand.
    E. sugar transferase.

13. A progenitor cell is:

    A. formed from mature cells.
    B. less differentiated than a stem cell.
    C. derived from a stem cell and can differentiate
       into only certain types of cells.
    D. formed before stem cells in developmental
       pathways.
    E. found only in the nervous system.

14. How many times is the Notch receptor cleaved?

    A. 0
    B. 1
    C. 2
    D. 3
    E. 4

15. Which of the following is not supported by the passage?

    A. The central nervous system has at least two
       protection mechanisms.
    B. Cerebrospinal fluid is produced by ependymal
       cells, which are a type of glial cell.
    C. Neural stem cells can produce neurons but not
       glial cells.
    D. The central nervous systems has three types of
       stem cells: neural, neuronal and glial.
    E. More than one of the above.

16. Which of the following is true?

    A. Manic is a Notch modifying enzyme.
    B. Lunatic is a Notch receptor.
    C. Notch1 is a plasma membrane receptor.
    D. Jagged2 is a plasma membrane ligand.
    E. More than one of the above.

17. Notch singling promotes the development of neurons
    from neuronal stem cells and neural progenitor cells.
    Notch signaling can either promote or inhibit cancer,
    depending on the tissue.

    A. Both statements above are supported by the
       passage.
    B. Neither statement is supported by the passage.
    C. The first statement is supported by the passage
       but the second is not.
    D. The second statement is supported by the
       passage but the first is not.

18. The author discusses the role of Notch singling in each
    of the following except:

    A. leukemia.
    B. prostate cancer.
    C. breast cancer.
    D. ovarian cancer.

19. Delta3 is a:

    A. receptor.
    B. ligand.
    C. modifying enzyme.
    D. protease.
    E. transcription factor.

ANSWERS AND EXPLANATIONS

Passage 1: Komodo Dragon

1. **D** In paragraph 8, the passage indicates that humans make Komodo dragons skittish and that this makes them more difficult to study. Choice (A) is wrong because only juveniles are mentioned as spending time in trees, no mention is made of camouflage, and no indication is given that this makes them harder to study. Choice (B) is wrong because paragraph 8 indicates that they are not normally aggressive towards humans. Choice (C) is wrong because it is not mentioned. Choice (E) is wrong because it is not mentioned; paragraph 3 mentions that there are around 5,000 in the wild, but it is not clear whether this is a large, small, or medium number, or how it compares to "nearly extinct."

2. **B** Paragraph 2 mentions the goanna and says that it is an enormous reptile species that is still alive. Choice (A) is wrong because paragraph 2 says that it did not go extinct. Choice (C) is wrong because it is not mentioned. Choice (D) is wrong (though hilarious) because that was actually *Bullockornis planei,* higher in the paragraph, not goanna. Choice (E) is wrong because that was a fact about Komodo dragons in paragraph 4.

3. **C** In paragraph 12, the passage says that Burden undertook his expedition in 1926 and (later in the same paragraph) published a book about it the following year. That's 1927. Note: This question has four answers, which is unusual but not unprecedented on the OAT.

4. **B** Paragraph 3 describes the Komodo dragons as living "on Komodo and other nearby islands." These are islands in Indonesia, but there is no indication that the dragons lives on the mainland in Southeast Asia or in Australia. While the passage discusses Australasian megafauna, there is no reason to believe that any particular type of such fauna (such as the dragon) was spread across all of the Australasian region.

5. **A** This is a New Information question. The new information is that the dragon egg was refrigerated. This must connect to something about warmth or cold somewhere in the passage. The only such mention in the passage is in Paragraph 3, which says that warmth is essential to the health of the dragons' eggs. Thus, a dragon hatched from an egg that was kept cold would probably not be very healthy. None of the other answers are mentioned in the passage.

6. **C** Paragraph 9 says that eggs are laid in September and hatch in the following April. That's 7 months later. The reference to the mating season in the previous sentence is irrelevant.

7. **C** Paragraph 4 says that the average length of a dragon is 2.5 meters, and half of their length is tail. Thus, the tail is typically about 1.25 meters.

8. **E** Since this is an "except" question, finding 4 things that are mentioned is as good as finding 1 that is not. Paragraph 8 mentions that dragons eat deer, birds, and other reptiles, and paragraph 9 mentions that adult dragons frequently eat young dragons. However, paragraph 8 says that only "a few" dragons will eat humans, and that the general tendency is that dragons are uncomfortable around humans. Thus, the answer is (E).

9. **E** This question is a quite tricky New Information question. The new information is the first part. We are to assume that a human father could reproduce parthenogenically in the way that a Komodo dragon mother can. (Never mind that in reality a father can't; this question asks what would happen if he could.) Paragraphs 10 and 11 talk about parthenogenesis, which, if you didn't already know what it is, is defined in paragraph 10. The answer choices to this question suggest that we're interested in the sex of the child, however, so look at paragraph 11.

For Komodo dragons, the mother creates an egg cell, and then the sex chromosome duplicates. The mother has W and Z chromosomes to give to the egg, so you can get a WW or a ZZ, and we're told that WW is unviable and ZZ is male. Now, relate this back to the new information in the question. A man has an X and a Y chromosome. Thus, if he creates a fertilized egg in the same way, he'll either get an XX (a female) or a YY (unviable). This makes the correct answer (E). If you guessed that mothers having boys among Komodo dragons would sort of be like fathers having girls among humans and ended up with (E), that's a good guess! It may not account for the full complexity of the question, however.

10.   C   Paragraph 6 mentions that dragon saliva is reddish from the dragon's own blood, so the saliva must contain blood. Paragraph 6 also mentions the virulent pathogens. However, mucus doesn't come up until paragraph 8, and in a context totally independent of saliva (instead, regurgitation). Thus, I and II are supported, but III is not.

11.   A   The author does not judge either of the two theories but simply presents them. That is neutral or unbiased, which is what "disinterested" means (it does not mean "uninterested"). There is no evidence of any of the other four answers. "Enthusiastic" would have to be supported with the kind of tone words that appear in the final paragraph on an unrelated subject, so it does not fit here. "Cynical" means "distrusting people's motives or things' value," which is unrelated. "Apathetic" means "not caring," and if the author didn't care, why would he write about the subject? (If the question asked what *your* attitude toward the theories was, the answer might be different.) "Sardonic" means "mocking" or "cynical" (see above), which also doesn't fit.

12.   E   Paragraph 7 mentions that Komodo dragons are thought not to see well at night. Thus, the answer is (E). The rest are not mentioned. Choice (D) refers to scent, not sight, which isn't what the question was asking about in the first place.

13.   D   This is a Purpose question with some vicious trap answers. Hypothetical human parthenogenesis is mentioned in paragraph 10. "Consider the analogous situation" introduces this portion. Right before this, the passage says that the parthenogenic offspring is "not a clone of the mother," so presumably this analogy, or comparison, is supposed to explain that. Thus, (D) is the answer. Choice (A) is wrong because this is not a reason that human children in fact differ from their parents; it is hypothetical. Choice (B) is wrong because this portion barely discusses eye color genetics (it doesn't even mention that the brown eye gene is dominant over the blue eye gene, or anything like that); it's all just a vehicle for explaining how parthenogenesis differs from cloning. Choice (C) is wrong because this is not a digression; it's an analogy. Choice (E) is wrong because we are simply told that an egg can act like a sperm and fertilize another egg, not how the egg does this.

14.   A   Paragraph 9 says that young dragons spend much of their time in trees and spread out from their hatching place. Choices (B) and (C) are not supported. Choice (D) is a bad reference, since paragraph 8 mentions that dragons "can" lie in the sun sometimes. Choice (E) is contradicted by paragraph 9, which says that dragons are normally solitary.

15.   D   Paragraph 5 says that Komodo dragon teeth are viciously serrated, like the great white shark's teeth. Thus, (D) is the answer. Choice (A) is wrong because while paragraph 3 says that dragons can swim, it does not say that great white sharks eat them. Choice (B) is wrong because while most of the passage is about Indonesian animals, it never says that great white sharks are Indonesian (and in fact they are not). Choice (C) is wrong because while paragraph 8 says that dragons do eat birds, there is no reason to believe that they compete with sharks (especially since great white sharks are not even from the same area). Choice (E) is wrong because it is not mentioned.

16. **B** In paragraph 12, the author describes Burden's book as "sensationalist" and "exciting," and says that they "inspired further scientific investigations." This suggests a positive tone, but nothing as somber as "reverential," which means "deeply respectful." Choice (B) is better. Choice (C) is wrong because there's no indication that he doubted any of these stories (they're all true, as far as we know). Choice (D) is wrong because it means "representing the interests of common or ordinary people," which is completely unrelated. Choice (E) is wrong because while exciting stories might provoke feelings of drama and tension when they are first heard, these stories are over and done and there's no indication that the author still feels anxiety.

17. **A** Paragraph 4 describes the color of the Komodo dragon. Choices (B), (C), (D), and (E) are unsupported.

Passage 2: Fission Yeast and Cell Cycle

1. **B** Paragraph 6 states that the fission yeast genome contains slightly over 5000 protein-coding genes ((B) is correct). According to the passage, the fission yeast genome is comprised of 3 chromosomes ((A) is incorrect), containing 12.5 megabases of DNA (or 12,500 kilobases, (C) is incorrect) with 400 replication origins ((D) is incorrect). The 5000 genes have an average length of 1400 base pairs. However, this does not necessary mean that every gene is this length ((E) is incorrect).

2. **A** This is a very challenging question, so you should save it for the end of the passage. It is similar to question 3, so answering these two questions together is a good idea. The passage states that Wee1 inhibits the activity of Cdc2, keeping the cell in G_2 and preventing mitosis. Cdc25 and Sal3 promote Cdc2 activation and therefore help push the cell through G_2 and into M-phase. Decreased expression of Wee1 would cause the cells to pass through G_2 and enter mitosis early; they would therefore be smaller than wild type cells ((A) is correct). In contrast, an activating mutation in Wee1 would cause the opposite: cell would stay in G_2 longer and would become elongated (eliminate (B)). A silent mutation by its very definition has no effect ((C) is incorrect). Decreased Sal3 levels would cause the cell to stay in G_2 phase longer and therefore the cells would be larger or elongated ((D) is incorrect). A nonsense mutation in Cdc25 would cause the same phenotype (also eliminate (E)) since the cells cannot progress into M-phase.

3. **D** This is a very challenging question, so you should save it for the end of the passage. It is similar to question 2, so answering these two questions together is a good idea. If a fission yeast cell over-expresses Sal3, it will be pushed through G_2 and will enter M-phase early. Less time in G_2 means the cells will be smaller ((D) is correct). Choice (A) describes cells that have less Sal3 (or Sal3 knock-out cells), and (B) and (C) are impossible (a cell cannot spend more time in a growth phase and be smaller than wild type cells, and vice versa).

4. **B** Paragraph 8 says that Cdc2 is expressed throughout the cell cycle ((B) is correct). Paragraph 9 states that Cdc13 levels start to increase in G_2 phase ((A) is incorrect). Proteins Rfc4, Chk1, and Cds1 are involved in sensing DNA damage or replication errors and controlling the progression from G_2 to M phase, therefore they would be expressed in the G_2 phase ((C), (D), and (E) are incorrect).

5. **D** Before the cell divides, it must check the integrity of the genome it is passing to the daughter cells. This includes making sure DNA replication is complete, DNA is stable, and mutations have been repaired ((D) is correct; eliminate (A) and (C)). Checking the levels of nucleotides in the cell is part of the G_1/S checkpoint (the other major checkpoint pathway mentioned in the passage), since these building blocks are required for DNA replication (eliminate (B) and (E)).

6. **C** Wee1 is mentioned in paragraph 9, where it states that Wee1 is responsible for phosphorylating Y15 on Cdc2 in order to keep Cdc2 active ((C) is correct).

7. **A** According to the passage (paragraph 16), fission yeast cells are exposed to various stressors including heat shock, osmotic and oxidative stress, and exposure to toxins (eliminate (B), (C), (D), and (E)). Yeast cells have developed molecular mechanism to stop cell cycle progression when exposed to those stressors, until the conditions improve. Apoptosis, also known as programmed cell death, is not mentioned as one of the stressors. In fact, single-celled organisms rarely undergo apoptosis ((A) is correct).

8. **A** A kinase adds a phosphate group to molecules (such as proteins, lipids, carbohydrates or nucleic acids), using ATP as the source of the phosphate ((B) describes a kinase, not a phosphatase and is therefore not the answer). The passage says that Cdc25 is a phosphatase and has the opposite effect as the kinases Wee1 and Mik1. A phosphatase must therefore remove phosphate groups ((A) is correct; eliminate (E)). Choice (C) is too specific; there is no information in the passage to support the fact that phosphatases work EXCLUSIVELY on proteins (eliminate (C)). Choice (D) is a false statement and mixes up concepts in reaction kinetics: enzymes function to DECREASE the activation energy barrier, this increasing the reaction rate ((D) is incorrect).

9. **A** The 911 complex is made up of three proteins, Rad9, Rad1 and Hus1, as stated in paragraph 13 of the passage ((A) is correct). The 911 complex is involved in sensing DNA damage or replication errors during the G_2 phase ((B) is incorrect). It binds to DNA ((C) is incorrect) and recruits Crb2 and Cut5/Rad4 proteins to send a downstream signal to the rest of the cell that the DNA is damaged ((D) is incorrect). Chk1 is phosphorylated by Rad3 ((E) is incorrect).

10. **D** The passage says that the activity of Cdc2, a CDK, is regulated by cyclin associations ((C) or (D) is correct) and phosphorylation, a type of post-translational modification ((A) or (D) is correct). There is no information in the passage on allosteric regulation of Cdc2 ((A) and (B) are incorrect) or proteolytic cleavage ((B) and (C) are incorrect).

11. **B** There are a few ways to answer this question. Yeast are part of the fungi kingdom, are eukaryotic, and have a cell wall ((D) is incorrect). The bacterial cell wall is made of peptidoglycan ((A) is incorrect), the fungal cell wall is made of chitin (see paragraph 5; (B) is correct), and the plant cell wall is made of cellulose ((C) is incorrect). Prokaryotes have a 70S ribosome, made from 30S and 50S subunits ((A), (C) and (E) are incorrect). Eukaryotes have an 80S ribosome, made from 40S and 60S subunits ((B) is correct).

12. **C** This is a tricky question that requires POE. Fungi have a cell wall made of chitin, so promoting chitin synthesis would not harm the fungus. In fact, many antifungal drugs target and DECREASE chitin biosynthesis ((A) is incorrect). Inhibiting the electron transport chain would also harm the patient ((B) is incorrect), as would inhibiting eukaryotic translation ((D) is incorrect) and inhibiting eukaryotic transcription (eliminate (E)). This leaves (C) as the best answer option; ergosterol is a steroid that fungi use in their plasma membrane, similar to how animals use cholesterol. Since animals do not use ergosterol, the patient would be fine, and the fungi would be harmed. This is the basis for many anti-fungal remedies.

13. **D** To answer this question, you should go to paragraph 3 and find this term in the passage. Then look for a phrase that would mean the same thing and have the same effect on the sentence and paragraph. Paragraph 3 mentions that cells can take "time-out" from undergoing the cell cycle. The only phrase that means the same thing in this context is (D), that is, a break or pause in activity.

14. **B** See paragraph 10 or 11. Both say that the interaction between Cdc25 and Rad24 requires Cdc25 to be phosphorylated, but that the kinase that accomplishes this is currently unknown ((B) is correct).

15. **C** This is a tricky two-part question, because you must infer something from the passage (instead of just finding something directly stated). The first sentence is true (see paragraph 10). The second sentence is false. Paragraph 11 says that at the end of mitosis, Cdc25 is phosphorylated and then associates with Rad24/25. Rad24 contains a nuclear export signal (NES), which facilitates the association of the exportin Crm1 and thus nuclear export. Although it doesn't directly say that Crm1 doesn't bind Cdc25, if Rad24 is the protein with the NES, it is most likely that Crm1 would bind Rad24. Overall then, (C) is correct.

16. **D** See paragraph 13; the checkpoint loading complex (CLC) contains Rad17 (eliminate (B)), Rfc2 (eliminate (A)), Rfc3 (eliminate C), Rfc4 and Rfc5 (eliminate (E)). Rad1 is part of the 911 complex ((D) is correct).

17. **D** Bear in mind that this is an except question. Paragraph 13 of the passage says that Rad3 phosphorylates Rad26 and forms a complex with it, not the other way around. This is important because Rad3 is acting as a kinase but Rad26 is not ((D) is correct). Paragraph 13 mentions that Rad3 is activated when DNA is damaged, and associates with the chromatin (eliminate (B)). The 911 complex gets recruited (eliminate (C)), and gets loaded onto the damaged DNA by checkpoint loading complex (eliminate (E)). Chk1, Crb2 and Cut5/Rad4 eventually send the downstream signal that DNA is damaged, halting cell cycle progression (eliminate (A)).

18. **C** Paragraph 16 said that Spc1 and Srk1 function together during osmotic stress, not oxidative stress (eliminate (A)). Paragraph 10 says that Cdc25 dephosphorylates tyrosine 15 of Cdc2, which is the opposite of what choice (B) says (eliminate this answer choice). Paragraph 12 says that Cdc25 can be degraded by the anaphase-promoting complex (APC) ubiquitin ligase ((C) is correct). Paragraph 7 says that fission yeast have only one CDK (Cdc2), which can bind to one of 7 different cyclin partners (eliminate (D)). Paragraph 10 says that Cdc25 is bound to the 14-3-3 protein Rad24 during interphase.

19. **C** According to paragraph 3 of the passage, non-dividing cells enter senescence or quiescence by exiting the cell cycle during G_1, which is the first part of the interphase. This means the first statement is correct, and you should therefore eliminate (B) and (D). Paragraph 3 also mentions that multicellular organisms have the ability for cells to undergo differentiation, such as a stem cell becoming a muscle cell or a neuron. However, fission yeast is a unicellular organism, and they therefore they lack the ability to undergo further differentiation. The second statement is false, and (C) is correct.

20. **B** Paragraph 9 says that kinases add phosphate groups. Cdc2 phosphorylates many proteins in the cell (see paragraph 9, eliminate (A)). Paragraph 11 says that Crm1 is an exportin protein; there is no information on the passage to support the fact that it has any kinase activity ((B) is correct). Both Mik1 and Wee1 phosphorylate Cdc2 (see paragraph 9, eliminate (C)). Rad3 phosphorylates Rad9 and Hus1 (see paragraph 13, eliminate (D)). Cds1 and Chk1 phosphorylate Cdc25 (see paragraph 15, eliminate (D)).

Passage 3: Affinity Chromatography

1. **D** Paragraph 15 describes a typical affinity chromatography experiment, and says that a large culture of cells is usually about 4L of growth media ((D) is correct).

2. **C** If you can't find this word right away, save this question for later. The term "versatile" is used at the beginning of paragraph 3. This paragraph implies that the basis of this versatility was the development of new types of chromatograph during the 1930s and 1940s (see sentence 1). This best matches (C), which is correct. Eliminate (A) and (D), because they are the opposite of what versatility means. The passage doesn't mention other fields like physics, or new technologies; (B) and (E) are beyond the scope of the passage (eliminate both).

3. **D** This is an Inference question; you need to apply information in the passage to the question stem. Both paragraphs 9 and 14 say that small tags (such as HA and FLAG tags) can usually be added to either terminus of a peptide ((D) is correct).

4. **A** Paragraph 5 says that Protein A, Protein G, and Protein L are isolated from microbes and are useful because they bind mammalian immunoglobulins (or antibodies). Therefore, the first statement is supported by the passage (eliminate (B) and (D)). Paragraph 6 says that in large scale purifications, the stationary phase is a column packed with solid resin. Paragraph 7 says that in smaller scale experiments, the solid phase is added to a small tube and later centrifuged to isolate the heavy solid resin at the bottom of the tube. Overall the second statement is also supported by the passage ((A) is correct; eliminate (C)).

5. **E** Paragraph 5 mentions Protein A, Protein G, and Protein L, and says that each can be linked to a solid. It goes on to say that each can be covalently linked to a solid support, such as agarose beads, magnetic beads, or polyacrylamide resin-linked solid (eliminate (A), (B) and (C)). Imidazole is mentioned in paragraph 11 (eliminate (D)). Paragraph 11 mentions nickel, zinc, copper, and cobalt-based resins. Iron-based resins are not mentioned in the passage ((E) is correct).

6. **A** Paragraph 12 says that Glutathione is a tripeptide (Glu-Cys-Gly) and the substrate for GST ((A) is correct). The rest of the answer choices are just common words from the passage, there to waste your time.

7. **B** Both paragraphs 7 and 15 say that the supernatant it the liquid layer formed after centrifugation ((B) is correct).

8. **E** Choices (A), (B), (C) and (D) are all mentioned in paragraph 13 as part of the TAP tag protocol. Instead of spending time on figuring out these answer choices, focus on finding something obviously NOT in paragraph 13. This paragraph doesn't mention pH conditions at all. In fact, elution at low pH conditions is in paragraph 11 on His tags. This means the answer to this question must be (E).

9. **A** Paragraph 12 says that the GST tag is 220 amino acids long; this is a pretty large tag compared to others in the passage. Paragraph 9 says that when working with large tags, the tag should be added to the less important end of the protein. For example, "Many proteins can be tagged on either end, but only one end works well on other proteins. If the C-terminus of a protein codes for the catalytic domain, and the N-terminus of the protein is mostly structural, it would be better to tag the N-terminus." Therefore, (A) is correct.

10. **D** The passage talks about five affinity tags:
    - His tags are 6–10 amino acids in length (paragraph 11)
    - GST tags are 220 amino acids long (paragraph 12)
    - TAP tags are 172 amino acids long (paragraph 13)
    - HA tags are 9 amino acids long (paragraph 14)
    - FLAG tags are 8 amino acids long (paragraph 14)

    The smallest of these is the His tag at 6 amino acids in length ((D) is correct).

11. **B** This is an open-ended question that will take you a while; save it for your second pass to avoid wasting time. The passage talks about centrifugation in a few parts (paragraphs 7 and 15, eliminate (A)). Electrophoresis is not mentioned in the passage, so is the correct answer ((B) is correct). Lysis is mentioned in paragraph 15, where the passage talks about how cells are lysed to release cellular lysate (eliminate (C)). Transfection and transformation are both mentioned in paragraph 10 (eliminate (D) and (E)).

12. **A** This is a challenging open-ended question. Save it for your second pass through the questions. Paragraph 1 says that Mikhail Tsvet started his work on chromatography in 1900, and that the chromatography experiments performed today are based on work done in the first five decades of the 20th century ((A) is supported by the passage and is the correct answer). Paragraph 13 says that TAP tags are purified in *two* steps (TEV and calmodulin-coated beads in the presence of calcium), not *three* steps (eliminate (B)). TEV protease cleavage is part of TAP purification, not GST purification (eliminate (C)). Paragraph 13 says that HA tags are from an influenza virus surface glycoprotein, while FLAG is a synthetic octapeptide (eliminate (D) because it says the opposite). While Martin and Synge *did* work on chromatography (see paragraph 3), it was Mikhail Tsvet who worked on plant pigments (eliminate (E)).

13.   C   Paragraph 11 says that His tags are eluted using 150-300 mM imidazole, or low pH (eliminate (A) and (E)). Paragraph 13 says that TAP tags use a two step purification strategy. First, protein A in the TAP tag binds an IgG matrix. The protein of interest is eluted using TEV cleavage. Next, the CBP tag binds calmodulin-coated beads in the presence of calcium. The passage never says how the second elution is performed. However, the conditions in (B) and (D) are used to isolate the protein of interest, not elute it out (eliminate both these choices). Paragraph 12 says that GST tags are eluted using reduced glutathione ((C) is correct). Make sure you're not wasting time on answer choices that have common words from the passage. Your goal on this question is to find the pair mentioned in the passage, so focus on that as you're doing POE.

14.   E   Paragraph 2 says that Mikhail Tsvet used chromatography to study plant pigments such as chlorophyll, carotenes, and xanthophylls. Note that fucoxanthin is not mentioned in the passage, but the best answer choice is still (E). If you picked (A) by accident: make sure you're at least skim reading the other answer choices to make sure you pick the best one!

15.   B   Paragraph 3 days that chromatography techniques developed substantially as a result of the work of Archer John Porter Martin and Richard Laurence Millington Synge during the 1940s and 1950s ((B) is correct).

16.   B   The passage talks about five affinity tags:
   • His tags are 6–10 amino acids in length (paragraph 11)
   • GST tags are 220 amino acids long (paragraph 12)
   • TAP tags are 172 amino acids long (paragraph 13)
   • HA tags are 9 amino acids long (paragraph 14)
   • FLAG tags are 8 amino acids long (paragraph 14)

   The largest of these is the GST tag at 220 amino acids in length ((B) is correct).

17.   D   Paragraph 9 says that making an antibody requires optimization, since it's characteristics (binding affinity, optimal concentrations, titer values) aren't known. Overall, (D) is correct.

18.   B   Paragraph 5 says that Protein A, Protein G and Protein L can be covalently linked to a solid support, such as agarose beads, magnetic beads, or polyacrylamide resin ((B) is correct).

19.   A   Paragraph 3 says that Martin and Synge contributed to development of all the methods listed except filtration chromatography, which is not in the passage and is the correct answer ((A) is correct).

20.   B   This is a challenging application question! Save it for near the end of this passage, or answer it using your letter of the day. Magnetic beads and a magnet are one option for a solid phase, but this doesn't directly answer the question on how TAP-tagged proteins are eluted (eliminate (C)). Imidazole and pH conditions are relevant to His tags, not TAP tags (eliminate (D) and (E)). Paragraph 13 says that TAP tags use a two step purification strategy. First, the protein A in the TAP tag binds an IgG matrix. The protein of interest is eluted using TEV cleavage. Next, the CBP tag binds calmodulin-coated beads in the presence of calcium. The passage never says how the second elution is performed. However, if calcium is required for the interaction between CBP and calmodulin, it is logical that to break this interaction and elute the protein, you would have to take away the calcium. This means you should eliminate

(A) and pick (B). A chelating agent is a molecule that binds metal ions such as calcium. Even without this knowledge you can find (B) as the correct answer by Process of Elimination.

Passage 4: Practical Applications of DNA Technology

1. E Paragraph 2 mentions all of the disease and treatment pairings except for the tumor necrosis factor as a treatment for stroke ((E) is correct).

2. B Paragraph 12 mentions gene therapy treatment as an option for all of the disease choices except hemophilia ((B) is correct).

3. D According to paragraph 2, the TI plasmid is obtained from a strain of soil bacteria is commonly used to genetically alter plants ((D) is correct).

4. C Paragraph 8 mentions that legumes can fix their own nitrogen ((C) is correct). In the same paragraph, it is stated that scientists are working on genetically engineering corn and rice to fix their own nitrogen but there is no mention that they have been successful ((B) and (D) are incorrect).

5. B Paragraph 5 states that plasmids containing the chymosin gene have been cloned and introduced into both prokaryotes (bacteria) and eukaryotes (yeast) ((B) is correct). Paragraph 6 states that the energy in biofuels comes from geologically recent carbon fixation ((A) is incorrect). The same paragraph says that bioethanol is derived from carbohydrates via fermentation, and biodiesel is from animal and plant fats ((C) and (E) are incorrect). Paragraph 8 mentions that corn and rice strains that are capable of nitrogen fixation would decrease the global fertilizer use ((D) is incorrect).

6. C The first statement is true (see paragraph 4). Cows are being used for breast milk production, not goats (see paragraph 5). The second statement is false.

7. A The author mentions in paragraph 9 that golden rice, which is genetically modified rice containing β-carotene, is used to treat vitamin A deficiency ((A) is correct).

8. A The author states in paragraph 1 that while biotechnology has great applications, there are ethical issues that should be considered ((A) is correct). Paragraph 2 refers to use of recombinant bacteria in drug production ((B) is incorrect), and paragraph 9 mentions genetically engineered crops that increase both shelf life and nutritional value ((C) is incorrect). There is no mention of safety issues with genetically modified foods in the passage ((D) is incorrect). The passage talks about various organisms being used for genetic engineering, ranging from bacteria, viruses, and yeast to multicellular organisms such as animals and plants, and there is no indication that the author believes that use of multicellular organisms is problematic ((E) is incorrect).

9. B Bear in mind that this is an "except" question. Paragraph 12 mentions retrovirus, adenovirus, and lentivirus being used for gene therapy but there is no mention of cytomegalovirus ((B) is correct).

10. **B** There are several different topics and examples in the passage, but the author doesn't really compare them (eliminate (A)). Choice (B) is a good match the purpose and writing style of the passage (and is the correct answer). The author supports genetic engineering and biotechnology, but (C) and (E) are too narrow. Choice (C) specifically talks about creating genetically modified foods, which is only a small part of the passage (eliminate (C)). Similarly, (E) focuses on the use of cloning and transgenic animals in medical research, which is also only a small part of the passage (eliminate (E)). There are no misconceptions mentioned in the passage (eliminate (D)).

11. **E** In paragraph 13, the diseases that are mentioned to have genetic testing available for detection are hemophilia, cystic fibrosis, Duchenne muscular dystrophy, and BRCA1 and BRCA2 mutations for ovarian and breast cancer. There is no mention of sickle cell anemia as being one of the diseases for which there is genetic testing available ((E) is correct).

12. **C** The author is generally supportive of genetic engineering and DNA technology. You can eliminate (A) and (D) because of their negative tone. Choices (B) and (E) describe information that is already in the passage (paragraphs 2 and 4/5, respectively). By Process of Elimination, the best answer is (C). The author mentions the importance of ethics in the first paragraph but then never expands on this topic. It is possible they would circle back to this in a future paragraph.

13. **A** Paragraph 4 says that transgenic potato plants are being developed to express proteins from the cholera bacterium and ingestion of these modified potatoes can cause production of anti-cholera antibodies. This is a similar mechanism to how traditional vaccines act to provide immunity against certain diseases ((A) is correct).

14. **D** Paragraph 11 says that certain genetically modified pigs can produce an enzyme called phytase in their saliva, which can break down indigestible phosphorus ((D) is correct).

15. **A** In paragraph 10, the only two animals specifically stated as being endangered are Puerto Rico parrot and orangutans ((A) is correct). There is no mention of any of the other animals in the passage.

16. **E** Both (A) and (C) are mentioned in paragraph 11, so (E) is the best answer. Pigs (not bacteria) break down indigestible phosphorus, thus reducing water pollution (eliminate (C)). Zebrafish (not bacteria) detect pollution in aquatic biomes (eliminate (D)).

Passage 5: Notch Cell Signaling

1. **C**   Paragraph 4 says that furin-like convertase enzymes are responsible for the first cleavage in the synthesis pathway of the Notch receptor proteins, and that Notch receptors are made through the secretory pathway involving the rough ER and Golgi apparatus. Therefore, it can be concluded that furin-like convertases would be found in the organelles involved in the secretory pathway ((C) is correct).

2. **E**   Paragraph 7 tells you that the Fringe family of proteins are sugar transferase enzymes that can modify Notch receptors or ligands via glycosylation (eliminate (B) and (C)). The passage also says that the Notch receptor is cleaved three times (paragraphs 4 and 5). This would require proteolytic cleavage, since Notch is a receptor protein (eliminate (A) and (D); (E) is correct). There is no information in the passage to suggest that Notch is phosphorylated (another reason to eliminate (B) and (D)).

3. **A**   Paragraph 8 states that astrocytes are part of the blood-brain barrier ((A) correct). Ependymal cells are involved in the production of the cerebrospinal fluid ((B) is incorrect). Microglial cells aid in waste removal ((C) is incorrect). Oligodendrocytes synthesize myelin in the CNS and Schwann cells synthesize myelin in the PNS ((D) and (E) are incorrect).

4. **B**   There is no information in the passage that the Notch signaling pathway is *the most* complex pathway found so far. Choice (A) is too extreme and thus is not the answer. Choice (B) is supported by paragraph 3 and is the best answer. Paragraph 11 says that Notch signaling has "has complex and tissue-dependent roles in cancer and other diseases" and that "elucidating roles for Notch in other cancers has been difficult: the effect of active Notch signaling seems to depend on tissue, cell, niche and timing." This seems to contradict (C). Paragraph 2 says that "while this basic setup seems straightforward, in an actual organism it is anything but!", which contradicts (D). The author seems interested in Notch signaling, so you can eliminate (E).

5. **C**   Paragraph 3 discusses the role of Notch signaling in fruit fly (insect) development and wing phenotypes (eliminate (A) and (E)). Paragraph 10 discusses the role of Notch in CNS development (eliminate (D)). Paragraph 11 says that Notch signaling is associated with cell growth and proliferation of the mammary gland (eliminate (B)). The musculoskeletal system is not discussed in the passage, so (C) is correct.

6. **E**   Paragraph 5 states that there are 5 Notch ligands ((E) is correct).

7. **B**   This is a difficult application question; save if for your second pass through the questions. Paragraph 10 explains how Notch signaling affects development of the CNS. Since this was discovered using knock-out and knock-in mice, these mice would have altered CNS development ((E) is incorrect). Paragraph 10 says that Notch signaling has three effects on cells in the nervous system: it inhibits the development of neuronal progenitor cells into neurons, inhibits the development of glial progenitor cells into oligodendrocytes, and promotes astrocyte differentiation. A Notch knock-out mouse would have less Notch signaling and therefore the opposite effects. Notch would not inhibit neuron development, so this mouse would have more neurons than a wildtype mouse (eliminate (A) and (C)). Notch would not inhibit oligodendrocyte development, so this mouse would also have more oligodendrocytes than a wildtype mouse (eliminate (A) and (D)). Finally, Notch would not promote astrocyte development, so this mouse would have fewer astrocytes than a wildtype mouse ((B) is correct).

8.　**C**　According to paragraph 7, Fringe proteins are sugar transferase enzymes that glycosylate (or add sugar molecules to) Notch receptors and their ligands. The statement that correctly describes their function is (C); they act as modifying enzymes.

9.　**A**　This is a difficult application question; save if for your second pass through the questions. Paragraph 10 explains how Notch signaling affects development of the CNS. Since this was discovered using knock-out and knock-in mice, these mice would have altered CNS development ((E) is incorrect). Paragraph 10 says that Notch signaling has three effects on cells in the nervous system: it inhibits the development of neuronal progenitor cells into neurons, inhibits the development of glial progenitor cells into oligodendrocytes, and promotes astrocyte differentiation. A Jagged knock-in mouse would have more or elevated Notch signaling. This means Notch would over-inhibit neuron development, so this mouse would have fewer neurons than a wildtype mouse (eliminate (B)). Notch would also over-inhibit oligodendrocyte development, so this mouse would also have fewer oligodendrocytes than a wildtype mouse ((A) is correct; eliminate (D)). Finally, Notch would over-promote astrocyte development, so this mouse would have more astrocytes than a wildtype mouse (eliminate (C); (A) is correct).

10.　**A**　In paragraph 4, it says that Notch receptors have a transmembrane domain and paragraph 5 mentions that Notch ligands are also transmembrane proteins ((A) is correct). There is no mention of Fringe proteins being transmembrane proteins (eliminate (B) and (C)).

11.　**E**　Paragraph 8 clearly states that oligodendrocytes have the same function as Schwann cells; both are involved in the synthesis of myelin ((E) is correct).

12.　**C**　Paragraph 5 says that the γ-secretase enzymes cleave the C-terminal end of the Notch receptor. This is the third and last cleavage event, also called S3, in the Notch pathway ((C) is correct). Fringe proteins mentioned in paragraph 7 function as sugar transferases ((E) is incorrect).

13.　**C**　This is a tricky question based on paragraph 9; you may want to leave it for your second pass. Progenitor cells are derived from stem cells and so are more differentiated than stem cells ((B) and (D) are incorrect). Progenitor cells differentiate into mature cells, not the other way around ((A) is incorrect). Paragraph 9 describes how stem cells can differentiate into many cells types (in this example, neurons, astrocytes and oligodendrocytes) and progenitor cells can differentiate into fewer cell types ((C) is correct). There is no information in the passage to support (E).

14.　**D**　The passage says that the Notch receptor is cleaved three times ((D) is correct). See paragraphs 4 and 5.

15.　**E**　Paragraph 8 describes how the CNS is protected by bones and floats in the CSF ((A) is supported and is not the answer). Choice (B) is supported by paragraph 8 (eliminate this option). Paragraph 9 describes how neural stem cells produce neuronal and glial progenitor cells, which produce mature neurons, and astrocytes and oligodendrocytes, respectively. This means (C) is false. Paragraph 9 also says that developmentally, the nervous system contains neural stem cells, but neuronal and glial progenitor cells. It also says that neural stem cells differentiate into progenitor cells. This means (D) is also false, and the correct answer is (E).

16.   **E**   Paragraph 7 says that the three Fringe modifying enzymes are Lunatic, Manic and Radical ((A) is true; eliminate (B)). Notch1 is a plasma membrane receptor (paragraph 4, (C) is correct) and Jagged2 is a ligand expressed on the plasma membrane ((D) is also correct). Overall then, the best answer is (E).

17.   **D**   The first statement is false: notch singling promotes the development of neurons from neural stem cells and neuronal progenitor cells (see paragraph 9, eliminate (A) and (C)). The second statement is true. Paragraph 11 describes how Notch signaling promotes cancer in T-ALL and breast cancer, but inhibits tumor development in the prostate ((D) is correct; eliminate (B)).

18.   **D**   Paragraph 11 discusses the role of Notch signaling in T-cell acute lymphoblastic leukemia (eliminate (A)), breast cancer (eliminate (C)) and prostate cancer (eliminate (B)). Ovarian cancer is not discussed in the passage ((D) is the correct answer).

19.   **B**   Paragraph 5 states that Delta3 is a ligand that binds to the Notch receptor ((B) is correct).

Quantitative Reasoning Test (QRT)

Chapter 18
Overview of the QRT

SECTION FORMAT AND STRATEGY

The Quantitative Reasoning Test (QRT) on the OAT contains 40 questions that you must complete in 45 minutes. The questions are not arranged in any useful order (for example, they are not in order of difficulty). Additionally, most students find that they do not have time to complete the section comfortably and must rush, at least to some extent, to complete the questions in the allotted time.

Two-Pass System

The above facts (time pressure and no order of difficulty) give rise to the first basic section strategy, the **Two-Pass System**. The Two-Pass System means to take two passes through a section. On the first pass, complete questions that you can answer quickly and easily. On the second pass, come back for questions that you know you can answer but are likely to take more time. By doing this, you will make sure that you get to all the questions that you definitely can answer; if you simply do the questions in the order that they are presented, you run the risk of putting too much time into an earlier but harder question (which you might get wrong anyway) and not getting to a question that you could have answered correctly if only you'd known it was there.

Generally, determining whether you know how to do a question quickly takes no more than a few seconds of reading, so skipping questions will not waste time; in fact, it will save you time. If you take the section in two passes, you'll get the easy questions right first, and then you'll have a very good idea how much time you have left for the harder questions. Thus, you will be able to allot your time more effectively.

The Two-Pass System takes some practice, so don't worry if it seems awkward at first. It will improve your score if you use it a few times.

Calculator

One change to the QRT in 2010 was the inclusion of an on-screen calculator that can be called up in the same way that you call up the periodic table in the Survey of the Natural Sciences. The calculator looks like this:

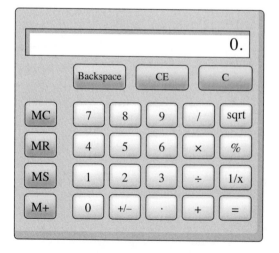

This is a basic four-function (not scientific or graphing) calculator. It can add, subtract, multiply, divide, take a square root, and take a reciprocal. However, it cannot do exponents, roots other than square roots, logs, or trig, and it does not know Order of Operations (it calculates as soon as you press buttons, rather than waiting for you to hit an "Enter" key).

Interestingly, this has not appeared to cause a major change in the test. The questions asked on the current QRT are not very different from the questions asked prior to the addition of the calculator.

Test Content

The questions cover arithmetic, algebra, geometry, and trigonometry. ADA describes the test content as follows:

I. **Mathematics Problems (30)**
    A. **Algebra (12)**
        1. Equations and expressions
        2. Inequalities
        3. Exponential notation and logarithms
        4. Absolute value
        5. Ratios and proportions
        6. Graphical analysis
    B. **Numerical calculations (5)**
        1. Fractions and decimals
        2. Percentages
        3. Approximations
        4. Scientific notation
    C. **Probability and statistics (3)**
    D. **Geometry (5)**
    E. **Trigonometry (5)**
II. **Applied Mathematics (Word) Problems (10)**

Note that this differs in emphasis from the content of the DAT. The OAT does not test Conversions. It also has more Algebra, slightly more Geometry and Trigonometry, and slightly fewer Numerical Calculations and Probability and Statistics. Also, the descriptions of the topics are rather vague. For example, "trigonometry" is tested, but what exactly that means is not specified. Does this just refer to the definitions of sine, cosine, and tangent? Does this also refer to more complex identities and laws? ADA is deliberately vague about this, which has provoked confusion and rumors among test takers. We have carefully studied the test and determined what it tests regularly. Those topics are covered in the later chapters that cover the content of the test.

It is certainly true, as you might expect from the specifications above, that knowing the content of the test is extremely important in order to do well. Much of the rest of our discussion of the math on the test will focus on content. However, content is not the only aspect of the test that you should be familiar with. While it is certainly impossible to do well on the QRT without knowing certain mathematical facts and formulas, it is also important to make effective use of the knowledge that you already possess. We will discuss some of the most crucial techniques for doing this now.

Plugging In

Many questions on the test ask you to work with variables for everyday quantities. This is highly artificial and potentially confusing. In daily life, you probably don't walk around with *d* dollars in your pocket or travel *f* feet in *t* seconds. You probably have five dollars, or ten dollars, or travel four feet in two seconds, or some actual, constant number. Since these are the numbers that you use every day, you're probably quite familiar with them and make few mistakes with them. On the other hand, you probably do algebra only when you're asked to do algebra problems, which is not nearly as often. No matter how good you are at algebra, it's easier to know whether you've made a mistake when you use regular old numbers than when you use algebraic expressions. But how can you use regular numbers when the test gives you an algebra problem? That's the magic of Plugging In.

Plugging In Your Own Number

Let's say you're given the following problem.

1. If a, b, c, d, and e are nonzero numbers such that a is b percent of c and c percent of the square of d is e, then what percent of e is a, in terms of b and d ?

(A) $\dfrac{100d^2}{b}$

(B) $100b$

(C) $\dfrac{d^2}{b}$

(D) $\dfrac{d^2}{100b}$

(E) $\dfrac{100b}{d^2}$

You might (if you weren't a savvy test taker) panic and guess on this question. It looks pretty horrible, after all. You could set up a whole bunch of equations with a whole bunch of variables, and if you make one little mistake anywhere, the whole problem is shot. However, take heart: you don't need to do any of that to solve this.

The whole point of algebraic formulas is that they relate variables that can have whatever value you could dream up. If the right answer is really right, it should work for *any* values of a, b, c, d, and e that fit the requirements they mention. Thus, you can just make up some values and run through the problem with those. If the answer doesn't work with the values that you chose, eliminate it.

Let's do that here. Since we're taking b percent of c to find a, let's make $b = 10$ and $c = 50$. This is easy enough: 10% of 50 is one-tenth of 50, which just removes the zero from the 50, so it's 5. With these numbers, then, $a = 5$.

The next portion of the problem says that c percent of the square of d is e. Now, c is already 50. Next, let's choose an easy square near these numbers, such as $d = 4$, so the square of d is 16. Thus, the question says that 50 percent of 16 is e. That means $e = 8$.

Now, the question is asking what percent of e is a, which might as well be saying what percent of 8 is 5. This is $\frac{5}{8}$, which you plug into the on-screen calculator to find that it is 62.5%. Thus, the answer to the question should be 62.5, if $a = 5$, $b = 10$, $c = 50$, $d = 4$, and $e = 8$.

At this point, the problem becomes pure calculation: plug these numbers into (A) and see if you get out 62.5. You don't. Choice (A) gives $\frac{100 \times 4^2}{10} = 160$. Likewise, (B) gives 1000, (C) gives 1.6, (D) gives 0.016, and (E) gives 62.5, so (E) is the right answer.

Okay, now for the bottom line. The point of this question is that on just about any question that asks for an algebraic expression, uses variables or unknown quantities, or uses the phrase "in terms of" (which, frankly, is meaningless here anyway—all of the answers are in terms of the right variables, so feel free to ignore that phrase entirely), you can make up your own numbers instead of working with their variables. The right answer should be right no matter what numbers you're using, so feel free to use the simplest, easiest numbers you can. Using regular numbers (constants) instead of variables is called Plugging In, and in this case, you're **Plugging In Your Own Number** (a number that you made up).

Notice, by the way, that this question is pretty darn hard unless you plug in. If you were to try to solve this with algebra, your first step would be to write down three equations: $a = \frac{b}{100}c$, $\frac{c}{100}d^2 = e$, and $\frac{x}{100}e = a$ (where x is the value you're actually solving for). From there, you would have to solve for x in terms of b and d by eliminating the other variables. This is challenging algebra. The only thing challenging about the plugging in solution is making sure that you use numbers that are easy enough to manipulate that you keep the problem from becoming even more unwieldy than it has to be.

On some other questions, it's not necessarily *hard* (in the sense of being complicated) to get the right answer, even if you don't plug in. However, such questions can be extremely *tricky*, since it's difficult to tell whether $\frac{x^2}{y}$ is okay or wildly wrong, whereas if you know that the answer should be about 20 and you get that the answer is 0.2, you know you've forgotten to multiply by 100 somewhere. The second crucial point is this: Plugging In will make some questions easier to *work*, but its true significance is that it makes most questions easier to *check*. You're less likely to get wrong answers—or more likely to catch wrong answers if you get them—if you plug in.

Plugging In More Than Once

In general, when you make up numbers, it's possible to choose numbers such that more than one answer works. You must check all five answer choices when Plugging In Your Own Number, because you have to make sure that the answer that works is the *only* answer that works. If more than one answer works, try another number. A few tips to avoid having more than one answer work:

- Do plug in numbers that fit the constraints in the question (if it says "even" numbers, use an even number).
- Do plug in numbers that make the math easy. On most problems, this means 2, 3, 5, 10, or 100.
- Don't plug in 0 or 1. These numbers have strange properties and tend to break things.
- Don't plug in numbers that appear in the question.
- Don't plug in the same number for more than one variable.

Bear in mind that these only apply to the first number you plug in. You may need to break several of these rules if you have to plug in again (discussed below).

Let's consider another example.

2. If x is an integer, which of the following must be an odd integer?

    (A) $x + 2$
    (B) $x - 3$
    (C) $2x$
    (D) $3x$
    (E) $2x - 3$

Applied Strategies

To solve this, you might plug in. The only constraint on x is that it be an integer (not a fraction or a decimal), so let's try $x = 2$. In that case, (A) would be 4, which is not odd, so eliminate it. Choice (B) would be -1, which is odd, so keep it. Choice (C) would be 4, which is not odd, so eliminate it. Choice (D) would be 6, which is also not odd, so eliminate it. Choice (E) would be 1, which is odd, so keep that as well. With $x = 2$, both (B) and (E) work. They're not both correct; it's just that while both of them *could* be an odd integer, only one of them *must* be an odd integer, as the question stem says.

So try a different number, and since we're talking about odd and even and tried an even number before, try an odd number. Let's say $x = 3$. In that case, we don't have to check (A), (C), or (D) again; we know that they don't *have* to be odd. Just check (B) and (E). (B) is 0, which is not odd (it's even), so eliminate it. (E) is 3, which is still odd, so it must be the right answer.

There are two points to this question. First, check all five answers when you're Plugging In Your Own Number! If you had just gone with the first answer that worked, you would've chosen (B) and gotten the question wrong.

Second, notice (and take seriously) words like "must" or "could." If a question asks what "must" be the case, then it's likely that many of the answers *could* work, given the right values of *x*, but only one of them *must* work with all values of *x*. On the other hand, if a question asks what "could" be the case, then it's likely that you need very particular values of *x* to make anything work at all, and with most values of *x* that you could choose, none of the answers will be right. You're just looking for an answer that *could ever* be right, which means that there might only be one value of *x* that ever makes it right, and your job is to find it. There's a pretty good chance you'll have to Plug In more than once on questions that ask what *must* or *could* be true, and there's nothing worse than Plugging In repeatedly but getting that (B) and (E) always work. You need to try different, weird numbers in order to differentiate between answers.

What are different, weird numbers? Well, for your second try at Plugging In on the same question, everything that we just said about not choosing numbers that break the question goes completely out the window. In fact, 0, 1, numbers in the question, and the same number for more than one variable are among the first things that you should try if you're working a question on which you have to Plug In a second time. The acronym **ZONE-F** may be useful: try zero, one, negatives, extremes (very large and very small), and fractions, if you're trying to find different numbers to Plug In that don't just give the same results as what you've already done.

Remember, this only applies when you're plugging in a second time on the same question, which you should only do if more than one answer worked on your first try.

Plugging In a Given Value

Sometimes questions will ask what the value of an expression is if a variable equals something (also known as **substitution**). For example, "What is the value of $x + 4$ when $x = 6$?" We substitute 6 for the *x* in the expression $x + 4$ and get $6 + 4$, which equals 10. This is plugging in, but the test has already given you the value to use. Consider the following examples.

3. Evaluate $2x + 7$ when $x = -3$.

    (A) −13
    (B) −1
    (C) 1
    (D) 8
    (E) 13

Once we substitute −3 for *x*, we get $2(-3) + 7 = -6 + 7 = 1$. Thus, the answer is (C).

4. If $f(x) = 3x^2 - x - 1$, what is $f(2)$?

    (A) 9
    (B) 11
    (C) 13
    (D) 15
    (E) 33

Once we substitute 2 for x, we get $f(2) = 3(2^2) - 2 - 1 = 12 - 2 - 1 = 9$. Thus, the answer is (A).

5. What is the value of $(3x)^2 - x - 1$ when $x = 2$?

    (A) 9
    (B) 11
    (C) 13
    (D) 15
    (E) 33

Be sure to notice the difference between this expression and the one in the previous example. Substitute 2 for x and evaluate: $(3 \cdot 2)^2 - 2 - 1 = 6^2 - 2 - 1 = 33$. Thus, the answer is (E).

6. Evaluate $2x + 3y$ when $x = 1$ and $y = -4$.

    (A) −14
    (B) −10
    (C) −5
    (D) 6
    (E) 14

We substitute 1 for x and −4 for y, then simplify: $2(1) + 3(-4) = 2 + (-12) = -10$. Thus, the answer is (B).

Plugging In Points

On a graphical question, sometimes you can choose points from the graph to plug into an equation, and this will help you eliminate answers. Consider the following example.

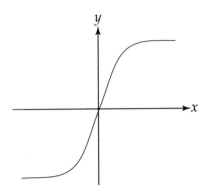

7. Which of the following equations represents the graph above?

(A) $y = \dfrac{10x - 1}{\sqrt{x^2 + 1}}$

(B) $y = \dfrac{10x^2 + 2}{\sqrt{x^4 + 1}}$

(C) $y = \dfrac{x^2 + 1}{\sqrt{x^2 + 2}}$

(D) $y = \dfrac{10x + 1}{\sqrt{x^2 + 1}}$

(E) $y = \dfrac{10x}{\sqrt{x^2 + 1}}$

Okay, these are not normal equations. There is no way you're supposed to know, off the top of your head, the shapes of the graphs of these equations. However, there is one point on the graph that you know: the origin. When $x = 0$ on this graph, $y = 0$. Thus, plug in this point! In (A), when $x = 0$, $y = \dfrac{-1}{1}$, which is definitely not 0. Eliminate (A). In (B), when $x = 0$, $y = \dfrac{2}{1}$, which is also not 0, so eliminate (B). In (C), when $x = 0$, $y = \dfrac{1}{\sqrt{2}}$, which is still not 0, so eliminate (C). In (D), when $x = 0$, $y = \dfrac{1}{1}$, which continues to not be 0, so eliminate (D). Presumably it's (E), and when you plug in $x = 0$, you get that $y = \dfrac{0}{1}$, which is indeed equal to 0, so (E) must be the answer. It's the only option that contains the one identifiable point in the graph.

Whenever you have any question that involves a graph, remember that you can plug in points.

Plugging In The Answers

For much the same reasons as making up a number can be useful, sometimes it can be useful to test answers to see if they are correct. This is called **Plugging In the Answers**. For example, consider the following problem.

> 8. The ratio of boys to girls in a certain club is 1:2. When 5 girls leave the club (but no boys leave), the ratio becomes 2:3. How many girls were originally in the club?
>
> (A) 2
> (B) 5
> (C) 10
> (D) 15
> (E) 20

Notice that the answer choices are arranged in order. This is typically the case. Thus, start in the middle (for reasons that will become apparent in a moment if they are not already). The question is how many girls were originally in the club, and if there were 10 originally in the club (as (C) indicates), then the 1:2 ratio says that there would have been 5 boys in the club. So there were 5 boys and 10 girls, and then 5 girls left. That means that there are now 5 boys and 5 girls. That's a 1:1 ratio, not a 2:3 ratio, so C is not the right answer.

Next, we can tell that (C) is too small. A 2:3 ratio means that there are more girls than boys, so because 10 girls gave a 1:1 ratio, there are not enough girls. Go for a larger number. If there were 15 girls originally, then the 1:2 ratio says that there would have been 7.5 boys. This seems pretty unlikely, but if you want to follow it all the way through, then after the 5 girls left, there would have been 7.5 boys and 10 girls; this is 3:4 ratio, which is still not right (but is closer than 1:1 was).

So presumably the answer is (E), if (C) is too small and (D) is unlikely. If you want to be sure, you can run this one through as well: 20 girls would mean 10 boys originally, and then after the 5 girls leave, there would be 10 boys and 15 girls, which is a 2:3 ratio. So (E) is in fact the right answer.

In general, regular numbers (not variables) in the answer choices are an indication that you can likely Plug In the Answers. That is, when you see variables in the answer, you can probably Plug In Your Own Number, and when you don't, you can probably Plug In the Answers.

Estimation

Answer choices on the test are often substantially different, so that even if you don't know exactly what the answer is, you can eliminate several that are not even close. A reasonable estimate is sometimes as good as an exact answer, so **estimation** is another major technique. Some questions explicitly ask for an estimate, as in the following.

9. Which of the following is the best approximation of the value of $\left(\sqrt{80} + \dfrac{11}{9}\right)^{3.01}$?

   (A) 1
   (B) 11
   (C) 108
   (D) 1075

To solve this, note first that the square root of 81 should be pretty close to the square root of 80, and the square root of 81 is an integer, so use that instead. That is, simplify $\sqrt{80} \approx \sqrt{81} = 9$. Also, 11 divided by 9 is going to be only slightly more than 9 divided by 9, and 9 divided by 9 is an integer, so use that instead. That is, $\dfrac{11}{9} \approx \dfrac{9}{9} = 1$. Thus, $\sqrt{80} + \dfrac{11}{9} \approx 9 + 1 = 10$, so the expression inside the parentheses should be pretty close to 10. (Since the square root of 80 is only *barely* less than the square root of 81, whereas 11 divided by 9 is somewhat more than 9 divided by 9, we can even say that it should be a little more than 10, although it makes no difference in this particular problem.) Now, that exponent is not a friendly one, but it is quite close to an integer, so just say that $3.01 \approx 3$, and you're left with $10^3 = 1000$. The only answer that is even close is (D).

In general, when approximating, try to make expressions into integers by changing as little as possible. The square root of 80 is almost exactly equal to the square root of 81 (it differs by less than 1%), but it's not nearly as close to the square roots of 64 or 100, so using those to approximate would be substantially less accurate.

In addition to questions that specifically ask for an estimate, some questions that don't mention approximating in any way can still be solved by this method. Consider the following example.

10. If $\log 2 = 0.301$, $\log 3 = 0.477$, and $\log 5 = 0.699$, then what is the value of $\log 900$?

   (A) 0.010
   (B) 0.100
   (C) 1.477
   (D) 2.186
   (E) 2.954

Okay, this looks like a monster. This is some sort of "rules of logarithms" question. Set that aside for a second, and focus on the end of the question, where it actually asks the important part. What is the value of log 900? That's the bit you have to answer.

Now, remember that a log is asking, "What power do I need to raise 10 to in order to get this number?" In other words, log 900 will be whatever the exponent has to be on a 10 to get 900. That is, if log 900 = x, then $10^x = 900$. So what do you have to raise 10 to in order to get 900? Well, to get 1000, you need to raise 10 to the 3. To get 900, you should raise 10 to somewhat less than 3 (not much less, since $10^2 = 100$, which is nowhere near 900). There's only one answer that's even close anyway: (E). If you're curious how to get an exact answer (why is it 2.954, not 2.955 or some other number that is somewhat less than 3?), we'll cover that in the section on logs. The point for right now is that an estimate can get you the answer just as well as anything else, and this will frequently be true on the test.

18.1   ARITHMETIC

Properties of Numbers Vocabulary

Integer: Not a fraction or decimal, including positives (1, 2, 3, …), negatives (–1, –2, –3, …), and zero.

Positive: greater than zero

Negative: less than zero

Sum: result of addition

Difference: result of subtraction

Product: result of multiplication

Quotient: result of division

Remainder: amount left over after division (for example, when 5 is divided by 2, the remainder is 1)

Factor: an integer that divides into another integer with no remainder

Multiple: the result of multiplying a number by an integer

Distinct: different; not equal

Prime: having exactly two distinct factors

Sum and Product Properties

positive × positive = positive

negative × negative = positive

negative × positive = positive × negative = negative

anything × 0 = 0

even + even = even

odd + odd = even

even + odd = odd + even = odd

even × even = even

odd × odd = odd

even × odd = odd × even = even

Fractions

Multiply fractions as follows:

$$\frac{a}{c} \times \frac{b}{d} = \frac{ab}{cd}$$

Divide fractions by multiplying by the reciprocal:

$$\frac{a}{c} \div \frac{b}{d} = \frac{a}{c} \times \frac{d}{b} = \frac{ad}{cb}$$

Add or subtract fractions as follows:

$$\frac{a}{c} + \frac{b}{d} = \frac{ad + bc}{cd}$$

Decimals

Use the calculator whenever possible for decimals.

To add or subtract decimals, line up the decimal points.

To multiply decimals, multiply without the decimal points and then count the number of spaces after each decimal point.

To divide decimals, convert to integers by multiplying by 10 and then divide normally.

Percents

Percent means "divide by 100." You may also use the following table for problems involving fractions, decimals, and percents.

Verbal statement	Equivalent algebraic expression/symbol
two-thirds of a number	$\frac{2}{3}x$ ("of" means multiply)
two out of three	$\frac{2}{3}$ ("out of" means divide)
five percent	$\frac{5}{100}$ or 0.05
is	=
what	x, y, or any other variable

Exponents and Roots

Exponents indicate repeated multiplication (for example, $2 \times 2 \times 2 = 2^3$).

A root undoes an exponent (for example, $2^2 = 4$, so $\sqrt{4} = 2$).

To multiply with the same base, add the exponents.

To divide with the same base, subtract the exponents.

To raise to another power, multiply the exponents.

Exponents distribute to multiplied or divided terms (e.g., $(4 \times 5)^2 = 4^2 \times 5^2$).

Anything to the zero is 1 (except 0^0, which is undefined).

Negative exponents are reciprocals (e.g., $2^{-3} = \dfrac{1}{2^3}$).

Fractional exponents are roots (e.g., $2^{\frac{1}{3}} = \sqrt[3]{2}$).

Scientific notation writes numbers in the form $a \times 10^b$, where $1 \leq a < 10$ and b is an integer.

Logarithms

A logarithm expresses an exponent differently, as follows:

If $a^b = c$, then $b = \log_a c$.

A log asks to what power (b) you raise the base (a) in order to get the number (c). Hence, the log (base 10) of 100 is 2, because you raise 10 to the 2 in order to get 100.

$\log(a) + \log(b) = \log(ab)$

$\log(a) - \log(b) = \log\left(\dfrac{a}{b}\right)$

$\log(a)^b = b\log(a)$

Order of Operations

Perform arithmetic operations in the following order (PEMDAS, or Please Excuse My Dear Aunt Sally):

- Parentheses
- Exponents
- Multiplication and Division
- Addition and Subtraction

Read from left to right to avoid ambiguity.

18.2 ALGEBRA

Solving Equations

To solve an algebraic equation, if you want to do something to one side of an equation, you must do it to the other as well.

The Distributive Law says that $a(b + c) = ab + ac$. In the same way, to multiply sums, multiply each term in one sum by each term in the other sum. For example, FOIL (Firsts Outsides Insides Lasts): $(a + b)(c + d) = ac + ad + bc + bd$.

Factoring is undoing distribution. That is, divide a common factor out of each part of a sum. You can simplify algebraic fractions or solve quadratics by factoring too.

$$(x + y)(x + y) = x^2 + 2xy + y^2$$

$$(x - y)(x - y) = x^2 - 2xy + y^2$$

$$(x + y)(x - y) = (x - y)(x + y) = x^2 - y^2$$

Solve simultaneous equations (multiple equations with multiple variables, such as x and y) by multiplying equations by integers (if necessary) and then adding or subtracting them from each other.

Absolute Value and Inequalities

The absolute value of a number is its distance from 0 (always a positive number).

An inequality is a relation that does not involve an equals sign. For example, $4 > 3$, $6 \leq 7$, or $1 \neq 2$.

Solve inequalities by the same means as you would solve equations, except that if you multiply or divide by a negative number, you must switch the direction of the inequality.

Functions

A function is a set of instructions for operations to perform on a number, often in function $f(x)$ notation, but sometimes with funny symbols.

Solve functions by plugging the given numbers into the equation defining the function.

18.3 WORD PROBLEMS

Translating a Verbal Statement into an Algebraic Expression

Verbal statement	Equivalent algebraic expression
a number increased by 2	$x + 2$
a number decreased by 5	$x - 5$
5 less than a number	$x - 5$
5 decreased by a number	$5 - x$ [*not* $x - 5$]
3 more than twice a number	$2x + 3$ [*not* $2(x + 3)$, which is "twice the sum of a number and 3"]
7 less than three times a number	$3x - 7$ [*not* $7 - 3x$, which is "7 decreased by three times a number"]
the square of 1 more than a number	$(x + 1)^2$ [*not* $x^2 + 1$, which is "1 more than the square of a number"]
two consecutive integers	n and $n + 1$
two consecutive even integers	n and $n + 2$ (where n is an even integer)
two consecutive odd integers	n and $n + 2$ (where n is an odd integer)
the sum of three consecutive integers	$n + (n + 1) + (n + 2)$
8 more than four times the cube of a number	$4x^3 + 8$

The following are common types of word problems:

- Counting and ratios
- Age
- Money
- Averages and rates
- Mixtures and weighted averages
- Groups

18.4   ADVANCED ARITHMETIC

Statistics, Probability, and Arrangements

Mean: Average.

Median: The middle of a list of numbers arranged in order.

Mode: The most frequently occurring number in a list of numbers.

Standard deviation and variance: Expressions of the spread of data. The higher the standard deviation or variance, the farther the data points are from the mean value.

Normal distribution: A bell curve.

$$\text{Probability} = \frac{\text{Number of outcomes you want}}{\text{Number of outcomes possible}}$$

Factorial: The product of all the integers from the starting down to 1. For example, $3! = 3 \times 2 \times 1$.

The number of ways of doing a series of things is the product of the number of ways of doing each thing.

If you are choosing things from the same set of options without replacement, the number of ways of choosing decreases by one with each decision.

If order doesn't matter, you must divide by the factorial of the number of choices you had.

18.5   PLANE GEOMETRY

Vocabulary

Acute angle: Less than 90°.

Right angle: Equal to 90°.

Obtuse angle: Greater than 90°.

Straight angle: Equal to 180°.

Complementary: Angles that add up to 90°.

Supplementary: Angles that add up to 180°.

When two lines cross (and are not perpendicular), they create two kinds of angles: big angles and small angles. All the big angles are equal, all the small angles are equal, and any big angles plus any small angles equals 180°. The same applies when parallel lines are added.

Polygons

Polygon: A closed figure with straight sides.

The sum of the interior angles of an n-sided polygon is $(n - 2)180$.

Perimeter: The sum of the lengths of the sides.

Area: The size of the region enclosed by the sides.

Congruent: Same size and same shape. The angles of one polygon are equal to the angles of the congruent polygon, and the sides of one are equal to the sides of the other as well.

Similar: Same shape, but not necessarily the same size. The angles of one polygon are equal to the angles of the similar polygon, and their sides are proportional.

Triangles

Triangle: A 3-sided polygon.

The sum of the interior angles is 180°.

$$A = \frac{1}{2}bh$$

Equilateral: Three equal sides and three equal angles.

Isosceles: Two equal sides and two equal angles.

Scalene: No equal sides and no equal angles.

Obtuse triangle: A triangle containing an obtuse angle.

Right triangle: A triangle containing a right angle.

Acute triangle: A training containing only acute angles.

Pythagorean Theorem: $a^2 + b^2 = c^2$ in a right triangle, where c is the length of the longest side (the hypotenuse) and a and b are the lengths of the shorter sides (the legs).

Quadrilaterals

Quadrilateral: A 4-sided polygon.

The sum of the interior angles is 360°.

Parallelogram: Opposite sides are parallel and equal. The perimeter is $2b + 2c$, if b and c are the side lengths, and the area is bh, if b is the base and h is the height.

Rectangle: All angles are 90°, and opposite sides are equal. The perimeter is $2b + 2h$, and the area is bh, if b and h are the side lengths.

Square: All angles are 90°, and all sides are equal. The perimeter is $4b$ and the area is b^2, if the side length is b.

Circles

Circle: The set of points in a plane that are a fixed distance from a center point.

Radius: The distance from the center to the outer rim of the circle.

Diameter: Twice the radius. A line segment with endpoints on the circle and passing through the center.

Tangent: A line that touches a circle at a single point. It is perpendicular to the radius at that point.

$A = \pi r^2$

Circumference: Like perimeter, the distance around the outside of the circle, given by $C = 2\pi r$.

Arc: A portion of the circumference. Proportional to the central angle defining the arc and also to the sector bounded by the arc.

Semicircle: Half a circle.

Solve geometric word problems by drawing diagrams of the situations they describe.

18.6 SOLID AND COORDINATE GEOMETRY

Solid Geometry

Volume is the amount of space enclosed in a 3D shape.

Surface area is the sum of the areas of its faces.

Box (rectangular prism): $V = l \times w \times h$ and $SA = 2lw + 2lh + 2wh$

Cube: $V = l^3$ and $SA = 6l^2$

Any prism: $V = Bh$, where B is the area of the base

Any cone or pyramid: $V = \dfrac{1}{3}Bh$

Coordinate Geometry

Find the distance between two points in the coordinate plane by making a right triangle. The general

formula is $d = \sqrt{\left(x_2 - x_1\right)^2 + \left(y_2 - y_1\right)^2}$.

The slope m of a line passing through (x_1, y_1) and (x_2, y_2) is $m = \dfrac{y_2 - y_1}{x_2 - x_1}$.

The equation of a line is $y = mx + b$.

Inequalities are represented with shading and sometimes dashed lines.

18.7 TRIGONOMETRY

SOHCAHTOA

$$\sin\theta = \frac{\text{opposite}}{\text{hypotenuse}} \qquad \cos\theta = \frac{\text{adjacent}}{\text{hypotenuse}} \qquad \tan\theta = \frac{\text{opposite}}{\text{adjacent}}$$

Reciprocal Trigonometry Functions

$$\csc\theta = \frac{1}{\sin\theta} = \frac{\text{hypotenuse}}{\text{opposite}} \qquad \sec\theta = \frac{1}{\cos\theta} = \frac{\text{hypotenuse}}{\text{adjacent}} \qquad \cot\theta = \frac{1}{\tan\theta} = \frac{\text{adjacent}}{\text{opposite}}$$

θ	$\sin\theta$	$\cos\theta$
0°	$\frac{\sqrt{0}}{2} = 0$	$\frac{\sqrt{4}}{2} = 1$
30°	$\frac{\sqrt{1}}{2} = \frac{1}{2}$	$\frac{\sqrt{3}}{2}$
45°	$\frac{\sqrt{2}}{2}$	$\frac{\sqrt{2}}{2}$
60°	$\frac{\sqrt{3}}{2}$	$\frac{\sqrt{1}}{2} = \frac{1}{2}$
90°	$\frac{\sqrt{4}}{2} = 1$	$\frac{\sqrt{0}}{2} = 0$

θ	$\tan\theta$	$\csc\theta$	$\sec\theta$	$\cot\theta$
0°	0	undefined	1	undefined
30°	$\frac{\sqrt{3}}{3}$	2	$\frac{2\sqrt{3}}{3}$	$\sqrt{3}$
45°	1	$\sqrt{2}$	$\sqrt{2}$	1
60°	$\sqrt{3}$	$\frac{2\sqrt{3}}{3}$	2	$\frac{\sqrt{3}}{3}$
90°	undefined	1	undefined	0

$A = \dfrac{1}{2}ab\sin\theta$ in a triangle with sides of a and b and θ the angle between them.

Inverse trig functions undo trig functions. For example, if $\sin\theta = a$, then $\theta = \sin^{-1}a$.

π radians $= 180°$

Use the unit circle to find values of trig functions of angles greater than $90°$.

$\sin^2\theta + \cos^2\theta = 1$

If given other identities in the text of a problem, use those identities, even if they are unfamiliar.

18.8

18.8 QUANTITATIVE COMPARISON AND DATA SUFFICIENCY

In 2018, the ADA introduced two new types of math questions, called "quantitative comparison" and "data sufficiency." These question types will only make up a handful of the questions on the QRT; however, knowing the format of these questions and how to approach them can help save time and improve accuracy when tackling them. Note that techniques of plugging-in and ballparking are applicable and often the best ways to approach these problems. It's not uncommon when plugging-in for these problems that you'll need to plug in multiple times. To help with your choice of value to plug in, consider the acronym FROZEN: fractions, repeats, one, zero, extremes, and negatives. For example, after trying a positive value you could try a negative value, and after trying an integer value, you could try a fraction.

Quantitative Comparison

These questions ask you to compare two quantities and pick an answer choice that appropriately describes the relationship between the two quantities. The answer choices consist of the following, potentially in varied order:

(A) A is always greater than B
(B) B is always greater than A
(C) A and B are always equal
(D) Cannot be determined from the information given

It's worth noting that you don't necessarily need to know the exact values of A and B; it's enough to know how the quantities compare to each other. For instance, if A is positive and B is negative, then A is always greater than B. In this case, you could confidently pick answer choice A even though you don't have specific values for quantities A and B. Furthermore, Plugging In and Ballparking (estimation) can be valuable techniques for these question types.

11. If you have $x^2 - 4x + 4 = 0$, and:

A	B
x	$+2$

(A) A is always greater than B
(B) B is always greater than A
(C) A and B are always equal
(D) Cannot be determined from the information given

Although Quantity A is listed as a variable, x, it can be solved for based on the equation in the question stem. Factoring the quadratic in the question stem gives

$$x^2 - 4x + 4 = 0 \rightarrow (x-2)^2 = 0 \rightarrow x = 2$$

If $x = 2$, then so does Quantity A. Therefore, Quantities A and B are always equal and (C) is correct.

12. If you have $x^2 - 9 = 0$, and:

A	B
x	$+2$

(A) A is always greater than B
(B) B is always greater than A
(C) A and B are always equal
(D) Cannot be determined from the information given

Again, Quantity A is a variable. Factoring the quadratic gives

$$x^2 - 9 = 0 \rightarrow (x+3)(x-3) = 0 \rightarrow x = 3 \ \ or \ \ x = -3$$

If $x = 3$, then Quantity A = 3 and A > B. But if $x = -3$, then A = -3 and A < B. Therefore, the relationship between Quantities A and B cannot be determined from the information given. Choice (D) is correct.

18.8

Data Sufficiency AD/BCE

These questions present you with two statements and ask you to assess what statement or statements, if any, are sufficient to answer the question. Note that you're not asked to actually answer the math problem; you're asked if you CAN solve the math problem. So, you don't need to spend time fully answering the problem. These questions are preceded by a paragraph on background information explaining how to answer them. Be sure to refer back to this information if you get confused about the question task or answer choices. The answer choices likely consist of the following

(A) Statement 1 alone is enough to answer the question, but statement 2 alone is not sufficient to answer the question

(B) Statement 2 alone is enough to answer the question, but statement 1 alone is not sufficient to answer the question

(C) Both statements 1 and 2 together are sufficient to answer the question, but neither statement alone is sufficient

(D) Each statement alone is sufficient to answer the question

(E) Statements 1 and 2 together are not sufficient to answer the question, and additional data are needed

These questions should be tackled in steps, using Process of Elimination. First, assess whether or not statement 1 alone provides sufficient information to answer the question. According to (B), (C), and (E), statement 1 alone doesn't provide sufficient information to answer the question. Therefore, if statement 1 does provide sufficient information to answer the question, then the correct answer must either be (A) or (D). Next, assess statement 2. If it is sufficient to answer the question on its own, the correct answer is (D); otherwise, the correct answer is (A). If, instead, statement 1 alone is insufficient to answer the question asked, you can eliminate (A) and (D), leaving you with (B), (C), and (E). Again, assess whether or not statement 2 alone provides sufficient information to answer the question asked. If it does, pick (B). Otherwise, you can eliminate (B), leaving you with (C) and (E). Finally, assess whether both statements 1 and 2 together provide sufficient information to answer the question. If they do, pick (C); otherwise, pick (E). We call this the AD/BCE approach since the assessment of statement 1 will leave you with either AD or BCE as remaining answer choices.

It's worth noting that sometimes there are only four answer choices on the QRT. If that happens with a data sufficiency question, it's likely that either (C) or (D), as described above, would be removed. Regardless, you should still approach the question in steps and apply Process of Elimination similar to what was just described in the previous paragraph.

13. If x and y are positive integers and $x/y = 3$, what is the value of x ?

    (1) $3 < y < 7$
    (2) y is odd.

Simplifying any algebraic expressions in the question is often a good way to start. For instance, rearranging $x/y = 3$ to state $x = 3y$ gives a slightly more straight-forward way to assess whether or not there is sufficient information to solve for x.

To find a unique, positive integer value for x, this expression requires a unique, positive integer value for y. Looking at statement 1 alone first, y is limited to the positive integer values of 4, 5, or 6. Three possible values for y means there are three possible values for x: statement 1 alone is insufficient to answer the question. Eliminate (A) and (D).

Next, looking at statement 2 alone, y is restricted to odd, positive integers meaning there are an infinite number of possible values for y. Remember, you're assessing statement 2 alone and ignoring statement 1. Statement 2 alone is insufficient to answer the question, so eliminate (B).

Looking at both statements together, the only odd, positive integer value between 3 and 7 is 5. Therefore, there is only one possible value for y, which is what is required to solve for x. Eliminate (E) and pick (C). Again, you don't need to know that $x = 15$ to know that there will be a unique, positive integer value for x; it's enough to know that you can solve for that unique, positive integer value for x that allows you to confidently pick (C).

Data Sufficiency: Question Types

There are two common question types for data sufficiency problems: value-based and yes/no. Value-based questions are ones that ask for a specific amount or value for the answer. The question stem for a value-based question will often contain the phrase "what is the value of" or "how much/many." Value-based question can be thought of as a jig-saw puzzle that you have to put together. A typical math problem will require the exact value for the answer, i.e., it will require the full puzzle to be put together. A value-based data sufficiency problem, however, will only require that you have the means to solve the problem, i.e., it will only require that you have the pieces needed to put the puzzle together. Following this analogy, we call the basic approach to value-based data sufficiency problems "pieces of the puzzle." Setup each value-based problem by first putting together what you **know** from the question and from your core math knowledge (the pieces you have) and use that to then figure out what you **need** to solve the problem (the pieces missing to complete the puzzle).

14. At a certain bakery, pecan pies cost $15. How many pecan pies did the baker sell on Wednesday?

    (1) On Tuesday, the bakery's pecan pie sales totaled $225.
    (2) On Wednesday, the bakery's pecan pie sales were $75 more than Tuesday's pecan pie sales.

Let's start by using pieces of puzzle and taking stock of what we know and what we need to solve this puzzle. We know the cost of pecan pie is $15/pie. What we need, given that we know pecan pies cost $15/pie, is the pecan pie sales for Wednesday: multiplying those two quantities together would give us the number of pecan pies sold on Wednesday.

Looking at statement 1 alone first, we are given the pecan pie sales for Tuesday. Be careful to read the full statement. This statement gives us the pecan pie sales for the wrong day, so it doesn't address the missing puzzle piece we need. Therefore, statement 1 on its own is insufficient to answer the question, so eliminate answer choices (A) and (D).

Looking at statement 2 alone, we are given the pecan pie sales on Wednesday relative to that of Tuesday. On its own, statement 2 is insufficient, so eliminate answer choice (B). Putting statements 1 and 2 together, we now have Wednesday's pecan pie sales, which was the missing piece to the puzzle we needed. Therefore, we have sufficient information to answer the question. Eliminate answer choice (E) and pick (C).

The other common data sufficiency question is the yes/no question. These questions are ones that are answered by either a "yes" or a "no." Sufficient information in these cases means you can confidently answer the question with either only a "yes" or only a "no." If, based on the information available, the question could be answered with a "yes" or a "no" depending on a few things, then there is insufficient information to answer the question. Plugging-in is often the best technique to employ to work through these types of problems. If your first choice of number gave a "yes" as an answer, try plugging-in again to find a "no" as an answer and vice versa. If you can find such a case, work the AD/BCE approach to eliminate answer choices. If you can't find such a case, take a step back from the problem to see if you must always get that answer.

15. Is $x + 7$ an odd integer?

    (1) $2x + 3$ is an odd integer.
    (2) $x + 11$ is an even integer.

The answer to this question won't be a specific value, but rather a "yes" or a "no." Let's consider statement 1 on its own. Let's plug in $x = 2$. In this case, $2x + 3 = 2(2) + 3 = 7$, which is an odd integer. This satisfies the statement, so let's see what answer it gives us. $x + 7 = 2 + 7 = 9$, which is an odd integer. Therefore, the answer to our question is "yes." Let's plug in again to see if that has to always be the case. Let $x = 3$. Now $2x + 3 = 2(3) + 3 = 9$, which is an odd integer. This satisfies the statement, so let's see what answer it gives us. $x + 7 = 3 + 7 = 10$, which is an even integer. Therefore, the answer to our question is "no." There is insufficient information based on statement 1 alone to answer the question because the answer could be a "yes" or a "no." Eliminate answer choices (A) and (D).

Let's consider statement 2 on its own. Again, let's plug in $x = 2$. In this case, $x + 11 = 2 + 11 = 13$, which is an odd integer. This doesn't satisfy the conditions of the statement, so we need to plug in something different. Let's plug in $x = 3$, which gives $x + 11 = 3 + 11 = 14$, which is an even integer. This satisfies the statement, and we know the answer to the question becomes a "no" having tried $x = 3$ already. Let's plug in again to see if that always has to be the case. If $x = 1$, then $x + 11 = 1 + 11 = 12$, which is an even integer, which satisfies the statement. The answer to the question is $x + 7 = 1 + 7 = 8$, which is an even integer, hence the answer to the question is again "no." This is a consistent answer, so let's take a step back to see if we must always get this answer. The only way for $x + 11$ to be an even integer, given that 11 is an odd integer, is for x to be an odd integer, too. Therefore, $x + 7$ will always be an even integer since an odd integer plus an odd integer is an even integer. The answer to the question will always be a "no" meaning we have sufficient information to answer the problem. Eliminate answer choices (C) and (E) and pick (B).

QUANTITATIVE COMPARISON DRILL

1. Set C: {2, 3, 5, 8, 9, 21, 25)
   List D: {5, 5, 6, 9, 10, 11)
   Quantity A: The median of Set C
   Quantity B: The median of List D

   (A) Quantity A is greater.
   (B) Quantity B is greater.
   (C) The two quantities are equal.
   (D) The relationship cannot be determined from the information given.

2. x, y, and z are three consecutive positive even integers.
   Quantity A: $x + z - 3$
   Quantity B: $y + 1$

   (A) Quantity A is greater.
   (B) Quantity B is greater.
   (C) The two quantities are equal.
   (D) The relationship cannot be determined from the information given.

3. x is directly proportional to y in a ratio of 3 to 1, and y is directly proportional to z in a ratio of 4 to 1.
   Quantity A: x
   Quantity B: y

   (A) Quantity A is greater.
   (B) Quantity B is greater.
   (C) The two quantities are equal.
   (D) The relationship cannot be determined from the information given.

4. Quantity A: The sum of the prime factors of 40.
   Quantity B: The product of the distinct prime factors of 75.

   (A) Quantity A is greater.
   (B) Quantity B is greater.
   (C) The two quantities are equal.
   (D) The relationship cannot be determined from the information given.

5. Quantity A: $\sqrt{0.25 \times 0.36}$
   Quantity B: $(0.25 \times 0.36)^2$

   (A) Quantity A is greater.
   (B) Quantity B is greater.
   (C) The two quantities are equal.
   (D) The relationship cannot be determined from the information given.

DATA SUFFICIENCY DRILL

1. Is the value of $a^3 + 3ab$ equal to 0 ?
   1. $a = 0$
   2. $b = 0$

   (A) Statement (1) ALONE is sufficient, but statement (2) alone is not sufficient.
   (B) Statement (2) ALONE is sufficient, but statement (1) alone is not sufficient.
   (C) BOTH statements TOGETHER are sufficient, but NEITHER statement ALONE is sufficient.
   (D) EACH statement ALONE is sufficient.
   (E) Statements (1) and (2) TOGETHER are NOT sufficient.

2. In what year was a certain study completed?
   1. The study's findings were published in 1988, exactly 6 months after the study was completed.
   2. The study began in 1985 and was completed exactly 3 years later.

   (A) Statement (1) ALONE is sufficient, but statement (2) alone is not sufficient.
   (B) Statement (2) ALONE is sufficient, but statement (1) alone is not sufficient.
   (C) BOTH statements TOGETHER are sufficient, but NEITHER statement ALONE is sufficient.
   (D) EACH statement ALONE is sufficient.
   (E) Statements (1) and (2) TOGETHER are NOT sufficient.

3. Integer z has how many factors?
   1. z is the square of a prime number.
   2. z and $\sqrt{16}$ each have the same number of factors.

   (A) Statement (1) ALONE is sufficient, but statement (2) alone is not sufficient.
   (B) Statement (2) ALONE is sufficient, but statement (1) alone is not sufficient.
   (C) BOTH statements TOGETHER are sufficient, but NEITHER statement ALONE is sufficient.
   (D) EACH statement ALONE is sufficient.
   (E) Statements (1) and (2) TOGETHER are NOT sufficient.

4. Is $y > 0$?
   1. $y^3 > 0$
   2. $|y| > 0$

   (A) Statement (1) ALONE is sufficient, but statement (2) alone is not sufficient.
   (B) Statement (2) ALONE is sufficient, but statement (1) alone is not sufficient.
   (C) BOTH statements TOGETHER are sufficient, but NEITHER statement ALONE is sufficient.
   (D) EACH statement ALONE is sufficient.
   (E) Statements (1) and (2) TOGETHER are NOT sufficient.

5. What is the value of the prime integer b ?
   1. $b^2 < 26$
   2. $b^3 < 26$

   (A) Statement (1) ALONE is sufficient, but statement (2) alone is not sufficient.
   (B) Statement (2) ALONE is sufficient, but statement (1) alone is not sufficient.
   (C) BOTH statements TOGETHER are sufficient, but NEITHER statement ALONE is sufficient.
   (D) EACH statement ALONE is sufficient.
   (E) Statements (1) and (2) TOGETHER are NOT sufficient.

ANSWERS AND EXPLANATIONS

Quantitative Comparison

1. **A** Set C contains an odd number of numbers and its elements are already in order. So, the median is the middle number, which is 8. So, Quantity A is 8. List D contains an even number of numbers. Again, those numbers are already in order, so take the average of the two middle numbers, 6 and 9. So, the median of List D is 7.5. Quantity B is, therefore, 7.5. Quantity A is greater.

2. **D** This is a Quantitative Comparison question with variables, so Plug In more than once. Start with an easy set of numbers, such as $x = 2$, $y = 4$, $z = 6$. Quantity A is $2 + 6 - 3 = 5$. Quantity B is $4 + 1 = 5$. The two quantities are equal, so eliminate (A) and (B). Plug In again using FROZEN numbers. Negatives, zero, one, and fractions are not allowed, so try extremes, such as $x = 100$, $y = 102$, $z = 104$. Quantity A is $100 + 104 - 3 = 201$. Quantity B is $102 + 1 = 103$. Quantity A is now greater. Eliminate (C). The correct answer is (D).

3. **D** There are variables in the quantities, so Plug In. Because y is in both ratios, try $y = 4$. If $y = 4$, then based on the ratios given in the problem, $x = 12$ and $z = 1$. Quantity A is greater, so eliminate (B) and (C). Now, try FROZEN numbers, such as negatives. If $y = -4$, then $x = -12$ and $z = -1$. Quantity B is now greater. Eliminate (A). The correct answer is (D).

4. **B** To compare Quantity A with Quantity B, start by drawing two factor trees. The prime factors of 40 are 2, 2, 2, and 5, so Quantity A equals $2 + 2 + 2 + 5$, which equals 11. The prime factors of 75 are 3, 5, and 5, but because the problem says "distinct," count 5 only once. Because the product of the distinct prime factors of 75 is $3 \times 5 = 15$, Quantity B equals 15. Thus, Quantity B is greater than Quantity A, making (B) the correct answer.

5. **A** Compare, don't calculate. Both quantities have (0.25×0.36). That product is a number between 0 and 1. Quantity A is the square root of that number and Quantity B is that number squared. Taking the square root of a number between 0 and 1 results in a number that is greater than the original number. Squaring a number between 0 and 1 results in a number that is less than the original number. Therefore, the value in Quantity A must be greater than the value in Quantity B. Choice (A) is the correct answer.

Data Sufficiency

1 **A** Since this is a Yes/No question, you can and should plug in values for the variables. Statement (1) tells you that a = 0. No matter what you plug in for b, the answer to the question is Yes. So, Statement (1) is sufficient; eliminate (B), (C), and (E). Statement (2) tells you that $b = 0$. If you plug in $a = 0$, the answer is Yes. If you plug in $a = 2$, the answer is No. Since you got both Yes and No, Statement (2) is not sufficient. Eliminate (D). The correct answer is (A).

2 **B** From Statement (1), if the findings were published in January 1988, then the study was completed in July 1987, but if the findings were published in December 1988, then the study was completed in June 1988, so you should write down BCE. From Statement (2), you know that the study was completed in 1988, so the answer is (B).

3 **D** For statement 1, plug in some values of z. If $z = \sqrt{16} = 4$, then z has 3 factors (1, 2 and 4). If $z = 32 = 9$, then z has 3 factors (1, 3 and 9). If $z = 72 = 49$, then z has 3 factors (1, 7 and 49). So, no matter what you plug in, you get a consistent answer of 3, which means that you should write down AD. For Statement 2, you don't have to do any math: you know that $\sqrt{16}$ has a certain, unchanging number of factors, and you know that z has the same number of factors, so the answer is (D).

4 **A** Since this is a Yes/No question, you can and should plug in values for the variable. (1) Start with an easy number, $y = 2$. This answers our question Yes. We can't plug in zero but can use $y = 1$, which also answers the question Yes. We can't plug in a negative number. Have we exhausted all of the possible numbers? Not yet, try a fraction between 0 and 1 such as $y = 0.5$, but yet again we get a Yes. Eliminate BCE. (2) $y = 2$ answers the question Yes and $y = -2$ answers the question No. Since you got both Yes and No, not sufficient. Eliminate (D). The correct answer is (A).

5 **B** If $b^2 < 26$ where b is a prime integer, then b can be 2, 3, or 5. But we need one value, so Statement (1) is not sufficient. Check Statement (2). This information means that b can only be 2. Therefore, the answer is (B).

Practice

PHYSICS DRILL

Energy and Momentum

1. An automobile with a certain shape experiences a drag force due to air resistance that is, in Newtons, equal to one-third the square of the car's speed, in meters per second. How much power would the engine have to supply to the wheels to balance this drag force when the car is moving at a constant speed of 30 m/s ?

   (A) 10 W
   (B) 300 W
   (C) 9 kW
   (D) 27 kW

2. A young child is sliding down a hill at an incline of 30 degrees on a sled with total combined mass of 10 kg. If the coefficient of friction between the hill and the sled is 0.3 m and the length of the hill is 50 m, how much work has been done by gravity when the child reaches the bottom of the hill?

   (A) 1000 J
   (B) 2500 J
   (C) 3535 J
   (D) 4330 J

3. An experiment is conducted where a cue ball (mass 0.25 kg) moves at 10 m/s towards an adjacent numbered ball (mass 0.25 kg) at rest. In Trial 1, the collision is elastic. In Trial 2, the collision is perfectly inelastic. What is the speed of the cue ball immediately after the collision in Trial 1 and Trial 2, respectively?

   (A) 0 m/s and 5 m/s
   (B) 0 m/s and 10 m/s
   (C) 5 m/s and 0 m/s
   (D) 5 m/s and 5 m/s

4. A 200 kg roller coaster starts from rest 50 m above the ground. It falls toward the ground without any friction, then once it reaches ground level, the brakes are applied over 30 m in order to bring the coaster to a complete stop. How much work is done by the brakes?

   (A) 10×10^4 J
   (B) 10×10^5 J
   (C) -10×10^4 J
   (D) -10×10^5 J

5. A 1000 kg car traveling at 60 km/h hits a stationary truck weighing 20,000 N. If the truck has a velocity of 1 m/s after the crash, what is the velocity of the car after the crash?

   (A) 14.5 m/s in the same direction it was initially traveling
   (B) 14.5 m/s in the opposite direction it was initially traveling
   (C) 19 m/s in the same direction it was initially traveling
   (D) 19 m/s in the opposite direction it was initially traveling

6. A 7 kg ball is dropped from 20 m. If the speed just before it hits the ground is 18 m/s, what is the work done by air resistance?

   (A) 266 J
   (B) 13 J
   (C) −13 J
   (D) −266 J

Fluid Statics

7. A person is leaning on his elbow on a table. If the amount of force the table must exert to keep the person upright is F, the area of contact between the person and the table is A, and the angle that the person's arm makes with the table's surface is $\square$, how much pressure is exerted by the person on the table?

   (A) $\dfrac{F}{A}$

   (B) $\dfrac{F \sin\theta}{A}$

   (C) $\dfrac{F \cos\theta}{A}$

   (D) Since the force exerted by the person on the table is not given, the pressure exerted by the person on the table cannot be determined.

8. If the density of a person is approximately the density of water, and the density of air is approximately 1 kg/m³, how many times greater is the weight of the person than the buoyant force from the air on the person?

   (A) 10
   (B) 100
   (C) 1000
   (D) 10000

9. Will an object with more mass but the same volume as another object sink faster in a non-viscous fluid?

   (A) No, because acceleration due to gravity is independent of the mass of the object being accelerated.
   (B) No, because the buoyant force is greater on an object with more mass.
   (C) Yes, because it weighs more, and the weight itself induces greater acceleration for the heavier object than for the lighter.
   (D) Yes, because the buoyant force impedes the downward acceleration of a greater mass less than it does a lesser mass.

10. A particular eucalyptus tree has a density of 667 kg/m³ and a mass of 6000 kg. What volume of the tree would float above the surface of water?

    (A) 3 m³
    (B) 5 m³
    (C) 6 m³
    (D) 9 m³

D.C. Circuits

11. Determine the total power dissipated through the circuit shown below in terms of V, R_1, R_2, and R_3.

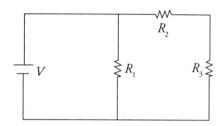

    (A) $\dfrac{V^2}{R_1 + R_2 + R_3}$

    (B) $\dfrac{R_1 + R_2 + R_3}{V^2}$

    (C) $\dfrac{R_1(R_2 + R_3)}{V^2(R_1 + R_2 + R_3)}$

    (D) $\dfrac{V^2(R_1 + R_2 + R_3)}{R_1(R_2 + R_3)}$

12. Lightning is an atmospheric discharge of electricity that can propagate at speeds of up to 60,000 m/s and can reach temperatures of up to 30,000°C. A single lightning strike lasts for approximately 250 ms and can transfer up to 500 MJ of energy across a potential difference of 2×10^7 volts. Estimate the total amount of charge transferred and average current of a single lightning strike.

    (A) 6.25×10^{-4} coulombs, 8×10^7 amps
    (B) 6.25×10^{-4} coulombs, 2.5×10^{-3} amps
    (C) 25 coulombs, 100 amps
    (D) 25 coulombs, 8×10^7 amps

13. Which of the following statements will increase the resistance of a closed circuit system?

    I. Replacing the wire with one that has a smaller cross sectional area
    II. Adding a voltmeter to the wire
    III. Doubling the wire length in the closed circuit

    (A) III only
    (B) I and III only
    (C) II and III only
    (D) I, II and III

14. If the resistance of a wire in a household appliance becomes 4 times its original value, which of the following statements is/are correct?

   I.   The voltage of the wire becomes quadrupled.
   II. The current through the wire becomes one-fourth the original value.
   III. The power consumed by the appliance becomes quadrupled.

   (A) I only
   (B) II only
   (C) I and III only
   (D) II and III only

Linear Kinematics

15. A runner begins his run by accelerating to the right from rest and achieves a speed of 6 m/s in 3 s. What is the runner's displacement during this time?

   (A) 2 m
   (B) 6 m
   (C) 9 m
   (D) 18 m
   (E) 36 m

16. A rock is thrown upward at 20 m/s at the edge of a cliff and strikes the ground with an impact speed of 45 m/s. How long was the rock in the air?

   (A) 2 s
   (B) 2.5 s
   (C) 4.5 s
   (D) 6.5 s
   (E) 10 s

17. Which one of the following statements is true concerning the motion of an ideal projectile launched at an angle of 45° to the horizontal?

   (A) The acceleration vector points opposite to the velocity vector on the way up and in the same direction as the velocity vector on the way down.
   (B) The speed at the top of the trajectory is zero.
   (C) The object's total speed remains constant during the entire flight.
   (D) The horizontal speed decreases on the way up and increases on the way down.
   (E) The vertical speed decreases on the way up and increases on the way down.

18. A rock is dropped off a cliff that's 180 m high. If it strikes the ground with an impact velocity of 60 m/s, what magnitude of acceleration did it experience during its descent?

   (A) 0.67 m/s^2
   (B) 3 m/s^2
   (C) 4.5 m/s^2
   (D) 6 m/s^2
   (E) 10 m/s^2

19. A 75 kg athlete runs once around an oval track of total distance 500 m. How much larger is the athlete's distance travelled compared to the athlete's displacement?

   (A) 0 m
   (B) 250 m
   (C) 500 m
   (D) The displacement is larger than the distance travelled.
   (E) Cannot be determined from the information given

Nuclear Physics

20. The reaction $^{218}_{85}\text{At} \rightarrow {}^{214}_{83}\text{Bi}$ is an example of what type of radioactive decay?

   (A) Alpha
   (B) $\square^-$
   (C) $\square^+$
   (D) Electron capture
   (E) Gamma

21. Tungsten-176 has a half-life of 2.5 hours. After how many hours will the disintegration rate of a tungsten-176 sample drop to $\frac{1}{10}$ its initial value?

   (A) 5
   (B) 8.3
   (C) 10
   (D) 12.5
   (E) 25

22. What's the missing particle in the following nuclear reaction?

$$^{2}_{1}H + ^{63}_{29}Cu \rightarrow ^{64}_{30}Zn + (?)$$

(A) Proton
(B) Neutron
(C) Electron
(D) Positron
(E) Deuteron

23. What's the missing particle in the following nuclear reaction?

$$^{196}_{78}Pt + ^{1}_{0}n \rightarrow ^{197}_{78}Pt + (?)$$

(A) Proton
(B) Neutron
(C) Electron
(D) Positron
(E) Gamma

24. Compared to the parent nucleus, the daughter of a β–decay has

(A) the same mass number but a greater atomic number.
(B) the same mass number but a smaller atomic number.
(C) a smaller mass number but the same atomic number.
(D) a greater mass number but the same atomic number.
(E) None of the above

Units and Vectors

25. Two vectors are added together and the resulting vector has a magnitude of 10 units. Which of the following must be true about the two vectors?

(A) The sum of their magnitudes is less than 10 units.
(B) The sum of their magnitudes is equal to 10 units.
(C) The sum of their magnitudes is greater than 10 units, but the difference of their magnitudes is less than 10 units.
(D) The sum of their magnitudes is greater than 10 units, but the difference of their magnitudes is equal to 10 units.
(E) None of the above can be determined about them unless their relative directions are known.

26. Each of the following contains at least one scalar quantity EXCEPT one. Which one is the EXCEPTION?

(A) Velocity, mass, power
(B) Momentum, displacement, speed
(C) Electric field, torque, impulse
(D) Acceleration, force, kinetic energy

27. A vector has a length of 4 and makes a 30° angle with the x-axis. Which of the following best expresses the x-component of the vector?

(A) 0.86
(B) 1
(C) 1.7
(D) 2
(E) 3.4

28. A vector and its equivalent scalar quantity have:

(A) the same magnitude and direction.
(B) the same magnitude and units.
(C) the same direction only.
(D) the same magnitude only.
(E) the same units only.

29. A vector has a magnitude of 5, and another vector has a magnitude of 2. The sum of the two vectors has a magnitude of 3. Which of the following must be true of the two vectors?

(A) They are parallel.
(B) They are antiparallel.
(C) They are perpendicular.
(D) They form an acute angle when put tip-to-tail.
(E) They form an obtuse angle when put tip-to-tail.

Thermal Energy and Thermodynamics

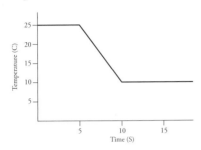

30. When a certain copper object is heated to 10 degrees Celsius, it gains 3,850 joules of energy. The graph above shows the temperature of the copper object as a function of time. How much heat was lost in the time from $t = 5$ seconds to $t = 10$ seconds?

    (A) 1925 J
    (B) 3850 J
    (C) 5775 J
    (D) 7700 J
    (E) It cannot be determined, because the mass of the object is not known.

31. The melting point of mercury is –39°C. Which of the following is most nearly the heat that must be added to a 1-kilogram block of solid mercury at –39°C to melt it and to raise its temperature to 1°C? (Heat of fusion of mercury = 1.2×10^4 joules per kilogram; specific heat of mercury = 140 joules per kilogram • °C)

    (A) 1.8×10^4 J
    (B) 1.3×10^4 J
    (C) 1.2×10^4 J
    (D) 6.8×10^3 J
    (E) 5.6×10^3 J

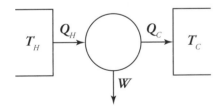

32. A heat engine draws thermal energy from a hot reservoir that is kept at a temperature of 400 Kelvins and exhausts thermal energy into a cold reservoir kept at a temperature of 200 Kelvins, as shown. If the heat engine takes in 4800 joules of thermal energy and does 1200 joules of work, which of the following is most nearly the efficiency of the heat engine?

    (A) 0.25
    (B) 0.33
    (C) 0.50
    (D) 0.75
    (E) 1.00

33. Which of the following properties must increase as the temperature of a gas increases, no matter the circumstances?

    (A) Average kinetic energy of the gas molecules
    (B) Molecular weight of the gas
    (C) Density of the gas
    (D) Pressure exerted by the gas
    (E) Volume of the gas

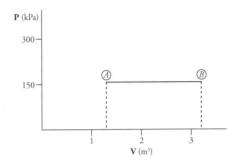

34. The pressure as a function of the volume of an ideal gas in a closed container is shown. The gas goes from state A, a pressure of 300 kilopascals at a volume of 1 cubic meters, to state B, a pressure of 300 kilopascals at a volume of 3 cubic meters. How much work is done by the expanding gas?

    (A) 1×10^5 J
    (B) 2×10^5 J
    (C) 3×10^5 J
    (D) 6×10^5 J
    (E) 9×10^5 J

35. An aluminum bar of length 2 meters is heated from –10° Celsius to 40° Celsius. If the coefficient of linear expansion of aluminum is 2.5×10^{-5}/°C, by how much will the bar lengthen?

    (A) 0.25 mm
    (B) 1.25 mm
    (C) 2.5 mm
    (D) 1.25 cm
    (E) 2.5 cm

Optics

36. What is the wavelength of an X-ray whose frequency is 1.0×10^{18} Hz?

    (A) 3.3×10^{-11} m
    (B) 3.0×10^{-10} m
    (C) 3.3×10^{-9} m
    (D) 3.0×10^{-8} m
    (E) 3.3×10^{26} m

37. When green light (wavelength = 500 nm in air) travels through diamond (refractive index = 2.4), what is its wavelength?

    (A) 208 nm
    (B) 357 nm
    (C) 500 nm
    (D) 700 nm
    (E) 1200 nm

38. A beam of light traveling in Medium 1 strikes the interface to another transparent medium, Medium 2. If the speed of light is less in Medium 2 than in Medium 1, the beam will

    (A) refract toward the normal.
    (B) refract away from the normal.
    (C) undergo total internal reflection.
    (D) have an angle of reflection smaller than the angle of incidence.
    (E) have an angle of reflection greater than the angle of incidence.

39. An object is placed 60 cm from a spherical convex mirror. If the mirror forms a virtual image 20 cm from the mirror, what's the magnitude of the mirror's radius of curvature?

    (A) 7.5 cm
    (B) 15 cm
    (C) 30 cm
    (D) 60 cm
    (E) 120 cm

40. The image created by a converging lens is projected onto a screen that's 60 cm from the lens. If the height of the image is 1/4 the height of the object, what's the focal length of the lens?

    (A) 36 cm
    (B) 45 cm
    (C) 48 cm
    (D) 72 cm
    (E) 80 cm

ANSWERS AND EXPLANATIONS

Energy and Momentum

1. **C** The word-equation given in the first sentence of the question stem can be expressed as F_{drag} = $\frac{1}{3}v^2$. (Ignore the dimensional incorrectness of the equation; the stem indicates that speed units of m/s will give force units of N here.) The question asks for power, and the relationship between force and power is $P = Fv$, so $P = (\frac{1}{3}v^2)(v) = \frac{1}{3}v^3$. Plug in the number given: $P = \frac{1}{3}(30)^3 = 9000$. Thus, the answer is 9 kW.

2. **B** There are a couple of ways to approach this problem:

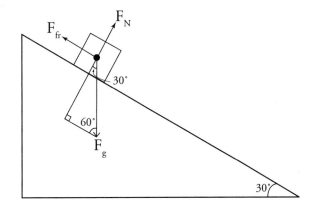

Number 1:

The formula for work is $W = Fd \cos\theta$, where W is the work, F is the force, d is the displacement, and θ is the angle between the force and displacement vectors. To determine the work done by gravity, we use gravitational force and length of the hill to get: $W = (mg)(d) \cos 60°$, where 60° is from the direction of gravitational force vertically down and d is along the ramp. Thus, $W = (10)(10)(50)(0.5) = 2500$ J.

Number 2:

We can resolve the F and d to be in the same direction, that is, take the component of the force acting in the same direction as the child's movement down the hill, eliminating the $\cos\theta$ (since $\cos 0° = 1$) from the equation. Then, we have $F = mg \sin\theta$, where $\theta = 30°$. Thus, $W = Fd = (mg \sin\theta)d = (10)(10)(0.5)(50) = 2500$ J.

3. **A** In a perfectly inelastic collision, recall that total momentum is conserved but not total kinetic energy, and that the balls all stick together. Initial momentum must be equal to final momentum. $p_{\text{initial}} = p_{\text{final}} = m_1 v_1 = (m_1 + m_2)v' \rightarrow v' = m_1 v_1 / (m_1 + m_2) = (0.25)(10) / (0.25 + 0.25) = 5$ m/s. This is the value for Trial 2, eliminating (B) and (C). For the elastic collision, kinetic energy must be conserved in addition to total momentum, and both objects can move at different velocities after the collision. Since momentum is conserved, $p_{\text{initial}} = p_{\text{final}} = m_1 v_1 = m_1 v_{1f} + m_2 v_{2f}$. Since $m_1 = m_2$, we have that $v_{2f} = v_1 - v_{1f}$. Similarly, if kinetic energy is conserved, then $KE_{\text{initial}} = KE_{\text{final}} = \frac{1}{2}m_1 v_1^2 = \frac{1}{2}m_1 v_{2f}^2 + \frac{1}{2}m_2 v_{2f}^2$. Therefore, $v_{2f}^2 = v_1^2 - v_{1f}^2$. In order for these two equations to hold true, v_{1f} must equal either 0 m/s or 10 m/s. Since 10 m/s would indicate the two balls did not collide at all (and 10 m/s for Trial 1 is not an option), the cue ball must have velocity of 0 m/s immediately following the elastic collision, transferring all kinetic energy to the numbered ball.

4. **C** This question requires you to use the Work-Kinetic Energy Theorem, which states that $W = \Delta KE$. The kinetic energy at the bottom is equal to the potential energy at the top, by Conservation of Energy, which is $mgh = (200)(10)(50) = 10^5$ J. The change in kinetic energy is the final kinetic energy minus the initial. Therefore, the work done by friction to bring the roller coaster to a stop is equal to $\Delta KE = -10^5$ J $= -10 \times 10^4$ J.

5. **A** For collisions, you must use Conservation of Momentum. Initially, the momentum is just of the car, and is equal to $m_c v_c = (1000$ kg$)(60$ km/h$) = (1000$ kg$)(16.5$ m/s$) = 16500$ kg·m/s. This is equal to the momentum after, which is $m_c v_f + m_t v_t$. Solving for v_f gives 14.5 m/s, and since it is a positive number, the car is traveling in the same direction as it was at the beginning.

6. **D** The initial energy is $mgh = (7)(10)(20) = 1400$ J. The final energy is completely kinetic, $1/2(mv^2) = 1134$ J. The equation for Conservation of Energy with frictional is $E_i + W_{\text{by friction}} = E_f$. Thus, the work done by friction is negative and equal to $1134 - 1400 = -266$ J.

Fluid Statics

7.   **B**   First, eliminate (D) because the force exerted by the table on the person, given as F, is equal in magnitude to the force exerted by the person on the table, according to Newton's Third Law. Next, the way that pressure, force, and area are related is $P = \dfrac{F_\perp}{A}$. Since the given angle is between the arm and the table, the vertical component of the force will be related to the sine of that angle. Thus, $P = \dfrac{F \sin\theta}{A}$. Choice (A) is wrong because it would be the pressure if the force were not at an angle, and (C) is wrong because it would be the pressure if the angle given were between the arm and a line perpendicular to the table's surface.

8.   **C**   The weight of a person, in terms of density, is $w_p = \rho_p V_g$, where V is the volume of the person. The buoyant force from air on the person is $F_B = \rho_{air} V_g$, where V is again the volume of the person because the whole person is submerged in air. This means that the only difference is the density of the person as compared to the density of air, and since we are told that the density of the person is approximately the density of water (1000 kg/m^3), and air has a density of approximately 1 kg/m^3, the relevant factor is 1000.

9.   **D**   Begin by setting up the forces and finding the acceleration. $F_{net} = ma$, as always, so (defining the sinking direction as positive) $w - F_B = ma$. Next, specify weight and the buoyant force: $mg - \rho_f V_{sub} g = ma$. Divide by m, which yields $a = g - \dfrac{\rho_f V_{sub} g}{m}$. For a larger mass, the subtracted buoyant force will be less, and subtracting less means ending up with a greater number. So, the acceleration is greater for an object with greater mass, provided that the compared objects are sinking in the same fluid on the same planet (that is, ρ_f and g are the same for the two objects), and they have the same volume (as the stem indicates they do). Notice that it is the buoyant force term that makes the difference here: mass canceled in the weight term. Objects fall at the same rate in vacuum, so it can't be the weight itself that is causing this effect, which is the reason that (C) is wrong. It is the buoyant force that is responsible for the difference in accelerations. Choices (A) and (B) are wrong for their "No" answers; (A) gives a true justification (acceleration due to gravity is independent of the mass of the object being accelerated), but it neglects the effect of the buoyant force, and (B) gives an incorrect reason, since equal volumes mean that the magnitude of the buoyant force on each object is the same.

10. **A** Recall that for floating objects $\dfrac{\rho_o}{\rho_f} = \dfrac{V_{sub}}{V}$. Since the density of the object is 667 kg/m³ and the density of water is 1000 kg/m³, two-thirds of the object will be submerged and one-third will be above the surface of the water. Since $\rho = \dfrac{m}{V}$, then $V = \dfrac{m}{\rho} = \dfrac{6000}{667} = 9$ m³. The total volume of the object is 9 m³, and one-third of that is 3 m³.

D.C. Circuits

11. **D** Power can be expressed as $P = V^2 / R$. Therefore, begin by determining total resistance of the circuit, R_{TOT}. In this circuit, R_2 and R_3 are connected in series, and are connected in parallel to R_1. R_2 and R_3 can be reduced to $R_{EQ} = R_2 + R_3$. This equivalent resistor connects in parallel to R_1, and it can be further reduced to $R_{TOT} = R_1 (R_2 + R_3) / (R_1 + R_2 + R_3)$. Use this equation for total resistance in the equation for power to yield $P = V^2 / R_{TOT}$, or (D).

12. **C** Change in electrical potential energy is given by the equation $\Delta PE = qV$. The problem states that there is an energy transfer of 500 megajoules across a potential difference of 20 megavolts. Solving for q yields a charge transfer of 500 MJ / 20 MV, or 25 coulombs. The problem states that the time over which the charge is transferred is 250 msec, or 0.25 seconds. Using the equation $I = Q / t$, the average current can be calculated as 25 coulombs / 0.25 seconds, or 100 amps.

13. **D** Item I is correct because the electrical resistance of a metal wire is inversely proportional to its cross sectional area ((A) and (C) can be eliminated). Note that since both remaining choices include Item III, Item III must be correct and we only need to evaluate Item II. Item II is also correct. The internal resistance of a voltmeter is very high, and thus adding a voltmeter will increase the resistance of the whole system ((B) can be eliminated, and (D) is correct). Item III is in fact correct. According to the formula $R = \rho L / A$, the resistance of the wire R, is directly proportional to its length L. Therefore, as the length of the wire increases, so does the overall resistance of the system.

14. **B** Item I is false. The voltage is the electromotive force that drives the current through the wire. Therefore, it remains constant and unaffected by the increase in resistance ((A) and (C) can be eliminated). Note that the remaining choices both include Item II, so Item II must be true: according to the equation $V = IR$, when V is constant, the current I is inversely proportional to the resistance R. Item III is false. The power P is expressed by the equation $P = IV$, where I is the current through the wire and V is the voltage that drives the current. Since V stays constant, and I becomes 1/4 of the original value, the power P would be $1/4\, I \times V = 1/4\, IV$, which is 1/4 the original power output ((D) is wrong, and (B) is correct).

Linear Kinematics

15. **C**   The question provides the initial and final velocities, the time, and asks for the displacement. Since acceleration is missing, use Big Five number 1.

$$d = \frac{1}{2}(v_0 + v)t = \frac{1}{2}(0+6)(3) = 9 \text{ m}$$

16. **D**   The question provides the initial and final velocities and asks for the time of flight. Given that this is a free-fall problem, the acceleration is due to gravity. Therefore, only the displacement is missing: use Big Five number 2. Setting up as positive gives the following:

$$v = v_0 + at$$

$$t = \frac{v - v_0}{a} = \frac{-45 - 20}{-10} = 6.5 \text{ s}$$

17. **E**   Since the acceleration of the projectile is always downward (because it's gravitational acceleration), the vertical speed decreases as the projectile rises and increases as the projectile falls. Choices (A), (B), (C), and D are false.

18. **E**   The rock is in free-fall, so it's acceleration must be due to gravity, i.e., $a = 10 \text{ m/s}^2$ in magnitude. Big Five number 5 can be used to solve this based on the information in the question, but that's ultimately not necessary.

19. **C**   Since the athlete's final and initial positions are the same, the displacement is zero. Therefore, the distance travelled is greater than the displacement by 500 m.

Nuclear Physics

20. **A**   Since the mass number decreased by 4 and the atomic number decreased by 2, this is an alpha decay.

21. **B**   After 3 half-lives, the activity will drop to $(1/2)^3 = 1/8$ its initial value, and after 4 half-lives, it will drop to $(1/2)^4 = 1/16$ its initial value. Since 1/10 is between 1/8 and 1/16, the time interval in this case is between 3 and 4 half-lives, that is, between $3(2.5 \text{ h}) = 7.5 \text{ h}$ and $4(2.5 \text{ h}) = 10 \text{ h}$. Only (B) is in this range.

22. **B**   In order to balance the mass number (the superscripts), we must have $2 + 63 = 64 + A$, so $A = 1$. In order to balance the charge (the subscripts), we need $1 + 29 = 30 + Z$, so $Z = 0$. A particle with a mass number of 1 and no charge is a neutron, $_0^1 \text{n}$.

23. **E** To balance the mass number (the superscripts), we must have 196 + 1 = 197 + A, so A = 0.

To balance the charge (the subscripts), we need 78 + 0 = 78 + Z, so Z = 0. The only particle

listed that has zero mass number and zero charge is a gamma-ray photon, $^0_0\gamma$.

24. **A** In □–decay, a neutron is transformed into a proton and an electron. Terefore, the total nucleon number (mass number) doesn't change, but the number of protons (the atomic number) increases by one.

Units and Vectors

25. **E** If one of the vectors had a magnitude of 9 and the other had a magnitude of 1, and they pointed in the same direction, then they would add to 10. In that case, (B) would be true. However, if one had a magnitude of 11 and the other had a magnitude of 1, but they pointed in opposite directions, their sum would still have a magnitude of 10 (as the stem describes), but the sum of their magnitudes would be 12. That would make (D) true. This makes the answer (E), since either (B) or (D) could be true and the other false. (Choice (A) is impossible, but (C) could be true: imagine perpendicular vectors with magnitudes of 6 and 8.)

26. **C** This previews some of the content that you'll see in later chapters, but this is a typical vector question on the OAT. Mass and power in (A) are scalars. Speed in (B) is a scalar. Kinetic energy in (D) is a scalar. All the quantities in (C) are vectors, however.

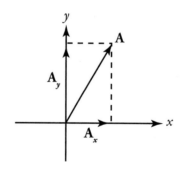

27. **D** Draw it! From the picture, you want 4 sin 30°, which is 2. That's (D).

28. **E** Direction is the easiest to get rid of; scalars don't even have direction, so eliminate (A) and (C). Vector and scalar equivalents don't always have the same magnitude, which you can see if you consider distance and displacement. Imagine moving to the left one meter and then back to the right one meter. Your net displacement is zero meters, but your total distance is two meters. Those are different magnitudes. Eliminate (B) and (D). The answer must be (E), as you can see from the above example (both displacement and distance have units of meters).

29. **B** Since 5 – 2 = 3, the only way for the two vectors to sum to 3 is for them to be in opposite directions. (B) expresses that. If they were parallel, as in (A), they would add to 7. If they were perpendicular, as in (C), they would add to approximately 5.4. If they formed an acute angle, they would add to something between 3 and 5.4, and if they formed an obtuse angle, they would add to something between 5.4 and 7.

Thermal Energy and Thermodynamics

30. **C**   The figure shows that from time $t = 5$ seconds to $t = 10$ seconds, the object drops from a temperature of 25°C to 10°C. This is a drop of 15°C. The question also mentions that when the object is heated 10°C, it gains 3850 J. To relate these, use $q = mc\Delta T$: since it's the same object in both the temperature increase and decrease, m and c are held fixed, so q is directly proportional to ΔT. A drop of 1.5 times as much in temperature (that is, 1.5 times as much ΔT) should release 1.5 times as much energy (that is, 1.5 times as much q). Take 3850 and multiply by 1.5, and you get (C).

31. **A**   First, to melt the mercury, use $q = mL$. In this case, that's $q = (1)(1.2 \times 10^4)$. Next, to raise the temperature from –39°C to 1°C, use $q = mc\Delta T$. In this case, that's $q = (1)(140)(40) = 5600$ J. Add the two together, and $12000 + 5600 = 17600$ J. Round, and you get (A).

32. **A**   The actual efficiency of a heat engine is $e = \dfrac{W}{Q_H}$ (not to be confused with the Carnot efficiency, the maximum possible efficiency). In this case, that's $e = \dfrac{1200}{4800} = 0.25$. That's (A). (It's taking 4800 J and only doing something worthwhile with 25% of them, hence an efficiency of 0.25.)

33. **A**   Given that $KE_{avg} = \dfrac{3}{2}k_B T$, if T increases, then KE_{avg} has to increase. Molecular weight shouldn't have anything to do with temperature. Density would most likely decrease with an increase in temperature, from $PV = nRT$ (an increase in T can increase V, decreasing density). Pressure and volume could increase with increasing temperature, but neither has to.

34. **D**   This is $W = P\Delta V$. Since P is fixed at 300,000 and V changes from 1 to 3, $W = (300,000)(2) = 600,000$ J. That's (D).

35. **C**   Apply $\Delta L = \alpha L_i \Delta T$. Here, that comes to $\Delta L = (2.5 \times 10^{-5})(2)(50) = 2.5 \times 10^{-3}$. Convert to millimeters, and you get (C).

Optics

36. **B**   Since light travels like a wave, we can use the equation $c = \lambda f$, where c = 3×10^8 m/s is the speed of light in vacuum.

$$\lambda = \frac{c}{f} = \frac{3 \times 10^8}{1.0 \times 10^{18}} = 3.0 \, 10^{-10} \, m$$

37.   A   The frequency is unchanged, but because the speed of light in diamond is less than in air, the wavelength of the light in diamond is shorter than its wavelength in air:

$$\lambda_{diamond} = \frac{v_{diamond}}{f} = \frac{c/n_{diamond}}{f} = \frac{c}{f}\left(\frac{1}{n_{diamond}}\right) = \frac{\lambda_{air}}{n_{diamond}} = \frac{500 \text{ nm}}{2.4} = 208 \text{ nm}$$

38.   A   If the speed of light is less in Medium 2 than in Medium 1, then Medium 2 must have a higher index of refraction, i.e., $n_2 > n_1$. Snell's Law then implies that $\theta_2 < \theta_1$: the beam will refract toward the normal upon transmission into Medium 2.

39.   D   Since the image is virtual, it has a negative image distance: $i = -20$ cm. Using $o = 60$ cm, the mirror equation gives

$$\frac{1}{f} = \frac{1}{i} + \frac{1}{o} = -\frac{1}{20} + \frac{1}{60} = -\frac{3}{60} + \frac{1}{60} = -\frac{2}{60} = -\frac{1}{30} \rightarrow f = -30 \text{ cm}$$

$$|f| = \frac{R}{2} \rightarrow R = 2|f| = 60 \text{ cm}$$

40.   C   Since the image is projected onto a screen, it must be real, and therefore inverted. The magnification must be negative, so $m = -1/4$, and the magnification equation gives

$$m = -\frac{i}{o} \rightarrow o = -\frac{i}{m} = -\frac{60}{-1/4} = 240 \text{ cm}$$

Now the lens equation gives

$$\frac{1}{f} = \frac{1}{i} + \frac{1}{o} = \frac{1}{60} + \frac{1}{240} = \frac{4}{240} + \frac{1}{240} = \frac{5}{240} \rightarrow f = 48 \text{ cm}$$

NATURAL SCIENCES DRILL

What follows is a small sample of problems that surveys some of the content that you will see in the Survey of Natural Sciences portion of the OAT. If, after reading the topic outlines in this book, you feel fairly confident that you know the stuff tested on the SNS, complete these problems to test your knowledge. If you get most of them right, great! You probably need only a light review of the science topics, and some combination of going over your old class notes and taking practice tests probably will suffice. If you get a sizable number wrong, or if you feel unsure about this content, you should review these topics in more detail. One way to do that is to purchase *Cracking the DAT,* which covers in detail the topics that the DAT and the OAT share.

Bear in mind, also, that what follows is not completely comprehensive. It's a sample of a few representative topics, not a survey of all possible topics. However, it covers Biology, General Chemistry, and Organic Chemistry, which are the three subjects on the SNS, and it covers a number of different topics within each subject, so you should be able to get a sense of where you are from working these problems.

Biology

1. Which of the following statements is NOT true?

    (A) Lipids are frequently found in the interior, hydrophobic regions of globular proteins.
    (B) Cholesterol is the precursor to steroid hormones.
    (C) Unsaturated fats have one or more double bonds.
    (D) Lipids are hydrophobic and lipophilic.
    (E) The cell membrane is made up of amphipathic phospholipids.

2. A nucleotide made of which of the following would be found in DNA?

    (A) Ribose, phosphate, and uracil
    (B) Ribose, phosphate, and thymine
    (C) Deoxyribose, ribose, and thymine
    (D) Deoxyribose, phosphate, and uracil
    (E) Deoxyribose, phosphate, and thymine

3. A red blood cell in a hypertonic salt solution will

    (A) swell up and explode.
    (B) shrivel up.
    (C) absorb the salt and explode.
    (D) absorb the salt and shrivel up.
    (E) remain the same.

4. During which phase of the cell cycle are the sister chromatids separated?

    (A) S phase
    (B) Telophase
    (C) Prophase
    (D) Metaphase
    (E) Anaphase

5. Which of the following statements about prokaryotes and eukaryotes is true?

    (A) Both prokaryotes and eukaryotes translate proteins in the cytosol.
    (B) Both prokaryotes and eukaryotes transcribe RNA in the nucleus.
    (C) Prokaryotes have a cell wall and eukaryotes have only a cell membrane.
    (D) Prokaryotes rely only on glycolysis for energy, while eukaryotes can get energy from the electron transport chain and oxidative phosphorylation (aerobic respiration).
    (E) Prokaryotes can exchange plasmids by conjugation, while eukaryotes exchange plasmids during sexual reproduction.

6. A reaction that would proceed quickly and spontaneously would have a

    (A) positive ΔG and a low energy of activation.
    (B) negative ΔG and a low energy of activation.
    (C) positive ΔG and a high energy of activation.
    (D) negative ΔG and a high energy of activation.
    (E) positive ΔG and a high ΔS.

7. Catalysts

    I. stabilize the transition state of a reaction.
    II. can drive a non-spontaneous reaction forward.
    III. reduce the energy of activation of a reaction.

    (A) I only
    (B) III only
    (C) I and II
    (D) I and III
    (E) I, II, and III

8. In fermentation, why is pyruvate reduced to ethanol or lactic acid?

   (A) To prepare pyruvate to enter the Krebs cycle
   (B) To oxidize NADH, so that glycolysis can continue to run in the absence of oxygen
   (C) So that yeast can produce the alcohol in wine and beer
   (D) So that the resulting drop in pH can increase the activity of the glycolytic enzymes
   (E) So that muscle cells can continue the Krebs cycle in the absence of oxygen

9. Which of the following is NOT true about DNA replication?

   (A) DNA gyrase unwinds the helix at the origin.
   (B) It is semiconservative.
   (C) The leading strand is polymerized in the same direction as the DNA is unwinding.
   (D) It occurs in the 5′ to 3′ direction.
   (E) It requires an RNA primer.

10. Which of the following is NOT a difference between replication and transcription?

   I. In replication, the new DNA is edited to correct mistakes, while in transcription there is no proofreading.
   II. In replication, DNA is synthesized in the 5′ to 3′ direction, while in transcription, RNA is synthesized in the 3′ to 5′ direction.
   III. Both strands of the DNA are replicated, while typically only one strand of the DNA is transcribed.

   (A) I only
   (B) I and II only
   (C) II only
   (D) II and III only
   (E) I, II, and III

11. If the frequency of the allele causing a dominant disorder is 0.1, what is the frequency of affected individuals in the population?

   (A) 0.01
   (B) 0.09
   (C) 0.19
   (D) 0.81
   (E) 0.90

12. A woman with blood type B− marries a man with blood type A+. They have a child with blood type O+. Which of the following is true?

   (A) The man is homozygous for blood type A (genotype $I^A I^A$).
   (B) The child is homozygous for the Rh factor (genotype RR).
   (C) The man must be the father of the child.
   (D) The man is not the father of the child.
   (E) The man might be the father of the child.

13. A pure-breeding white mouse is crossed with a pure-breeding black mouse. All offspring are grey. This is an example of

   (A) codominance.
   (B) incomplete dominance.
   (C) epistasis.
   (D) classical dominance.
   (E) recombination.

14. A man who is colorblind marries a woman who does not carry the colorblindness allele. His daughter marries a man with normal vision. What is the probability that the man's grandson is colorblind?

   (A) 0
   (B) $\frac{1}{4}$
   (C) $\frac{1}{2}$
   (D) $\frac{3}{4}$
   (E) 1

15. All chordates have several features in common. Which of the following is NOT a shared feature of chordates?

   (A) Notochord
   (B) Postanal tail
   (C) Pharyngeal gill slits
   (D) Bony skeletons
   (E) Dorsal hollow nerve cord

16. Which of the following is NOT an example of a prezygotic barrier to speciation?

   (A) The sperm of a hamster cannot fertilize the egg of a rabbit.
   (B) A mule, the offspring of a horse and a donkey, is sterile.
   (C) Birds have different mating seasons; some mate in the spring and some mate in the fall.
   (D) Elephants and mice are physically incompatible and cannot mate.
   (E) Swans do not know the mating rituals of geese.

17. Large evergreen trees that use cones as reproductive structures, and whose dominant life stage is the sporophyte are classified as

    (A) monocots.
    (B) dicots.
    (C) ferns.
    (D) gymnosperms.
    (E) angiosperms.

18. Which of the following is true of a cardiac muscle cell action potential but NOT a neuronal action potential?

    (A) The initial depolarization is caused by the influx of sodium.
    (B) Na$^+$/K$^+$ ATPases maintain resting potential for the cell.
    (C) Repolarization in a cardiac muscle cell is caused by the efflux of calcium.
    (D) Cardiac muscle action potentials have a plateau phase caused by the influx of calcium.
    (E) Repolarization is caused by the efflux of potassium.

19. Which of the following hormones is NOT made by the pituitary gland?

    (A) Thyroid stimulating hormone (TSH)
    (B) Prolactin
    (C) Oxytocin
    (D) Adrenocorticotropic hormone (ACTH)
    (E) Growth hormone

20. The kidney uses three main processes to make urine: filtration, reabsorption, and secretion. When compared to plasma concentration, the urine concentration of a secreted substance is

    (A) higher, because secretion moves substances from the blood to the filtrate.
    (B) lower, because secretion moves substances from the blood to the filtrate.
    (C) higher, because secretion moves substances from the filtrate to the blood.
    (D) lower, because secretion moves substances from the filtrate to the blood.
    (E) equal, because secretion is the process that originally filters substances out of the blood.

21. Each of the following are functions of the pancreas except:

    (A) secrete bicarbonate.
    (B) produce bile.
    (C) release insulin.
    (D) secrete digestive enzymes.
    (E) release glucagon.

22. Which of the following would be expected to occur if blood pressure was too low?

    I.   Aldosterone secretion would be increased.
    II. Antidiuretic hormone would be inhibited.
    III. Renin would be released.

    (A) I and II only
    (B) II only
    (C) I and III only
    (D) II and III only
    (E) I, II, and III

23. During which step of the sliding filament theory is ATP hydrolyzed?

    (A) Myosin pulls actin toward the center of the sarcomere (power stroke).
    (B) Myosin releases actin.
    (C) Myosin binding sites on actin are exposed.
    (D) Myosin binds to actin (crossbridge formation).
    (E) Myosin is reset to its high-energy conformation.

24. All of the following are characteristics of protostomes except:

    (A) they are all coelomates.
    (B) they undergo spiral and determinate cleavage.
    (C) the first opening (blastopore) develops into the mouth and the second opening into the anus.
    (D) the fates of the embryonic cells are decided very early in development.
    (E) the group includes echinoderms and chordates.

25. After transforming a plasmid into bacteria, cells were plated onto an agar plate containing glucose, amino acids and ampicillin. Why were the bacteria grown in the presence of ampicillin?

    (A) To enhance the growth of bacteria which have not taken up the plasmid.
    (B) To prevent growth of bacteria which have taken up the plasmid.
    (C) To prevent growth of bacteria which have not taken up the plasmid.
    (D) To prevent contamination of the population by a bacteriophage.
    (E) To prevent contamination of the population by fungi.

26. The elephant shark (*Callorhinchus milii*) is a holocephalan with approximately one billion base pairs in its genome. If cytosine represents 24% of the genome, which of the following is true?

    (A) Purines make up 52% of this Chondrichthyes' genome.
    (B) A = T pairs make up 50% of this prokaryote's genome.
    (C) Pyrimidines make up 50% of this Osteichthyes' genome.
    (D) C Ξ G make up 52% of this cartilaginous fish's genome.
    (E) Adenine nucleotides make up 26% of this animal's genome.

27. Which of the following would be the best experimental technique to transfer a plasmid into *E. coli*?

    (A) Conjugation
    (B) Transduction
    (C) Transfection
    (D) Transformation
    (E) Centrifugation

28. You can make a cDNA and a genome library in yeast. cDNA libraries give more useful information on gene expression than libraries made from gDNA.

    (A) Both statements above are true.
    (B) Both statements above are false.
    (C) The first statement is true but the second one is false.
    (D) The first statement is false but the second one is true.

29. Eukaryotic cells are used for cell fractionation after they are lysed. Which of the following would be in the first pellet?

    (A) Centriole
    (B) Nucleus
    (C) Lysosome
    (D) Mitochondria
    (E) Ribosome

30. Which of the following is the most important reason plasmids are important to recombinant technology?

    (A) Plasmids can be used to transfer and manipulate DNA.
    (B) Plasmids are essential for the conjugation between F+ and F– bacteria.
    (C) Plasmids are made of circular double-stranded DNA.
    (D) Eukaryotes can host a plasmid if a transfection protocol is used.
    (E) Both low copy and high copy plasmids are readily available.

31. A microcentrifuge tube contains three fragments of DNA, which are 1500 bp, 3200 bp, and 4500bp in size. If these fragments are separated by gel electrophoresis, which of the following would be observed?

    (A) The 1500 bp fragment migrates the farthest.
    (B) The 3200 bp fragment migrates the farthest.
    (C) The 4500 bp fragment migrates the farthest.
    (D) All the fragments migrate to the same location.

32. Which of the following techniques involves antigen-antibody interactions as a basis for its procedure?

    (A) RNA-Seq and ELISA
    (B) RT-PCR and western blots
    (C) Sanger sequencing and immunohistochemistry
    (D) ELISA and western blots
    (E) *In situ* hybridization and immunohistochemistry

33. A researcher is trying to determine the structure of a regulatory protein called p85. Which of the following would not be useful in this case?

    (A) NMR
    (B) Mass spectrometry
    (C) X-ray crystallography
    (D) The primary structure of p85
    (E) Flow cytometry

General Chemistry

34. What is the correct electron configuration for Zn^{2+}?

   (A) $[Ar]3d^8$
   (B) $[Ar]3d^{10}$
   (C) $[Ar]4s^2\,3d^8$
   (D) $[Ar]4s^2\,3d^9$
   (E) $[Ar]4s^1\,3d^{10}$

35. Bismuth-212 undergoes α decay followed by β decay. What is the resultant nucleus?

   (A) ^{210}Po
   (B) ^{208}Tl
   (C) ^{208}Bi
   (D) ^{208}Pb
   (E) ^{207}Hg

36. Which of the following atoms will have the smallest atomic radius?

   (A) Oxygen
   (B) Sodium
   (C) Carbon
   (D) Sulfur
   (E) Iron

37. What is the shape of chlorine trifluoride?

   (A) T-shaped
   (B) Square planar
   (C) Trigonal bipyramid
   (D) Trigonal pyramid
   (E) Bent

38. Which of the following best describes why the temperature of a pot of boiling water remains constant despite the continual addition of heat?

   (A) The heat is increasing the internal kinetic energy of the water rather than increasing the temperature.
   (B) The heat is decreasing the internal kinetic energy of the water rather than increasing the temperature.
   (C) The heat is used to break hydrogen bonds between water molecules rather than increasing the temperature.
   (D) The heat is used to form hydrogen bonds between water molecules rather than increasing the temperature.
   (E) None of the above

39. There are an unknown number of moles of Argon in a steel container. A chemist injects two moles of nitrogen into the container. The temperature and volume do not change, but the pressure increases by ten percent. Originally the container held:

   (A) 16 moles of Ar.
   (B) 18 moles of Ar.
   (C) 20 moles of Ar.
   (D) 22 moles of Ar.
   (E) 24 moles of Ar.

40. Air is a mixture of many gases. Yet, N_2 (78%) and O_2 (21%) comprise 99% of its composition. If the pressure of air at sea level is 760 torr, what are the approximate partial pressures of N_2 and O_2, respectively?

   (A) 590 torr, 160 torr
   (B) 590 torr, 380 torr
   (C) 160 torr, 590 torr
   (D) 160 torr, 380 torr
   (E) 380 torr, 380 torr

41. The packaging and storage of carbonated liquids (such as soda) is largely predicated on the properties of gas solubility in liquids. Which of the following best describes the relationship between solubility, pressure, and temperature for gases in liquids?

   (A) Gases (such as CO_2) are most soluble in liquids at high pressures and high temperatures.
   (B) Gases (such as CO_2) are most soluble in liquids at low pressures and low temperatures.
   (C) Gases (such as CO_2) are most soluble in liquids at low pressures and high temperatures.
   (D) Gases (such as CO_2) are most soluble in liquids at high pressures and low temperatures.
   (E) Gases (such as CO_2) are not soluble unless combined with other compounds.

42. A chemist is attempting to identify an unknown salt. When she adds a solution of silver nitrate, a white precipitate forms. Which of the following may be the identity of the unknown salt?

   I. Li_2CO_3
   II. $Ba(CH_3COO)_2$
   III. $NaCl$

   (A) I only
   (B) II only
   (C) III only
   (D) I and II
   (E) I and III

43. Which of the following statements is always true about the kinetics of a chemical reaction?

   (A) The rate law includes all reactants in the balanced overall equation.
   (B) The overall order equals the sum of the reactant coefficients in the overall reaction.
   (C) The overall order equals the sum of the reactant coefficients in the slow step of the reaction.
   (D) The structure of the catalyst remains unchanged throughout the reaction progress.
   (E) The units of the rate constant are $M^{-1}s^{-1}$.

44. Based on the reaction mechanism shown below, which of the following statements is correct?

$$2\,NO + O_2 \rightarrow 2\,NO_2$$

   1) $2\,NO \rightarrow N_2O_2$ (*fast*)
   2) $N_2O_2 + O_2 \rightarrow 2\,NO_2$ (*slow*)

   (A) Step 1 is the rate-determining step and the rate of the overall reaction is $k[N_2O_2]$.
   (B) Step 1 is the rate-determining step and the rate of the overall reaction is $k[NO]^2$.
   (C) Step 2 is the rate-determining step and the rate of the overall reaction is $k[NO_2]^2$.
   (D) Step 2 is the rate-determining step and the rate of the overall reaction is $k[N_2O_2][O_2]$.
   (E) The rate-determining step cannot be determined from the data provided.

45. Given the following equilibrium:

$$N_2(g) + 3H_2(g) \rightleftharpoons 2NH_3(g) \quad \Delta H = -91.8\,kJ$$

   How would an increase in temperature affect the concentration of N_2 at equilibrium?

   (A) The concentration of N_2 will increase because of an increase in K_{eq}.
   (B) The concentration of N_2 will decrease because of an increase in K_{eq}.
   (C) The concentration of N_2 will increase because of a decrease in K_{eq}.
   (D) The concentration of N_2 will decrease because of a decrease in K_{eq}.
   (E) The concentration of N_2 will remain unchanged.

46. Which of the following salts is least soluble in water?

   (A) PbI_2 ($K_{sp} = 7.9 \times 10^{-9}$)
   (B) $Mg(OH)_2$ ($K_{sp} = 6.3 \times 10^{10}$)
   (C) $Zn(IO_3)_2$ ($K_{sp} = 3.9 \times 10^{6}$)
   (D) SrF_2 ($K_{sp} = 2.6 \times 10^{-9}$)
   (E) Ag_2CrO_4 ($K_{sp} = 1.1 \times 10^{-12}$)

47. A graph depicting a titration of a weak acid with a strong base will start at a

   (A) high pH and slope downwards with an equivalence pH equal to 7.
   (B) high pH and slope downwards with an equivalence pH below 7.
   (C) low pH and slope upwards with an equivalence pH equal to 7.
   (D) low pH and slope upwards with an equivalence pH above 7.
   (E) neutral pH and slope upwards with an equivalence pH above 7.

48. List the following compounds by increasing pK_a:

   I. H_2SO_4
   II. NH_3
   III. CH_3CH_2COOH
   IV. HF

   (A) I < III < II < IV
   (B) I < IV < III < II
   (C) III < I < IV < II
   (D) II < III < IV < I
   (E) I < II < III < IV

49. Which of the following best explains why disorder tends to favor spontaneity?

   (A) First Law of Thermodynamics
   (B) Second Law of Thermodynamics
   (C) Third Law of Thermodynamics
   (D) Hess' Law
   (E) None of the above

50. Which of the following should have the highest enthalpy of vaporization?

   (A) N_2
   (B) Br_2
   (C) Hg
   (D) Al
   (E) He

51. If a chemist needed to measure 12.52 mL of a solution, the best piece of laboratory equipment to use would be:

   (A) an Erlenmeyer flask.
   (B) a beaker.
   (C) a pipette.
   (D) a buret.
   (E) a weighing bottle.

52. Which of the following pieces of glassware is NOT designed to measure solution volumes accurately?

(A) Buret
(B) Volumetric flask
(C) Graduated cylinder
(D) Beaker
(E) Volumetric pipette

53. In order to make a 1.5 M H_2SO_4 solution from 10.0 mL of 15 M H_2SO_4 solution, you should:

(A) add 10.0 mL of 15 M H_2SO_4 to a beaker, then add 100 mL of distilled water and stir.
(B) add 10.0 mL of 15 M H_2SO_4 to a beaker, then add 90 mL of distilled water and stir.
(C) add ~80 mL of distilled water to a beaker, add 10.0 mL of 15 M H_2SO_4 with stirring, then add enough distilled water to measure exactly 100 mL.
(D) add 90 mL of distilled water to a beaker, then add 10.0 mL of 15 M H_2SO_4 and stir.
(E) add 100 mL of distilled water to a beaker, then add 10.0 mL of 15 M H_2SO_4 and stir.

54. A chemist uses a volumetric pipette to transfer exactly 10.00 mL of water into a tared flask, which she then weighs on an electronic balance four separate times. The masses are determined to be 9.82 g, 9.80 g, 9.83 g, and 9.79 g. Assuming the density of water is 1 g/mL at the temperature in question, what can be said about the balance used?

(A) It was precise, but not accurate.
(B) It was accurate, but not precise.
(C) It was both precise and accurate.
(D) It was neither precise nor accurate.

55. In order to successfully separate a mixture of two solids via recrystallization, what should be true about the compounds?

(A) They should have the same solubility at high and low temperatures in a given solvent.
(B) One should be more soluble at high temperatures than the other.
(C) One should be less soluble at high temperatures than the other.
(D) One should be more soluble at low temperatures than the other.
(E) One should have a higher melting point than the other.

56. A chemist determines the specific heat of a piece of iron to be 0.39 J/g °C through a calorimetry experiment. If the accepted value for the specific heat of iron is 0.45 J/g °C, what is the percent error for the experiment?

(A) $\dfrac{0.39}{0.45}$

(B) $\dfrac{0.45}{0.39}$

(C) $\dfrac{(0.39-0.45)}{0.45} \times 100$

(D) $\dfrac{(0.39-0.45)}{0.39} \times 100$

(E) $\dfrac{(0.39-0.45)}{\frac{1}{2}(0.39+0.45)} \times 100$

Organic Chemistry

57. In the molecule below, what are the hybridizations of C_1, C_2, C_3, and C_4, respectively?

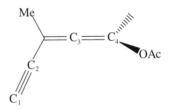

(A) sp, sp, sp^2, sp^2
(B) sp, sp, sp, sp^2
(C) sp^2, sp^2, sp, sp
(D) sp^2, sp, sp, sp
(E) sp^2, sp^3, sp^3, sp

58. Which of the following describes epimeric compounds?

I. Contain multiple chiral centers
II. Are non-superimposable, mirror images
III. Differ in absolute configuration at a single chiral center

(A) I only
(B) II only
(C) I and III
(D) I, II, and III
(E) I and II

59. Rank the conformations of 2-aminoethanol by increasing stability.

   (A) anti < gauche < eclipsed
   (B) eclipsed < anti < gauche
   (C) gauche < anti < eclipsed
   (D) eclipsed < gauche < anti
   (E) anti < eclipsed < gauche

60. Which of the following is the strongest nucleophile?

   (A) CN⁻
   (B) OH⁻
   (C) CH₃OH
   (D) NH₃
   (E) NH₄⁺

61. Which reaction proceeds the fastest?

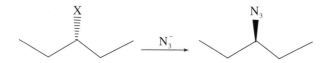

   (A) When X = Br
   (B) When X = F
   (C) When X = Cl
   (D) When X = I
   (E) When X = CH₃

62. Which of the following is associated with an S$_N$2 reaction?

   (A) sp^2 hybridized intermediate
   (B) A unimolecular rate law
   (C) An antiperiplanar conformation
   (D) Inversion of configuration
   (E) Formation of a carbocation

63. Which step of the radical process does the following reaction represent?

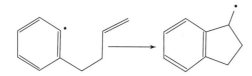

   (A) Initiation
   (B) Propagation
   (C) Termination
   (D) Elimination
   (E) Substitution

64. Which of the following reactions may involve a carbocation rearrangement?

   (A) S$_N$1 only
   (B) S$_N$2 only
   (C) S$_N$1 and E1 only
   (D) S$_N$2 and E2 only
   (E) S$_N$1, S$_N$2, and E1

65. If an alkyne is treated with two equivalents of hydrogen in the presence of platinum, what is the net change in bonds?

   (A) − 1 pi bond, + 4 sigma bonds
   (B) − 2 pi bonds, + 2 sigma bonds
   (C) − 2 pi bonds, + 4 sigma bonds
   (D) − 2 pi bonds, + 6 sigma bonds
   (E) − 4 pi bonds, + 6 sigma bonds

66. If benzene is treated with two equivalents of bromine in the presence of a FeBr₃ catalyst and elevated temperatures, what is the maximum number of disubstituted isomeric products that could be produced?

   (A) 1
   (B) 2
   (C) 3
   (D) 4
   (E) 5

67. The acid-catalyzed Markovnikov addition of H₂O to 1-butene should give a(n):

   (A) primary alcohol.
   (B) secondary alcohol.
   (C) tertiary alcohol.
   (D) cis-diol.
   (E) aldehyde

68. Which of the following of the following substituents is most likely to be meta directing?

   (A) –OH
   (B) –OCH₃
   (C) –Cl
   (D) –NO₂
   (E) –CH₂CH₃

69. Rank the protons from least acidic to most acidic.

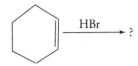

(A) $H_a < H_b = H_d < H_c$
(B) $H_c < H_d < H_b < H_a$
(C) $H_c < H_b = H_d < H_a$
(D) $H_c < H_b < H_d < H_a$
(E) $H_a = H_b < H_c < H_d$

70. Which of the following carbonyl compounds cannot undergo a symmetrical aldol condensation?

(A) 2,2,4,4-tetramethylpentan-3-one
(B) 1,2,2-triphenylethanone
(C) tert-butyl acetate
(D) pentan-2-one
(E) 2-methylpentan-3-one

71. The ^{13}C NMR spectrum for Compound X shows one peak at 128 ppm. If elemental analysis shows that the compound has an empirical formula of CH, how many possible stereoisomers could Compound X have?

(A) 0
(B) 1
(C) 2
(D) 4
(E) 8

72. For the following reaction, how would the R_f value of the product compare to that of the starting material if monitored by TLC on a normal silica gel plate?

HBr ⟶ ?

(A) The R_f value of the product would be greater than that of the reactant because the product is more polar.
(B) The R_f value of the product would be greater than that of the reactant because the product is less polar.
(C) The R_f value of the product would be smaller than that of the reactant because the product is more polar.
(D) The R_f value of the product would be smaller than that of the reactant because the product is less polar.
(E) The R_f values of the reactants and products would be the same, because their polarities are similar.

73. What will the 1H NMR spectrum of isobutane show?

(A) One 6 H triplet and one 4 H quartet
(B) Two 3 H triplets and two 2 H quartets
(C) One 9 H doublet and one 1 H multiplet
(D) One 6 H triplet, one 2 H multiplet, and one 2 H triplet
(E) Two 3 H triplets and one 4 H multiplet

ANSWERS AND EXPLANATIONS

1. **A** While lipids are hydrophobic, they are not frequently found in the interior of globular proteins, hydrophobic or not. They could be—for example, some carrier proteins in the blood are designed to transport lipids (the lipoproteins)—but they are not *frequently* found there ((A) is not true and the correct answer choice). All other statements are true.

2. **E** Nucleotides contain only one sugar, either deoxyribose or ribose ((C) is wrong), and for DNA, the sugar is deoxyribose ((A) and (B) are wrong). Uracil is a base found in RNA ((D) is wrong), while thymine is a base found in DNA ((E) is correct).

3. **B** A salt solution that is hypertonic to the red blood cell will have a tendency to draw water out of the cell by osmosis, causing the cell to shrivel up ((B) is correct, and (A) and (E) are wrong). The salt cannot cross the cell membrane ((C) and (D) are wrong).

4. **E** The replicated chromosomes (sister chromatids) are separated during anaphase. DNA replication occurs in S phase ((A) is wrong), cytokinesis and the reformation of the nucleus occur in telophase ((B) is wrong), creation of a spindle and dissolution of the nuclear membrane occur in prophase ((C) is wrong), and alignment of the replicated chromosomes at cell center occurs during metaphase ((D) is wrong).

5. **A** Protein synthesis (translation) occurs in the cytosol in both prokaryotes and eukaryotes. However, only eukaryotes transcribe RNA in the nucleus because prokaryotes lack cellular organelles. Prokaryotic transcription takes place in the cytosol as well ((B) is wrong). Prokaryotes do have a cell wall, but eukaryotes do not have ONLY a cell membrane; some have cell walls also (plant cells, fungi; (C) is wrong). Prokaryotes can also participate in aerobic respiration (and eukaryotes can perform glycolysis; (D) is wrong). Eukaryotes do not usually carry plasmids, and if they do, do not exchange them during sexual reproduction. Sexual reproduction in eukaryotes involves the fusion of egg and sperm ((E) is wrong).

6. **B** A spontaneous reaction must have a negative DG ((A), (C), and (E) are wrong). A reaction with a low energy of activation will proceed more quickly than one with a high energy of activation ((B) is correct, and (D) is wrong).

7. **D** Statement I is true: catalysts stabilize the transition state of a reaction ((B) can be eliminated). By stabilizing the transition state, the energy of activation (energy required to produce the transition state) is lowered, so Statement III is also true ((A) and (C) can be eliminated). However, Statement III is false: catalysts cannot make a non-spontaneous reaction spontaneous. All they can do is make an already spontaneous reaction go faster ((E) can be eliminated, and (D) is correct).

8. **B** Fermentation occurs in the absence of oxygen, when the PDC and the Krebs cycle are shut down ((A) and (E) are wrong). In order to continue running glycolysis, NADH must be oxidized back to NAD^+, and the reduction of pyruvate, to either ethanol or lactic acid, allows the oxidation of NADH. Fermentation in yeast does produce the alcohol in wine and beer, but this is not the reason that fermentation occurs ((C) is wrong). A drop in pH would reduce enzyme activity, not increase it ((D) is wrong).

9. **A** The enzyme that unwinds DNA at the origin to begin replication is called helicase. DNA gyrase is the enzyme that supercoils prokaryotic DNA ((A) is not true and is the correct answer). All of the other statements are true.

10. **C** Statement I is a valid difference: there is no proofreading or editing of newly made RNA transcripts ((A), (B), and (E) can be eliminated). Statement II is NOT a difference: both DNA and RNA are synthesized 5′ to 3′. Statement III is a valid difference: replication strives to produce two identical DNA strands from a single parent molecule, while the goal of transcription is to create a single RNA molecule from the DNA. Because the two strands of DNA are complementary, each DNA strand would produce a different strand of RNA, thus, typically only one of the DNA strands is transcribed (called the template strand). Choice (D) can be eliminated, and (C) is correct.

11. **C** The Hardy-Weinberg equation for allele frequency is $p + q = 1$. If the frequency of the dominant allele (p) is 0.1, then the frequency of the recessive allele (q) must be 0.9. Plugging these values into the equation for genotype frequency ($p^2 + 2pq + q^2 = 1$), we find that the frequency of homozygous dominant individuals (p^2) is 0.01, the frequency of heterozygous individual ($2pq$) is 0.18, and the frequency of homozygous recessive individuals (q^2) is 0.81. Individuals affected by the dominant allele include homozygous dominants and heterozygotes; 0.01 + 0.18 = 0.19.

12. **E** The child with blood type O must be homozygous ii, thus, both the man and woman must be heterozygous; the woman I^Bi and the man I^Ai ((A) is wrong). Since the child is Rh+, it could be either homozygous RR or heterozygous Rr; however, since the mother is Rh−, she must have the genotype rr. Thus all she could donate to the child is r, and the child must be heterozygous Rr ((B) is wrong). The man could be the father of the child, his genotype could be I^AiRR and could have donated i and R to the child ((D) is wrong). However, this does not absolutely establish paternity, as other men could also have the necessary blood types to produce an O+ child with this woman (for example, men with blood types O+ and B+). Choice (C) is wrong, and (E) is correct.

13. **B** If a pure-breeding (homozygous) white mouse (WW) is crossed with a pure-breeding (homozygous) black mouse (BB), then all offspring mice will be heterozygous (WB). If their phenotype is a blended version of the parental phenotypes, then this is an example of incomplete dominance. Codominance is when both alleles are expressed, but independently of each other (i.e., not blended, like blood typing; (A) is wrong). Epistasis is when the expression of one gene prevents the expression of another (e.g., the gene for baldness prevents the expression of hair shape genes; (C) is wrong). Classical dominance is when one allele is expressed and one is silent; if this were the case, all the heterozygous offspring would look like one of the parents (the one expressing the dominant phenotype; (D) is wrong). Recombination occurs between two different genes on the same chromosome, e.g., fur color and whisker length. Since only one gene is involved here, it cannot be recombination ((E) is wrong).

14. **C** Colorblindness is an X-linked disorder, so the man's genotype must be X^CY. His daughter inherits X^C from him and X^N (the normal allele) from her mother (the man's wife does not carry the colorblindness allele). The daughter's husband's genotype is X^NY. For the daughter to have a boy, her husband had to donate the Y chromosome. The probability that the boy is colorblind depends on what the daughter donates, either X^C (colorblind) or X^N (normal), one-half.

15. D Not all chordates have bony skeletons, some are cartilaginous as in sharks ((D) is not a shared feature and is the correct answer choice). All other choices list shared features.

16. B Prezygotic barriers to speciation prevent the union of sperm and egg into a zygote. They include species-specific sperm recognition ((A) is a prezygotic barrier and can be eliminated), temporal barriers such as different mating seasons ((C) is a prezygotic barrier and can be eliminated), mechanical barriers such as size differences ((D) is a prezygotic barrier and can be eliminated), and behavioral barriers, such as mating rituals ((E) is a prezygotic barrier and can be eliminated). Only (B) describes a postzygotic barrier; in this situation the sperm and egg fuse, and the hybrid develops, but is sterile and the line cannot continue ((B) is not a prezygotic barrier and the correct answer choice).

17. D The question describes conifers, tall pine trees that produce pinecones for reproduction. The seeds are not enclosed, and the plants are described as "naked seed" plants, or gymnosperms. Angiosperms are flowering plants and have enclosed seeds; monocots and dicots are subclasses of angiosperms ((A), (B), and (E) are wrong). Ferns are short, shrubby plants, not tall trees (their dominant stage is the sporophyte, however). Choice (C) is wrong.

18. D Cardiac muscle cells have voltage-gated calcium channels that open shortly after the action potential is initiated. The resulting influx of calcium greatly prolongs the cardiac action potential (200–300 msec), producing the characteristic plateau phase seen in these cells. Neuronal action potentials are about 100 times shorter (only 2–3 msec) and are not dependent on the influx of calcium. In both cardiac muscle cells and neurons the initial depolarization is caused by the influx of sodium, Na^+/K^+ ATPases maintain resting potential, and repolarization is caused by the efflux of potassium ((A), (B), and (E) are true of both and can be eliminated, and (C) is not true of either and can be eliminated).

19. C Oxytocin is released by the posterior pituitary, but is actually made by neuron cell bodies the hypothalamus and transported into the posterior pituitary for release. This is also true of ADH, the other posterior pituitary hormone. All other hormones listed are synthesized and released by the anterior pituitary.

20. A Secretion is the process used to move substances from the blood into the filtrate ((C), (D), and (E) are wrong). This helps eliminate substances faster than by filtration alone, because not only is the substance filtered, additional molecules of the substance are added to the filtrate as it is processed into urine. The concentration of the substance in the initial filtrate will be equal to plasma concentration of that substance, but as the substance is secreted, its concentration in the plasma will fall and its concentration in the filtrate will rise. Thus, the final urine concentration of the substances will be higher than plasma concentration ((A) is correct and (B) is wrong). Substances that are typically secreted include drugs and toxins.

21. B The pancreas is a major source of digestive enzymes for the GI tract ((D) is a function and can be eliminated). It also secretes bicarbonate along with those enzymes; this helps neutralize acidic chyme coming from the stomach and keeps the intestines at a more neutral pH of about 6–7 ((A) is a function and can be eliminated). The pancreas is also an endocrine organ, releasing insulin or glucagon to help regulate blood glucose levels ((C) and (E) are functions and can be eliminated). Bile, however, is made by the liver, not the pancreas ((B) is not a function and is the correct answer).

22.   C   Statement I would occur: aldosterone acts to increase sodium reabsorption at the distal tubule of the nephron. The resulting increase in blood osmolarity triggers the release of antidiuretic hormone that causes increased reabsorption of water, an increase in blood volume, and an increase in blood pressure ((B) and (D) can be eliminated). Statement II is false: the inhibition of antidiuretic hormone would lead to increased loss of water through the urine with a subsequent drop in blood volume and blood pressure ((A) and (E) can be eliminated and (C) is correct). Statement III is true: renin is released by the kidney when blood pressure falls. It catalyzes the conversion of angiotensinogen into angiotensin I, which is further converted to angiotensin II. Angiotensin II is a powerful vasoconstrictor that increases blood pressure.

23.   E   Returning myosin to its high-energy state (also referred to as "cocking" the myosin head) requires the hydrolysis of ATP. The power stroke, where myosin pulls actin toward the center of the sarcomere is simply myosin returning to its low-energy state, and does not require ATP hydrolysis ((A) is wrong). The release of actin by myosin requires the binding of ATP, but not ATP hydrolysis ((B) is wrong). Exposing the myosin binding sites requires calcium, but not ATP ((C) is wrong) and the actual binding of actin to myosin does not require anything special ((D) is wrong).

24.   E   "Proto" means "first" and "stoma" means "mouth," so in protostomes the first opening (the blastopore) develops into the mouth, and the second opening into the anus ((C) is true and can be eliminated). They are all coelomates (have a fluid-filled cavity separating their digestive tract from their body wall, (A) is true and can be eliminated). They undergo spiral (smaller cells lie in grooves between larger cells) and determinate cleavage (the fate of the embryonic cells is decided early in development ((B) and (D) are true and can be eliminated). However, the group includes annelids, mollusks, and arthropods; echinoderms and chordates are classified as deuterostomes ((E) is not true and is the correct answer).

25.   C   Ampicillin is a selection agent and antibiotic; it kills bacteria. In order for a bacterial cell to survive growth media containing ampicillin, it must contain a gene for ampicillin resistance (Amp^R). This gene is common in plasmids and allows researchers to select for bacteria that contain a plasmid. Any bacteria which take up the plasmid (i.e., become transformed) acquire resistance to ampicillin and can grow in its presence. Bacteria which have not transformed with the plasmid die in the presence of ampicillin (eliminate (A); it is the opposite of the correct answer). Using media containing ampicillin thus ensures that the only bacteria growing are those which contain the plasmid (eliminate (B); (C) is correct). A bacteriophage is a virus which infects bacteria, and antibiotics are ineffective at preventing viral infection (eliminate (D)). Antibiotics such as ampicillin (as well as tetracycline, penicillin or streptomycin) are also ineffective at killing fungi (eliminate (E)).

26.   E   This question is tricky because it tests a combination of diversity of life and molecular biology. Let's deal with the molecular biology first. A genome is always made of 50% pyrimidines and 50% purines, since pyrimidines always bind to purines (eliminate (A); keep (C) on your first pass). Cytosine is complementary to guanine, and thymine is complementary to adenine. Therefore, if a genome contains 24% cytosine, it also contains 24% guanine. This means C Ξ G pairs make up a total of 24% + 24% = 48% of the genome (eliminate (D)). This leaves 100 – 48% = 52% of the genome as T = A pairs (eliminate (B)). This means 52%/2 = 26% of the genome is thymine and 26% of the genome is adenine (also keep (E) on your first pass). Finally, sharks are cartilaginous fish, or Chondrichthyes. (Also remember that fish are animals, chordates, vertebrates.) They are not bony fish or Osteichthyes (eliminate (C); (E) is correct).

27. **D**   Conjugation is genetic exchange between two bacterial cells (eliminate (A)). Transduction is genetic exchange between bacterial cells, via a virus ((B) is wrong). Transfection is a lab technique where DNA is taken up from the environment into a eukaryotic cell (eliminate (C)). Transformation is another lab technique that involves the uptake of DNA from the environment by a prokaryotic cell ((D) is correct). Centrifugation is the process of spinning a sample at high speed. This pellets cells and precipitates at the bottom of the tube, and leaves everything else in the liquid layer above the pellet; this liquid layer is called the supernatant. Centrifugation would not be a useful technique to transfer DNA into a cell (eliminate (E)).

28. **A**   A cDNA library is made by harvesting mRNA molecules from a cell, reverse transcribing them into cDNA, cloning each molecule into a plasmid and then transferring the plasmids into host cells. A genomic DNA library is made by harvesting genomic DNA from a cell, fragmenting it into smaller pieces, cloning each piece into a plasmid and then transferring the plasmids into host cells. In both cases, bacteria and yeast are commonly used host cells (the first statement is true, eliminate (B) and (D)). Because cDNA libraries are made from the transcripts in a cell, they give information on what genes are being expressed or actively transcribed (the second statement is also true, (A) is correct, eliminate (C)).

29. **B**   Cell fractionation is when cell components are harvested into different samples via centrifugation, based on their size and density. The first sample contains whole cells and nuclei, because these components are large and heavy ((B) is correct). Organelles such as mitochondria, chloroplasts, lysosomes, and peroxisomes are collected in the second pellet (eliminate (C) and (D)). The endoplasmic reticulum, Golgi apparatus and vesicles usually break up to form small membrane-bound microsomes, which are collected in the third pellet. Finally, ribosomes, centrosomes, and other cytosolic components are collected last (eliminate (A) and (E)).

30. **A**   Plasmids are important because they can be used to transfer and manipulate DNA ((A) is correct). All the other statements are true but are irrelevant to the importance of plasmids to recombinant technology. Make sure you pay attention to what the question stem is asking, and that you pick the answer that is true and best answers the question.

31. **A**   Gel electrophoresis separates macromolecules by size and charge, using an electric current. Smaller molecules migrate quickly because they fit more easily through the pores of the gel. They are found near the bottom of the gel, close to the positive electrode. Larger molecules migrate more slowly because they don't easily fit through the pores of the gel. They are found near the top of the gel, near the negative electrode. In this example, the 1500 base pair fragment is smallest and will migrate the farthest ((A) is correct).

32. **D**   RNA sequencing does not require the interaction of an antigen and antibody, although ELISA does (eliminate (A)). No antibodies are used in polymerization reactions, so eliminate RT-PCR (B) and Sanger sequencing (C). Both ELISA and western blots require the interactions between an antigen and antibody ((D) is correct). Note that immunohistochemistry and flow cytometry also require antibodies. In situ hybridization studies nucleic acids, and so uses a probe instead of an antibody (eliminate (E)).

33. **E**   The major techniques that are used to determine protein structure are X-ray crystallography, mass spectrometry, NMR spectroscopy, and electron microscopy (eliminate (A), (B) and (C)). Each of these relies on knowing the primary structure of the protein (eliminate (D)). Flow cytometry gives information on which antigens are expressed at which level in a population of cells. It is not relevant to determining or studying protein structure.

General Chemistry

34. B The electron configuration for Zn (non-ionized) is $[Ar]4s^2\,3d^{10}$. Transition (*d*-block) elements always lose electrons from their highest energy *s* orbital first, meaning that the correct answer takes two electrons away from the $4s$ orbital.

35. D The only type of decay that changes the mass number of an atom is α decay, which results in the loss of two protons and two neutrons, meaning that the mass number is decreased by 4. Thus, the daughter nucleus must have a mass number of $212 - 4 = 208$, eliminating (A) and (E). The atomic number is affected by both α and β (which when present without a modifier refers to β^- decay) decay, with α decay decreasing the atomic number by 2, and β decay increasing it by 1. The atomic number of bismuth is 83, so $83 - 2 + 1 = 82$, which is the atomic number for lead, Pb.

36. A Remember that atomic radius increases as you go from right to left (since you decrease the number of protons in the nucleus providing an attractive force on the valence electrons) and as you go from up to down (since you increase the number of filled shells which provide a repulsive force on the valence electrons). Thus, the trend for smallest is the opposite; the smallest elements are found the upper right of the periodic table. Of the elements listed, oxygen is the one that is furthest towards the upper right hand corner, and thus is the smallest.

37. A To determine the shape of a molecule (which takes into account the number of lone pairs), we must first determine the geometry (which takes into account the total number of electron groups around the central atom, including both lone pairs and bonds). First, count the number of valence electrons on each atom. Since all are halogens, each will have seven valence electrons. With the chlorine as the central atom, there is a single bond between it and each of the fluorine atoms. Thus, each of the fluorine atoms has its valences satisfied. This leaves two lone pairs on the central chlorine, making a total of five electron groups. Five electron groups gives a geometric family of trigonal bipyramid. Since the geometry is trigonal bipyramid, but there are two lone pairs, the shape is T-shaped.

38. C During a phase transition such as boiling, the temperature of the substance does not change because the heat provided is used to disrupt the intermolecular forces between molecules (eliminating (D)). Since the temperature of a substance is a measure of its internal kinetic energy and is not changing, (A) and (B) may also be eliminated.

39. C At constant V and T, the pressure of an ideal gas reflects the number of particles (regardless of their identity). It is a simplification of the Ideal Gas Law from $PV = nRT$ to $P \propto n$. So, if the addition of two moles of N_2 into the chamber results in an increase in P of 10 percent, then the moles added must be 10 percent of the initial number of Ar moles. Two moles are 10 percent of 20 moles.

40. A According to Dalton's Law, the sum of the partial pressures of gases must equal to the total pressure of the system. Therefore, (B) and (D) may be eliminated, as they do not add up to approximately 760 torr. In addition, since the mole fractions of the two gases are not equal, (E) may also be eliminated. Therefore, since the proportion of nitrogen greatly exceeds that of oxygen, (A) must be correct.

41.   D   Based upon phase solubility rules, the solubility of gases increases with increasing pressure and decreases with increasing temperature. This is why carbonated beverages are maintained under pressure and are best stored at lower temperatures.

42.   E   Silver salts are generally insoluble unless they contain nitrate, perchlorate, or acetate ions. Since nitrate salts are always soluble, there is no cation among the items that would result in precipitation. Therefore, at least one of the anions must result in an insoluble salt. Based upon the solubility rules of silver salts, only the acetate ion (Item II) would result in a soluble salt, therefore both Items I and III would make insoluble salts.

43.   C   Choice (A) is incorrect because rate laws are dependent on the slowest step. If a reactant does not participate in the slow step, it will not be included in the overall rate law. Choice (B) is incorrect because rate laws of overall reactions can only be determined experimentally. Choice (D) is incorrect because while it is true that a catalyst comes out of a reaction unchanged, it can undergo temporary transformations during the reaction and revert back into its original form at the end. Choice (E) may be eliminated because the units of the rate constant are dependent upon the order of the reaction. Therefore, (C) is the best option because rate laws can be determined from elementary steps of a reaction mechanism by simply raising the reactants to their respective coefficients.

44.   D   The rate-determining step of a reaction mechanism is the slowest step of that mechanism, eliminating (A) and (B). The rate law of an elementary step can be determined from the coefficients of the reactants in the elementary step. Because Step 2 is the rate determining step, the overall rate law will be equivalent to the rate law for the step. Therefore, rate = $k[N_2O_2][O_2]$.

45.   C   Since the reaction is exothermic, an increase in temperature will shift the equilibrium to the left, and the concentration of N_2 will increase, eliminating (B), (D), and (E). For exothermic reactions, an increase in temperature will decrease the K_{eq}, eliminating (A) and making (C) the correct answer.

46.   E   All of the compounds are composed of three ions, so comparing K_{sp} values will give relative solubility. Since the question asks for an extreme, the middle values of the variable cannot be correct, eliminating (A), (B), and (D). The compound with the lowest K_{sp} value will have the lowest solubility according to the K_{sp} expression, $K_{sp} = [cation]x[anion]y$, where x and y represent the coefficients and total 3. Therefore, (E) is correct.

47.   D   A graph showing the titration of a weak acid will start at a low pH and slope upward as the titrant (in this case, a strong base) is added. Therefore, (A) and (B) cannot be true. As the weak acid and titrant strong base react, water and salt are formed as products. The salt will determine the pH at the equivalence point. The conjugate acid of a strong base has no acidic properties and will be neutral in solution. However, the conjugate base of the weak acid will be weakly basic. Because of this, the pH at the equivalence point will be above 7.

48.   B   A higher pK_a means a weaker acid, while a lower pK_a means a stronger acid. Since this is a ranking question, start with the extremes. Compound I is a strong acid and will have the lowest pK_a, eliminating (C) and (D). Compound II is the only base, so it will have the largest pK_a; (A) and (E) can be eliminated.

49. **B** The Second Law of Thermodynamics explains that the entropy of the universe must increase for a spontaneous reaction or that disorder favors spontaneity, making (B) the best answer. Hess' Law (D) relates to the enthalpy of the reaction rather than the entropy and may be eliminated. The First Law of Thermodynamics explains that energy can neither be created nor destroyed, but does not explain the impact of disorder, eliminating (A). The Third Law of Thermodynamics relates to the entropy of a substance rather than its impact on spontaneity, eliminating (C).

50. **D** Enthalpy of vaporization is the heat energy required per mole to change from the liquid to gas phase. He and N_2 are gases at room temperature, Br_2 and Hg are both liquids at room temperature, and Al is a solid at room temperature. Therefore, it is expected that Al will have the highest enthalpy of vaporization, making (D) correct.

51. **D** A buret allows for the highest level of precision of the given pieces of glassware (eliminate (A), (B) and (E)), and it is more versatile than a pipette (C), which are typically calibrated to dispense only specific preset volumes of a liquid.

52. **D** Beakers have very few graduated markings on them, so they do not provide a high degree of precision or accuracy for measurement. While not all other glassware allows for measuring a variety of different volumes, they will all measure at least one volume to a very high degree of accuracy.

53. **C** Dilution of a strong acid with water releases large amounts of heat, causing the concentrated acid to spatter dangerously. Therefore, remember the triple A rule of thumb—*a*lways *a*dd *a*cid to water when doing an acid dilution (eliminate (A) and (B)). The excess water can better absorb the energy released and minimizes spattering. The final volume of the dilute solution should be 100 mL (eliminate (E)) since it is a ten-fold dilution from 15 M to 1.5 M and the initial volume is 10.0 mL. Remember, molarity is defined as the number of moles of solute in a liter of total solution. In certain cases, volumes of liquids are not additive, so adding less distilled water, then bringing the solution to the correct total volume is best (eliminate (D)).

54. **A** Precision can be defined as reproducibility in measurement, or how little multiple measured values vary from each other. Since the four measurements agree within 0.04 g, the balance is precise (eliminate (B) and (D)). Since 10.00 mL of water should weigh exactly 10.00 *g*, this balance was not accurate. Accuracy is defined as how close a measured value is to a true or accepted value, and it is generally considered to be ± 1 or 2 in the last place value of the measurement (eliminate (C)). In this case, 10.00 ± 0.02 g would indicate both precision and accuracy. However, the measurements differed from the true value in the tenths place rather than the hundredths place, meaning the variation was greater than the uncertainty associated with the balance itself.

55. **D** Recrystallization is a separation technique that takes advantage of the different solubilities of the compounds to be separated over a range of temperatures (eliminate (A) and (E)). During a successful recrystallization, a mixture of compounds is dissolved in a solvent to form a saturated solution at a high temperature (usually the boiling point of the solvent). The solution is then cooled, and the compound that is less soluble at lower temperatures will precipitate out of solution while the compound that is more soluble stays dissolved, making (D) the best answer.

The compounds can then be separated by filtering off the precipitate from the rest of the solution. Note that if one compound is more soluble than the other at high temperatures, that means the other is less soluble, so (B) and (C) are identical, and therefore both incorrect.

56. **C** Since the question asks for a *percent* error, the first fraction term should be multiplied by 100 (eliminate (A) and (B)). Percent error compares the difference between a measured value and the accepted value to the accepted value. Since the real value of specific heat is given as 0.45 J/g °C, the 0.45 should be in the denominator (eliminate (D)). Note that (E) compares the difference between the two values to the average of the values, and as such would be called the percent *difference* between the two values, not the percent *error*.

Organic Chemistry

57. **B** Both C_1 and C_2 make up the triple bond. They are both *sp* hybridized, so you can eliminate (C), (D), and (E). C_3 is part of an allene. The bonds that it forms with its neighbors are linear (180°), so it is also *sp*. You can eliminate (A), which leaves (B) as the correct answer. C_4 has a double bond and two single bonds, so it is *sp²*.

58. **C** Epimeric compounds are diasteromers that differ in configuration at a single chiral center (recall the relationship between sugar molecules). Subsequently, Items I and III are correct. Item II may be eliminated because diasteromers are non-superimposable AND non-mirror images of one another.

59. **B** Since this is a ranking question, look for obvious extremes and eliminate answers. Choices (A), (C), and (E) should be eliminated because the eclipsed conformation is always the least stable due to sterics and electron repulsions in aligned bonds. Choice (D) is the more enticing answer of the remaining two because the general rule of thumb is that the anti conformation is the most stable because the bulky groups are farthest apart, while they are 60° apart in a *gauche* conformation. This question is tricky, however, because in this case there is intramolecular hydrogen bonding which can occur in the *gauche* conformation, making it the most stable one (eliminate (D)).

60. **A** Nucleophiles are electron dense: since (E) is positively charged, it would make a poor nucleophile. While neutral compounds that have lone pairs can be nucleophilic, negatively charged nucleophiles tend to be stronger (eliminate (C) and (D)). The stronger nucleophile is the more reactive nucleophile; more reactive corresponds to less stable. Therefore, the nucleophile that is less able to stabilize a negative charge will be the stronger nucleophile. For (A) and (B), the negative charge resides on the C and O, respectively. Since carbon is less electronegative than oxygen, it is therefore less able to stabilize a negative charge, making cyanide the best nucleophile (eliminate (B)).

61. **D** This is an S_N2 reaction, since it occurs with inversion of stereochemistry. Therefore the rate of the reaction is determined by both the nucleophile and the haloalkane. Since alkyl groups are not able to stabalize a negative charge well, (E) may be eliminated. The halogen that can best stabilize a negative charge will be the best leaving group and give the fastest reaction. Acidity of HX acids increases going down the periodic table because the larger halogens can

spread the negative charge over a larger surface area to stabilize it. Because iodine is the largest of the halogens, it is also the best leaving group.

62. **D** In an S_N2 reaction, the starting substrate undergoes a backside attack where the nucleophile attacks opposite the leaving group, causing a complete stereochemical inversion. Choice (A) can be eliminated because the there is no intermediate in this reaction. Choice (B) can be eliminated because S_N2 is a bimolecular process, as the name implies. Choice (C) can be eliminated because the conformation of the groups is not an important factor for the S_N2 reaction. Choice (E) may be eliminated because the formation of a carbocation is an important step during a S_N1 reaction.

63. **B** In a propagation step of a radical mechanism, there is no net change in the number of radicals in the reaction, as shown in this example. An initiation step results in a net increase in the number of radicals in the reaction (eliminate (A)). A termination results in a net decrease in the number of radicals in the reaction (eliminate (C)). Elimination and substitution reactions are not part of a typical radical reaction. Lastly, eliminate (D) since in this reaction a pi bond is broken.

64. **C** S_N1 and E1 reactions both involve the initial formation of a carbocation and therefore may involve carbocation rearrangements. Type 2 reactions cannot form carbocations, as their mechanism involves 1 concerted step.

65. **C** When an alkyne is treated with two equivalents of hydrogen in the presence of platinum, it is reduced to an alkane. This results in the loss of both pi bonds from the triple bond, so eliminate (A). The two pi bonds are converted to four C—H sigma bonds, so (B) and (D) can be eliminated.

66. **B** Although a minor product, given enough catalyst, heat, and time, the disubstituted products can form. In this reaction, two atoms of bromine will replace two hydrogens previously attached to the benzene ring. The bromine atoms can have either an *ortho* or *para* relationship to each other. This makes two possible isomers.

67. **B** The addition of water to 1-butene will only add one OH group, so it cannot form a diol (eliminate (D)). Since there are no tertiary carbons on the starting material, a tertiary alcohol cannot be formed (eliminate (C)). Markovnikov addition results in the addition of the hydroxyl group to the most substituted carbon of a double bond. Choice (A) can be eliminated because it represents addition of the hydroxyl group to the least substituted carbon. (E) may be eliminated because does not represent an addition reaction.

68. **D** Of the answers, only the nitro substituent is meta-directing and therefore, (D) is the best answer.

69. **C** Because H_a is bound to a carbon that is adjacent to two carbonyl groups, it is the easiest proton for a base to abstract since the conjugate base has the most resonance structures. Therefore, you can eliminate (A). Because this molecule has a mirror plane, H_b and H_d are equivalent, so you can eliminates (B) and (D), which leaves (C) as the correct answer. H_c is on a carbon that is not adjacent to any electron withdrawing groups or pi electrons, so it is the least acidic.

70. **A** A symmetrical aldol condensation is the same thing as a self-condensation reaction; it is an aldol condensation between two of the same molecule. In order for an aldol condensation to occur, at least one of the carbonyl compounds must be able to form an enolate through deprotonation of an a-carbon. Since 2,2,4,4-tetramethylpentan-3-one contains no a-hydrogens, it cannot form an enolate, and therefore cannot undergo a self-condensation reaction. All of the other molecules listed to have at least one a-hydrogen, and therefore can undergo self-condensation reactions.

71. **A** One signal on the ^{13}C NMR spectrum implies that either the molecule has only one carbon, or that all carbons in the molecule are equivalent. Since the empirical formula of Compound X is CH and the molecule contains no electronegative elements to shift the signal downfield, the single peak, located in the region common for alkenes and aromatic carbons (128 ppm), must represent some sort of sp^2-hybridized carbon(s). Any compound with only sp^2 hybridized carbons will have no stereoisomers, and in this case, the compound is benzene (C_6H_6).

72. **C** TLC separates compounds based on their polarities. The more polar a compound is, the more it adheres to the silica gel plate, giving it a smaller R_f value. Choices (A) and (D) are inconsistent with this type of interaction. The product for this reaction is bromocyclohexane, which is more polar than the reactant due to the presence of the halogen.

73. **A** The structure of isobutane is shown below. All three terminal CH_3 groups are chemically identical, and will show up as one resonance. More specifically, they will correspond to a doublet as they are split by the sole proton on the central carbon. The proton on the central carbon will show up as a multiplet, as it is split by 9 equivalent H atoms. Thus, one 9H doublet and one 1H multiplet is the correct answer, (A), which corresponds to *n*-butane.

QUANTITATIVE REASONING DRILL

Math Introduction

1. Which of the following is the best approximation of $\frac{7}{4} - 3\frac{3}{16}$?

   A. $-\frac{27}{16}$

   B. $-\frac{6}{4}$

   C. $-\frac{5}{4}$

   D. $-\frac{19}{16}$

   E. $-\frac{4}{4}$

2. Simone buys a car that costs d dollars. She pays p dollars immediately and the rest in x equal subsequent payments. How much greater is the cost of the car than each of her subsequent payments?

   A. $\dfrac{dx + p}{x}$

   B. $\dfrac{dx - p}{x}$

   C. $\dfrac{dx - 2p}{x}$

   D. $\dfrac{d(x - 1) + p}{x}$

   E. $\dfrac{d(x + 1) - p}{x}$

3. What is the value of $x^2 - 3x + 5$ if $x = -5$?

   A. -35
   B. -5
   C. 5
   D. 15
   E. 45

4. Kevin is twice as old as Jessica. Ten years ago, he was four times as old as she was. How old is Jessica now?

   A. 5
   B. 10
   C. 15
   D. 20
   E. 30

5. Which of the following is the closest to $\sqrt{997 \times 0.0012 \times 0.0001}$?

   A. 0.1
   B. 0.01
   C. 0.001
   D. 0.0001
   E. 0.00001

6. If $y = 3 + \dfrac{4}{x}$, then what is the value of x in terms of y ?

   A. $\dfrac{4}{y - 3}$

   B. $-\dfrac{4y}{3}$

   C. $\dfrac{7}{y}$

   D. $\dfrac{3}{4 - y}$

   E. $3 + \dfrac{4}{y}$

7. If x and y are both integers, which of the following must be an even integer?

   A. $x + y$
   B. xy
   C. $2x + y$
   D. $x^2 + 2y$
   E. $2x^2 + 6y^2$

8. Which of the following is the greatest for which $|2 - 3x| > 7$ is true?

   A. -5
   B. -2
   C. 2
   D. 5
   E. 10

9. The average of x, y, and z is 7. If $w = 3$, what is the average of w, x, y, and z ?

   A. 3
   B. 4
   C. 5
   D. 6
   E. 7

Arithmetic

10. Which of the following would change the most in value if rounded to three digits?

    A. 97.56
    B. 123.178
    C. 165.51
    D. 678.8824
    E. 1000.001

11. The fraction $\dfrac{4}{11}$ is between which of the following?

    A. $\dfrac{1}{3}$ and $\dfrac{3}{8}$

    B. $\dfrac{1}{4}$ and $\dfrac{7}{20}$

    C. $\dfrac{3}{13}$ and $\dfrac{5}{18}$

    D. $\dfrac{2}{9}$ and $\dfrac{3}{10}$

    E. $\dfrac{1}{5}$ and $\dfrac{9}{25}$

12. Approximate the representation in scientific notation of $6333 \times 35 + 123 - 580 + 1.2 \times 10^4$.

    A. -2.6×10^7
    B. 3.3×10^4
    C. 1.9×10^5
    D. 2.3×10^5
    E. 2.2×10^9

13. $\dfrac{9xy^3}{12x^4y^2} =$

    A. $\dfrac{2}{3}x^{-4}y^{-6}$

    B. $\dfrac{2}{3}x^{-3}y$

    C. $\dfrac{3}{4}x^{-4}y^{-6}$

    D. $\dfrac{3}{4}x^{-3}y$

    E. $\dfrac{3}{4}x^4y^6$

14. If $\log_x 6 = 2.585$, which of the following is closest to x ?

    A. 1.5
    B. 2
    C. 2.5
    D. 3
    E. 3.5

15. $1200^{\frac{1}{4}} =$

    A. 5.9
    B. 10.6
    C. 34.6
    D. 300

16. What is the value of $\left(\dfrac{4\times10^5}{3\times10^2}\right)\left(\dfrac{6\times10^3}{5\times10^4}\right)$?

    A. 2.4×10^1
    B. 4.0×10^1
    C. 1.6×10^2
    D. 4.0×10^2
    E. 1.6×10^3

Algebra

17. If $\sqrt[3]{3x + 9} + 3 = 0$, then what is the value of x ?

    A. −12
    B. 0
    C. 6
    D. 9
    E. 12

18. At what value of x do the graphs of $xy = -6$ and $y = -2x - 1$ intersect?

    A. −6
    B. −2
    C. −1
    D. 2
    E. 3

19. Which of the following describes the values of x that satisfy $|x + 6| < 7$?

    A. $x < -13$ or $x > -1$
    B. $x < -1$ or $x > 1$
    C. $-13 < x < 1$
    D. $-1 < x < 1$
    E. $-13 < x < 7$

20. If $x = 2 + \dfrac{1}{y}$ and $y = 1 + \dfrac{3}{z}$, then which of the following expresses x in terms of z ?

   A. $z + 2$

   B. $z + 3$

   C. $3 + \dfrac{z}{3}$

   D. $\dfrac{2z + 3}{z + 3}$

   E. $\dfrac{3z + 6}{z + 3}$

21. What is $4x^{\frac{3}{2}}$ if $x = \dfrac{25}{81}$?

   A. $\dfrac{625}{6561}$

   B. $\dfrac{125}{729}$

   C. $\dfrac{500}{729}$

   D. $\dfrac{500}{2916}$

   E. $\dfrac{20}{9}$

22. If a is negative and b is positive, which of the following must be positive?

   A. $a + b$

   B. $a - b$

   C. $|a| - b$

   D. $a + |b|$

   E. $|a| + b$

Word Problems

23. Kris has only dimes and quarters in his pocket, and these coins total to a value of $3.20. He has three more quarters than dimes. How many quarters does he have?

   A. 7
   B. 8
   C. 9
   D. 10
   E. 11

24. In Drytown this year, there were fifteen days in which it rained. On those days, an average of 6 inches of rain fell per day. In Drytown last year, there were only five days in which it rained, but on those days, an average of 14 inches of rain fell per day. On rainy days in Drytown for the past two years, what has been the average rainfall per day?

   A. 8
   B. 9
   C. 10
   D. 11
   E. 12

25. In a sporting arena with 500 people, 150 people are wearing red shirts, and 300 are wearing gold hats. If 100 people are not wearing red or gold, how many people are wearing both red shirts and gold hats?

   A. 0
   B. 50
   C. 100
   D. 150
   E. 2000

26. Which of the following equations represents the statement, "Two times the sum of x and y is equal to four less than z" ?

   A. $2x + y = 4 - z$
   B. $2(x + y) = 4 - z$
   C. $2x + y = z - 4$
   D. $2(x + y) = z - 4$

27. Joanna has two large bars of chocolate. Bar A consists of 4 grams of cacao and 8 grams of milk and other ingredients, and Bar B consists of 5 grams of cacao and 15 grams of milk and other ingredients. How much of each bar should she mix together to create 10 grams of chocolate that is 30% cacao?

    A. 9 grams of Bar A; 1 gram of Bar B
    B. 6 grams of Bar A; 4 grams of Bar B
    C. 5 grams of Bar A; 5 grams of Bar B
    D. 2 grams of Bar A; 8 grams of Bar B
    E. 1 gram of Bar A; 10 grams of Bar B

28. Grace's mother is four times as old as Grace is. Seven years ago, Grace's mother was eleven times as old as Grace was. How old is Grace now?

    A. 3
    B. 4
    C. 10
    D. 11
    E. 33

29. In a parking lot with 84 cars, each of which is either green or blue, there is a 5:7 ratio of green cars to blue cars. How many green cars are there?

    A. 24
    B. 35
    C. 42
    D. 49
    E. 60

30. A graduate has two student loans, one at an annual interest rate of 4% and the other at an annual interest rate of 6%. He has a total of $8,000 of debt, and his annual payments on the interest alone total $440. How large is the loan at the 4% interest rate?

    A. $2,000
    B. $3,000
    C. $4,000
    D. $5,000

Advanced Arithmetic

31. What is the approximate number of seconds between February 10th, 10:45:11 am, and February 14th, 2:10:05 pm?

    A. 271000
    B. 315000
    C. 358000
    D. 401000
    E. 444000

32. In a certain population, the probability of having genetic trait X is $\frac{1}{4}$. Three people are chosen at random from the population. What is the probability that at least one of them will have the trait?

    A. $\frac{1}{64}$
    B. $\frac{3}{64}$
    C. $\frac{3}{16}$
    D. $\frac{37}{64}$
    E. $\frac{63}{64}$

33. If the temperature is 50° Fahrenheit, what is the temperature in Celsius? (Note: $C = \frac{5}{9}(F - 32)$.)

    A. −4.2°
    B. 10°
    C. 59.7°
    D. 90°
    E. 122°

34. In a laboratory, three containers are marked with the amounts of sodium that they contain. The first has 8,000 micrograms of sodium. The second has 0.47 grams of sodium. The third has 55 milligrams of sodium. In total, how much sodium is in the three containers?

    A. 0.423 g
    B. 0.523 g
    C. 0.533 g
    D. 1.100 g
    E. 9.220 g

35. Jellybeans are to be drawn out of a jar, one at a time and without replacement. The jar contains 6 blueberry jellybeans, 9 mango jellybeans, and 5 raspberry jellybeans. What is the probability of drawing out a blueberry followed by a raspberry?

A. $\dfrac{3}{40}$

B. $\dfrac{3}{38}$

C. $\dfrac{9}{80}$

D. $\dfrac{27}{200}$

E. $\dfrac{27}{190}$

36. A miniature model of a house is being built to scale. An inch in the model represents 70 inches in the real house. Approximately what is the ratio of the volume of the real house to the volume of the model?

A. 10^2:1
B. 10^3:1
C. 10^4:1
D. 10^5:1
E. 10^6:1

37. In a large family, if a member is chosen at random, the probability that he or she will like ice cream is 0.60, and the probability that he or she will like cookies is 0.55. In the family, 10% of the members like neither ice cream nor cookies. What is the probability that a randomly selected member will like both ice cream and cookies?

A. 0.10
B. 0.15
C. 0.25
D. 0.35
E. 0.40

Plane Geometry

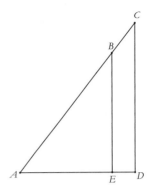

38. In the figure above, line segment $\overline{BE}$ is parallel to line segment $\overline{CD}$. The distance between point A and point E is 8, and the distance between point A and point D is 10. If the distance between point B and point E is 10, what is the distance between point C and point D?

A. 8
B. 10
C. 11.5
D. 12
E. 12.5

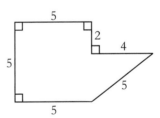

39. What is the area of the figure above?

A. 26
B. 31
C. 34
D. 37
E. 38

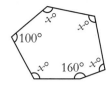

40. In the figure above, what is the value of x ?
(Note: Figure is not necessarily drawn to scale.)

 A. 25
 B. 70
 C. 108
 D. 115
 E. 160

41. The area of a rectangle is 300, and its length is five more than its width. What is its perimeter?

 A. 70
 B. $40\sqrt{3}$
 C. 75
 D. 80
 E. $24\sqrt{15}$

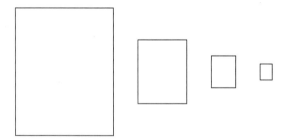

42. In the figure above, each rectangle has sides of half the length of the corresponding sides in the rectangle to its left. What is the ratio of the area of the first rectangle to the area of the fourth rectangle?

 A. 4
 B. 8
 C. 16
 D. 64
 E. 256

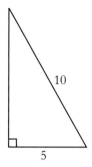

43. In the figure above, what is the area of the right triangle?

 A. 12.5
 B. $12.5\sqrt{3}$
 C. 25
 D. $25\sqrt{2}$
 E. $25\sqrt{3}$

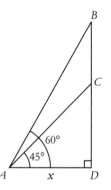

44. In the figure above, the distance between point B and point C is approximately 0.7. Which of the following is closest to the value of x ?

 A. 0.4
 B. 0.5
 C. 0.7
 D. 0.8
 E. 1.0

Solid and Coordinate Geometry

45. In square *ABCD*, point *A* is located at (1, 1) and point *B* is located at (2, 5). What is the area of the square?

A. 17
B. 25
C. 32
D. 45
E. 81

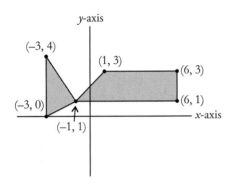

46. In the figure above, what is the area of the shaded region?

A. 12
B. 14
C. 15
D. 16
E. 20

47. A company is designing a label for the cylindrical portion of a bottle. The radius of this portion of the bottle is 6 centimeters, and the height is 8 centimeters. What is the area of the label, in square centimeters? (The label does not cover the neck, top, or bottom of the bottle.)

A. 48π
B. 96π
C   192π
D. 288π

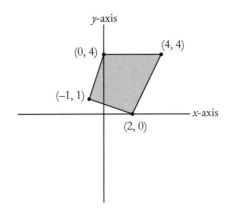

48. What is the area of the shaded region shown above?

A. 8
B. 10
C. 12
D. 13
E. 20

49. A cube has a volume of 64. If each of the twelve edges has its length divided by two, what is the new volume of the cube?

A. 1
B. $\dfrac{8}{3}$
C. 8
D. 16
E. 32

50. A cube with edge length 3 is painted red over all of its faces and then sliced into smaller cubes of edge length 1. How many of the smaller cubes have exactly 2 faces painted red?

A. 4
B. 6
C. 8
D. 10
E. 12

51. The vertex of a parabola is at (2, 4), and one root has a non-zero coordinate of 6. What is the non-zero coordinate of the other root?

A. –2
B. 2
C. 4
D. 8
E. 10

Trigonometry

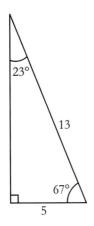

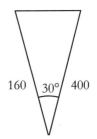

52. Which of the following is arccos $\dfrac{12}{13}$?

    A.   0°
    B.   23°
    C.   67°
    D.   90°

53. Given that csc $\theta = 2$ for $\dfrac{\pi}{2} < \theta < \dfrac{3\pi}{2}$, what is the value of cos θ ?

    A. $-\dfrac{\sqrt{3}}{2}$

    B. $-\dfrac{1}{2}$

    C. $\dfrac{1}{2}$

    D. $\dfrac{\sqrt{3}}{2}$

    E.   2

54. If $\cos(x) = \dfrac{3}{5}$ and $0° < x < 90°$, then what is the value of $\tan(x)$?

    A. $-\dfrac{4}{3}$

    B. $-\dfrac{3}{4}$

    C. $\dfrac{3}{4}$

    D. $\dfrac{4}{3}$

    E. $\dfrac{5}{3}$

55. What is the area of the triangle above? (Note: Figure is not necessarily drawn to scale.)

    A.   16000
    B. $16000\sqrt{2}$
    C. $16000\sqrt{3}$
    D.   32000
    E. $32000\sqrt{2}$

56. If $0° < \theta < 45°$, then which of the following is equal to cos θ ?

    A. $\cos(180° - \theta)$
    B. $\cos(90° + \theta)$
    C. $\cos(45° + \theta)$
    D. $\sin(180° + \theta)$
    E. $\sin(90° - \theta)$

57. What is the value of $\sin\left(\dfrac{3\pi}{4}\right)$?

    A. $-\dfrac{\sqrt{3}}{2}$

    B. $-\dfrac{\sqrt{2}}{2}$

    C. $-\dfrac{1}{2}$

    D. $\dfrac{1}{2}$

    E. $\dfrac{\sqrt{2}}{2}$

ANSWERS AND EXPLANATIONS

Math Introduction

1. **B** Since the question says to approximate, let's approximate. The first fraction is in fourths, so the second fraction can be approximated as $3\frac{1}{4}$. To subtract, convert this to an improper fraction, which is $\frac{13}{4}$. Now perform the subtraction: $\frac{7}{4} - \frac{13}{4} = -\frac{6}{4}$. This matches answer (B). (The exact answer is $-\frac{23}{16}$, which is closer to (B) than to any other answer.)

2. **D** This question has complicated algebraic expressions in the answer choices, so let's Plug In. Let's say that the car costs 100 dollars, she pays 10 dollars immediately, and the rest in 3 equal subsequent payments, so $d = 100$, $p = 10$, and $x = 3$. In that case, after the immediate payment, she still owes 90 dollars, so the three payments would be 30 dollars each. Be careful with the question, though! It asks how much greater the cost of the car is (and it was 100 dollars) than each of the subsequent payments (and they are each 30 dollars), so the answer that we're looking for is 70. With the numbers we chose, (A) gives about 103, not 70. (B) gives about 97, not 70. Choice (C) gives about 93, not 70. Choice (D) gives 70, so keep it. (E) gives 130, not 70. Thus, the answer is (D).

3. **E** Just plug in the given value. The expression becomes (–5)2 – 3(–5) + 5, which becomes 25 + 15 + 5, which is 45. Thus, the answer is (E).

4. **C** It would be possible to set up some algebraic expressions to answer this, but let's just Plug In The Answers instead. Start with (C), in the middle. If Jessica is 15 now, then Kevin is twice as old, which is 30. Ten years ago, she would have been 5 and he would have been 20. The question says that he was four times as old as she was, and 20 is four times as old as 5, so this works. Choice (C) is the answer.

5. **B** First, since the answer choices are factors of ten apart (that is, (B) is (A) divided by ten, and (C) is (B) divided by ten, and so on), the solution to this question does not have to be very precise. Approximate instead. This means that we really need to calculate $\sqrt{1000 \times 0.001 \times 0.0001}$. Since $1000 \times 0.001 = 1$, this becomes $\sqrt{0.0001}$. This is equal to 0.01; just use the calculator's square root button. Either way, the answer is (B).

6. **A** Algebraic expressions in the answer choices means Plug In. Let's say that $x = 2$. In that case, $y = 3 + \frac{4}{2}$, which simplifies to 3 + 2, or 5. Thus, the question is asking for the value of x, and we know that $y = 5$. Given this, (A) is $\frac{4}{5-3}$, which is 2. Choice (B) is $-\frac{20}{3}$, not 2.

Choice (C) is $\frac{7}{5}$, not 2. Choice (D) is $\frac{3}{4-5}$, which is –3, not 2. Choice (E) is $3+\frac{4}{5}$, not 2.

Thus, the answer is (A).

7. E Algebra in the answers? Plug In! Let $x = 2$ and $y = 3$. In that case, Choice (A) is 5, which is not even. Choice (B) is 6, which is even. Choice (C) is 7, which is not even. Choice (D) is 10, which is even. Choice (E) is 62, which is even. At this point, (A) and (C) are eliminated, because they weren't even, but (B), (D), and (E) are all still possible. Let's try different numbers. Since the question asks about even and odd numbers, try a different pairing (not even with odd, as with 2 and 3). In that case, let $x = 1$ and $y = 3$. (B) gives 3, which is not even, and (D) gives 7, which is not even, so they are both eliminated. (E) gives 56, which is still even, so (E) is the answer.

8. E Just Plug In The Answers. Since it asks for the greatest number, start with the greatest number, namely 10. In the inequality, this would become $|2 - 3(10)| > 7$. This simplifies to $|-28| > 7$, which becomes $28 > 7$, which is certainly true. So 10 works, and (E) is the answer.

9. D Given crazy variables, let's Plug In. Let $x = 6$, $y = 7$, and $z = 8$, so that their average is indeed 7. In that case, add them up and divide by 4. The sum of 3, 6, 7, and 8 is 24, and 24 divided by 4 is 6. Thus, the answer is (D).

Arithmetic

10. C Round each answer choice to three digits and see how much it changes. Choice (A) becomes 97.6, which is 0.04 larger. Choice (B) becomes 123, which is 0.178 smaller. Choice (C) becomes 166, which is 0.49 larger. Choice (D) becomes 679, which is 0.1176 larger. Choice (E) becomes 1000, which is 0.001 smaller. Thus, (C) is the answer, since it has the greatest difference.

11. A Change all to decimals (with a calculator if necessary: for example, divide 4 by 11 to find that the value we want is approximately 0.364). Choice (A) is between 0.333 and 0.375. The value in question is between those two, so you do not have to check the rest. However, for the sake of clarity, (B) is between 0.25 and 0.35, (C) is between 0.231 and 0.278, (D) is between 0.222 and 0.3, and (E) is between 0.2 and 0.36, with all answers rounded to three digits where applicable. Choice (E) is the only one that is close, but its upper limit is 0.360, and the number in question is slightly larger than that.

12. D With the calculator, you can find that 6333 times 35 is 221655, and by moving the decimal point right four times, you can find that 1.2 times 104 is 12000. Now just add and subtract from right to left, and you will get 233198. This is approximately equal to (D).

13. D Divide each portion individually (that is, evaluate this as $\frac{9}{12} \times \frac{x}{x^4} \times \frac{y^3}{y^2}$). Then 9 divided by 12 reduces to $\frac{3}{4}$, so eliminate (A) and (B). Next, x divided by x^4 is x^{-3}. (The exponent

rule to subtract the exponents when dividing is one way to see this: $\dfrac{x^1}{x^4} = x^{1-4} = x^{-3}$.)

Finally, y^3 divided by y^2 is just y, so (D) is the answer.

14. **B** It may be easier to see what the question is asking if you rephrase the log as an exponent. This means that $6 = x^{2.585}$. That is, 6 is something that is a little more than squared. Now, plug in the answers. Consider what happens when 2.5 is squared, namely that $2.5^2 = 6.25$. This is already greater than 6, so $2.5^{2.585}$ would be even greater. Go smaller. Since 2^2 is 4, $2^{2.585}$ should be somewhat greater than 4, which could be 6. To verify that this is the only possibility, try 1.5. Since $1.5^2 = 2.25$, and since $1.5^3 = 3.375$ (which you can verify on the calculator by doing $1.5 \times 1.5 \times 1.5$), $1.5^{2.585}$ should be between 2.25 and 3.375, which means that it can't equal 6. Only 2 is in the right area.

15. **A** One way to do this is to multiply each answer choice by itself four times. Start towards the middle with 10.6, and 10.6^4 can be calculated as $10.6 \times 10.6 \times 10.6 \times 10.6 \approx 12624$, which is nearly ten times as large as the desired value. Go smaller, and $5.9^4 \approx 1211$, so (A) is the right answer. (The value is not exactly 1200 because the answer choice has been rounded off. A more precise answer would be 5.886, but this rounds to 5.9.) Another way to do this is to calculate the square root of the square root of 1200, since $\sqrt{\sqrt{1200}} = \left(1200^{\frac{1}{2}}\right)^{\frac{1}{2}} = 1200^{\frac{1}{4}}$. Appeal to the on-screen calculator, and you get (A).

16. **C** Do some cross-canceling before you do anything else. Remove the parentheses, and the expression becomes $\dfrac{4 \times 10^5 \times 6 \times 10^3}{3 \times 10^2 \times 5 \times 10^4}$. Rearrange this to $\dfrac{6 \times 4 \times 10^5 \times 10^3}{3 \times 5 \times 10^2 \times 10^4}$, and divide the 6 by the 3 to get that the coefficients (not the powers of 10) are $\dfrac{2 \times 4}{5}$. This is 8 divided by 5, or 1.6. Next, add the exponents on the 10's (since multiplying with the same base means add the exponents) in the numerator and denominator to get $\dfrac{10^8}{10^6}$. Now, dividing with the same base means subtracting the exponents, so you get 10^2 for the power of 10. Thus, the answer is (C).

Algebra

17. **A** Just solve. Subtract 3 from both sides of the equation to get $\sqrt[3]{3x + 9} = -3$. Cube both sides, and get $3x + 9 = -27$. Subtract 9 from both sides, which yields $3x = -36$. Then divide by 3, and $x = -12$. Note that after subtracting 3 from both sides, we are left with a cube-root on the left-hand side and a negative number on the right-hand side. This guarantees that x must also be a negative number, which allows us to eliminate (B), (C), (D), and (E), leaving only (A), which must be correct.

18. **B** For the graphs to intersect, the values of x and y have to be the same in both equations. Either plug in the answers or plug one equation into the other. PITA would go as follows, starting with (C): If $x = -1$, then from the first equation, $-y = -6$, so $y = 6$. Then, from the second equation, $y = -(-2) - 1$, which becomes $2 - 1 = 1$. Since y would equal different things given $x = -1$ (either 6 or 1), the graphs do not intersect here. Making x more negative (as in –2) would decrease y in the first equation and increase it in the second, which would bring the values closer together, so go to (B) next. If $x = -2$, then $(-2)y = -6$ implies that $y = 3$, and $y = -2(-2) - 1$ implies that $y = 4 - 1 = 3$. These y-values are equal, so (B) is the answer, since the x-value is –2. Alternatively, the somewhat messy algebraic solution is to take the second equation, which already has y isolated, and plug that into the first equation, so that $(-2x - 1)x = -6$. Now expand the left-hand side to get $-2x^2 - x = -6$. Add 6 to both sides to get $-2x^2 - x + 6 = 0$. Factor this quadratic to find $(-2x + 3)(x + 2) = 0$. The two possible solutions of this are $x = 1.5$ and $x = -2$. Since 1.5 isn't an answer choice, the answer must be (B).

19. **C** Either plug in a few values of x or solve. Of the answers, (A), (B), and (E) allow x to equal 2, so try $x = 2$. Since $|2 + 6| = 8$, and since 8 is not less than 7, x can't equal 2, so (A), (B), and (E) are eliminated. Of (C) and (D), (C) allows x to equal –2 but (D) doesn't, so try $x = -2$. This results in $|-2 + 6| = 4$, which is less than 7, so eliminate (D), and (C) is the answer. Alternatively, if $|x + 6| < 7$, then $x + 6 < 7$ and $x + 6 > -7$. If $x + 6 < 7$, then $x < 1$, and if $x + 6 > -7$, then $x > -13$. Thus, $x < 1$ and $x > -13$, so $-13 < x < 1$, as in (C).

20. **E** Plugging In is the best bet here. If $z = 3$, then $y = 1 + 1 = 2$, so $x = 2 + 0.5 = 2.5$ Then the right answer should yield 2.5 when $z = 3$. Choice (A) gives 5, (B) gives 6, (C) gives 4, (D) gives 1.5, and (E) gives 2.5, so (E) must be the right answer.

21. C To evaluate $4\left(\dfrac{25}{81}\right)^{\frac{3}{2}}$, remember that the denominator of the exponent is a root, so the expression becomes $4\left(\sqrt{\dfrac{25}{81}}\right)^{3}$. The square root applies to the numerator and denominator, so this becomes $4\left(\dfrac{5}{9}\right)^{3}$. Now cube numerator and denominator to get $4\left(\dfrac{125}{729}\right)$. Finally, multiply the numerator by 4, and you get (C).

22. E Plug In! Let's say that $a = -3$ and $b = 2$. In that case, (A) is -1, (B) is -5, (C) is 1, (D) is -1, and (E) is 5. Only (C) and (E) are positive, so the others are eliminated. To eliminate (C), plug in $a = -2$ and $b = 3$, in which case (C) is -1.

Word Problems

23. D This is a money problem (and not of the mo money mo problems variety). You could plug in the answers or set up equations. PITA would go as follows: If he has 9 quarters, as in (C), then he has 6 dimes (since he has three more quarters than dimes). This adds up to $2.85, so this is too small. Try (D) next. If he has 10 quarters, he has 7 dimes, which is $3.20. Thus, (D) is the answer. Alternatively, if d is the number of dimes and q the number of quarters, then $10d + 25q = 320$ from the fact that he has $3.20, and $d + 3 = q$ from the fact that he has three more quarters. Multiply the second equation by 10 to get that $10d + 30 = 10q$, and bring it into the same format as the first equation by subtracting 30 and subtracting $10q$ from both sides to get $10d - 10q = -30$. Then subtract the second equation from the first to get $35q = 350$. Divide both sides by 35 to get $q = 10$. As a third option, you could note that the three extra quarters he has amount to $0.75, so without them, he would have $3.20 - $0.75 = $2.45 from an equal number of quarters and dimes. For each quarter-and-dime pair, he has $0.35, and $2.45 divided by $0.35 is 7. Thus, he has 7 pairs of quarters and dimes, plus 3 more quarters, which comes out to 10 quarters.

24. A This is a weighted average problem. Fifteen days of 6 inches of rain is 90 inches altogether. Five days of 14 inches of rain is 70 inches of rain altogether. Thus, in the two years, there were 160 inches of rain, in a total of 20 rainy days. Thus, the average is 160 divided by 20, which is 8, or (A). (Following the weighted average equation, think $\dfrac{(6)(15) + (14)(5)}{15 + 5} = 8$.)

25. B This is a group problem. From the group equation, $500 = 150 + 300 - B + 100$, where B represents the number of people wearing both red shirts and gold hats. This equation simplifies to $500 = 550 - B$, so the answer is 50, which is (B).

26. **D** This is a translation problem. Since the sum of x and y is $x + y$, two times that would be $2(x + y)$. Four less than z is $z - 4$ (not $4 - z$; Consider that "4 less than 5" would be $5 - 4 = 1$, not $4 - 5 = -1$). Thus, (D) represents the correct equation.

27. **B** This is a weighted average problem. One approach uses estimation and POE. While (A), (B), (C), and (D) add up to 10 grams of chocolate total, (E) adds up to 11, so it is impossible. Bar A has 4 grams of cacao out of a total of 12 grams, so it is approximately 33% cacao. Bar B has 5 grams of cacao out of a total of 20 grams, so it is approximately 25% cacao. The goal is 30% cacao, which is slightly closer to 33% than to 25%, so we want more of Bar A than of Bar B. This eliminates (C) and (D), and since it is only slightly closer to 33% than to 25%, the extreme imbalance of (A) looks unlikely. Thus, the answer must be (B). Alternatively, Plug In The Answers with the weighted average formula. With (C), the formula would yield a percentage in the final bar of $\dfrac{(33\frac{1}{3})(5) + (25)(5)}{10}$, which is approximately 29.1% cacao. This is slightly too little, so we need more of the higher percentage. Try (B) next, which gives $\dfrac{(33\frac{1}{3})(6) + (25)(4)}{10}$, which in turn reduces to 30%. This is the right percentage, so (B) is the answer. As a third option, if x represents the number of grams of Bar A, then the number of grams of Bar B is $10 - x$, and the weighted average equation could then be set up as $\dfrac{(33\frac{1}{3})(x) + (25)(10 - x)}{10} = 30$, which could be solved for x, but this is probably clunky.

28. **C** This is an age problem. Either PITA or set up algebraic equations. In the former, if Grace is 10, then Grace's mother is 40. Seven years ago, Grace would have been 3 and Grace's mother would have been 33, which fits the description in the second sentence, namely that the mother is eleven times as old as Grace. Thus, (C) is the answer. Alternatively, if g is Grace's age and m is Grace's mother's age, the first sentence says that $m = 4g$ and the second that $m - 7 = 11(g - 7)$. Plug the second equation into the first to get that $4g - 7 = 11(g - 7)$. Distribute the right, and $4g - 7 = 11g - 77$. Add 77 to both sides and subtract $4g$, and $7g = 70$. Divide both sides by 7, and $g = 10$. Thus, (C) is the answer again.

29. **B** This is a ratio problem. A 5:7 ratio means that in each group of 12, there are 5 green cars and 7 blue cars. In 84 cars, there are 7 such groups of 12. Thus, there are 35 green cars and 49 blue cars, making the answer (B).

Thus, there are 35 green cars and 49 blue cars, making the answer (B). This becomes a little bit more obvious when we organize the information in the ratio box. (A ratio box is used to organize data and solve the problem. Using the information provided to you, you can guess what the unknown quantities are based on proportions.) Let's look at this one below.

Green Cars	Blue Cars	Total Cars	
5	7		Ratio
			Multiplier
		84	Actual

Recall that we add the numbers in the "ratio" row to find the total parts involved in the ratio: 5 + 7 = 12. Next, connect the total ratio of 12 to the actual number of cars, 84, with a multiplier of 7. That same multiplier applies to each of the green and blue cars. Therefore, there must be 5 ×7 = 35 green cars, which is enough for us to choose (B). The completely filled out table is shown below.

Green Cars	Blue Cars	Total Cars	
5	7	12	Ratio
7	7	7	Multiplier
35	49	84	Actual

Alternatively, Plug In The Answers. If there were 42 green cars out of 84 cars total, there would be 42 blue cars, which is a 1:1 ratio, not a 5:7 ratio. There need to be fewer green cars, so try (D) next. If there are 35 green cars out of 84 total, there are 49 blue cars. The ratio 35:49 reduces to 5:7 (if you divide both by 7), so this is the desired number.

30. **A** This is a weighted average problem. Either PITA or set up the weighted average equation. In PITA, if the loan at the 4% interest rate is $4,000, then the payment for this loan is $160. The remaining money is $4,000, and it would be in the 6% interest rate, which gives a payment of $240. The total payment would then be $400, which is too small. Put more in the greater interest rate, so try (B) next. $3,000 at an interest rate of 4% is a payment of $120, and the remainder of $5,000 at an interest rate of 6% is a payment of $300, totaling $420. This is still too small but getting closer, so presumably (A) is the right answer. If you have copious amounts of extra time in the test when you get to this problem, you could check it. $2,000 at an interest rate of 4% is a payment of $80, and the remainder of $6,000 at an interest rate of 6% is a payment of $360, totaling $440, as desired.

Advanced Arithmetic

31. **C** Notice that there are about 4 days (and 4 hours) between the two times. First, calculate the number of seconds in 4 days, and then you can worry about the details. The number of seconds in 4 days is given by $4 \text{ days} \times \dfrac{24 \text{ hours}}{1 \text{ day}} \times \dfrac{60 \text{ minutes}}{1 \text{ hour}} \times \dfrac{60 \text{ seconds}}{1 \text{ minute}}$, and (appeal to the calculator) $4 \times 24 \times 60 \times 60 = 345600$. Thus, we need an answer that is about 4 hours greater than 345,600 seconds. Add the 4 hours by calculating $4 \text{ hours} \times \dfrac{60 \text{ minutes}}{1 \text{ hour}} \times \dfrac{60 \text{ seconds}}{1 \text{ minute}}$, which is 14,400 seconds. The total is 360,000 seconds. The only answer that is even close is (C).

32. **D** Either at least one of them has the trait (possibly more than one), or no one has the trait. It is easier to calculate the probability that no one has the trait, so calculate that first. The probability that the first person selected doesn't have the trait is $\dfrac{3}{4}$, and the probability remains the same for the second and third people, so the probability of never selecting someone with the trait is $\dfrac{3}{4} \times \dfrac{3}{4} \times \dfrac{3}{4} = \dfrac{27}{64}$. Since the total probability of all outcomes must be 1 $\left(\text{or } \dfrac{64}{64} \right)$, the probability of not getting someone with the trait plus the probability of getting someone with the trait at least once must sum to 1, as in $\dfrac{27}{64} + x = \dfrac{64}{64}$, where x is the probability of selecting at least one person with the trait. Thus, the probability in question is $\dfrac{64}{64} - \dfrac{27}{64} = \dfrac{37}{64}$, which matches (D).

33. **B** Just plug into the given equation. The temperature in Celsius should be given by $C = \dfrac{5}{9}(50 - 32)$. Appeal to the calculator, and you get (B).

34. **C** Watch your powers of 10. The first has 8,000 micrograms, which in grams is $8000 \times 10^{-6} = 0.008$. The second is still 0.47 in grams, and the third is $55 \times 10^{-3} = 0.055$. Add these decimals together, and you get 0.533 grams, as in (C).

35. **B** Since there are 6 blueberry jellybeans out of 20 total jellybeans, the probability of drawing out a blueberry is $\dfrac{6}{20}$. If one is successfully drawn out, there are 5 raspberry jellybeans out of 19 total jellybeans (since one blueberry was drawn out already). Thus, the probability of a raspberry is $\dfrac{5}{19}$. The probability of doing these two things consecutively is $\dfrac{6}{20} \times \dfrac{5}{19}$, which reduces to (B).

36. **D** Imagine that the model is a 1 inch by 1 inch by 1 inch cube. In that case, the real house would be a 70 inch by 70 inch by 70 inch cube. (Not much of a dwelling, admittedly, unless you're tiny, but this is just for mathematical simplicity.) In this case, the volume of the model is 1 cubic inch, and the volume of the real house is 70^3 cubic inches, which is 343,000 cubic inches. This is closest to (D).

37. **C** This is a group problem in disguise as a probability problem. The group equation says that total = group 1 + group 2 − both + neither. In this case, group 1 is the ice cream group, 0.6, and group 2 is the cookie group, 0.55. The neither group is expressed as a percent, but convert that to a decimal to get that it is 0.1. Now, to find the "both" category, we need the total. Well, the total probability must be 1 for any probability of any kind. Thus, the group formula in this case reads 1 = 0.6 + 0.55 − both + 0.1, or in reduced form, 1 = 1.25 − both. Thus, the "both" group must be 0.25.

Plane Geometry

38. **E** Since line segment $\overline{BE}$ is parallel to line segment $\overline{CD}$, triangle ABE and triangle ACD are similar (they contain all equal angles). This means that their sides are proportional, so that if the sides of ACD are in the numerators and ABE in the denominators, $\dfrac{10}{8} = \dfrac{x}{10}$, where x is the side we want. Multiply both sides by 10, and $x = \dfrac{100}{8} = 12.5$. Thus, (E) is the answer.

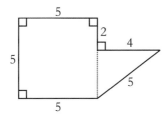

39. **B** If you add an extra line as shown, you see two familiar shapes in this one unfamiliar one. The left shape is a square. A 5 by 5 square has an area of 25. The right shape is a right triangle. Since one side is 4 and the hypotenuse is 5, you can recognize a 3-4-5 right triangle (or, alternatively, solve for the third side by determining the square root of $5^2 - 4^2$). Thus, with a base of 3 and a height of 4, the triangle has an area of 6. The total area is therefore 31, as in (B).

40. **D** Recall that the sum of the interior angles of a polygon is given by $(n - 2)180°$, where n is the number of sides of the polygon, so the sum of the angles in a hexagon (with 6 sides) must be 720°. Alternatively, remember that the pattern of adding 180° to get from a triangle (180°) to a quadrilateral (360°) continues to a pentagon (540°) and so forth. Either way, the total of the interior angles is 720°. Since the interior angles are $x + x + x + x + 100 + 160$, this means that $4x + 260 = 720$. Thus, $x = 115$, as in (D).

41. **A** With such nice integer numbers, it's probably not terribly labor intensive to guess and check to determine that the sides must be 15 and 20. However, if this doesn't immediately strike you, you can also say that $(x + 5)(x) = 300$, where x is the width. Thence $x^2 + 5x - 300 = 0$, which factors to $(x + 20)(x - 15) = 0$. Since $x = -20$ is a nonsensical solution (what would a width of -20 mean?), the width must be 15, which makes the length 20. Then the perimeter is $20 + 15 + 20 + 15 = 70$, as in (A).

42. **D** You can probably estimate from the picture that it's going to be pretty big, either choice (D) or (E). To find the exact value, start on the right with a 1 by 1 square. Then the third square is 2 by 2, the second is 4 by 4, and the first is 8 by 8. That means that the area of the first square is 64 and the fourth is 1, so it's a 64:1 ratio, as in (D).

43. **B** If it's a right triangle, the Pythagorean Theorem applies, so the unknown height is given by the square root of $10^2 - 5^2$. This is approximately 8.66. A base of 5 with a height of 8.66 yields an area of $A = \dfrac{1}{2}bh = \dfrac{1}{2}(5)(8.66) = 21.65$. This is equal to (B).

44. **E** Notice the two special right triangles, the 45-45-90 and the 30-60-90. These have sides in ratios of $x : x : x\sqrt{2}$ and $x : x\sqrt{3} : 2x$, respectively. The distance between C and D is one of the x sides of the 45-45-90, and the distance between B and D is the $x\sqrt{3}$ side of the 30-60-90. (This side marked x is, appropriately, the x side of the 30-60-90 and one of the **x** sides of the 45-45-90.) Since the length of $\overline{BC}$ is the difference between the lengths of $\overline{BD}$ and $\overline{CD}$, and since it was given as 0.7, this comes together as $0.7 = \sqrt{3}x - x$. Since $\sqrt{3} \approx 1.7$, this reduces to $0.7 \approx 1.7x - x$, or $0.7 \approx 0.7x$. Thus, x is approximately equal to 1, as in (E).

Solid and Coordinate Geometry

45. **A** Since the points are consecutively lettered (B comes right after A), we know that the length of a side of the square is the distance between $(1, 1)$ and $(2, 5)$. The difference in x is 1 and in y is 4, so, from the Pythagorean theorem, the side of the square s should be given by $s^2 = 1^2 + 4^2$, or $s^2 = 17$. Since s^2 is also the area of a square with side length s, the area is 17, which is (A).

46. **D** On the left is a trapezoid with bases of lengths from $(-1, 1)$ to $(6, 1)$ and from $(1, 3)$ to $(6, 3)$, which have lengths of 5 and 7, respectively, and height from $(6, 1)$ to $(6, 3)$, which is a length of 2. Its area could be calculated directly from $A_{\text{trapezoid}} = \left(\dfrac{b_1 + b_2}{2}\right)(h)$, which in

this case yields $A = \left(\dfrac{5+7}{2}\right)(2) = 12$. Alternatively, the area of the trapezoid could be figured from breaking it up into a triangle with base 2 and height 2 and a rectangle of base 5 and height 2. Either way, the shaded region on the right has an area of 12. The triangle on the right is a little stranger. The distance from (–3, 0) to (–3, 4) is 4 units, which should be interpreted as the base. Then the height is the distance between this line at an x of –3 and the point at (–1, 1), which is 2 away. Thus, a base of 4 and height of 2 gives an area of 4. Add this to the previously found area, and you get (D).

47. **B**   The label needs to wrap around the circumference of the cylinder, which from $C = 2\pi r$ is 12π, and stretch along its height, which is 8. That is, if the label were torn off the bottle and laid flat, its length would be the circumference of the cylinder and its width would be the height of the cylinder. Thus, the area of the label is $12\pi \times 8 = 96\pi$, as in (B). (Alternatively, just calculate the surface area of the cylinder, but leave off the top and bottom, so the lateral surface area is just $2\pi rh$).

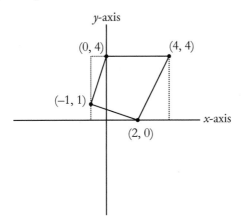

48. **D**   There is no formula for the area of a general quadrilateral, so you have to find some way to add or subtract standard shapes in order to find the area of this quadrilateral. For example, in this case, you could draw a 5 by 4 rectangle around this quadrilateral and then subtract three triangles to get the area of the quadrilateral, as shown above. The area of the rectangle is 20. The triangle in the upper-left has a base of 3 and height of 1, so its area is 1.5. The same is true of the triangle in the lower-left. In the lower-right, the triangle has a base of 2 and a height of 4, for an area of 4. Thus, subtract a total of 1.5 + 1.5 + 4 = 7 from the rectangle. The area of the shaded region is 20 – 7 = 13, as in (D).

49. **C**   If the cube has a volume of 64, then its edges are 4 by 4 by 4 (since $4 = \sqrt[3]{64}$). Divide the edge length by 2, and you get a 2 by 2 by 2 cube, which has a volume of 8, as in (C).

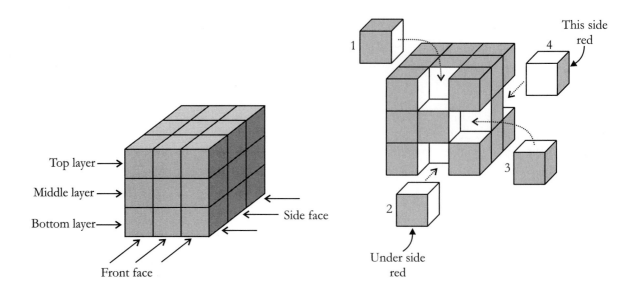

Top layer →
Middle layer →
Bottom layer →
← Side face
↗ ↗ ↗
Front face

1
4
This side
red

2
Under side
red

3

50.　E　Flex those Perceptual Ability muscles! There will be a top layer, a middle layer, and a bottom layer. In the top layer, the middle cubes on the front face, the two side faces, and the back face will have 2 faces painted (for a total of 4 cubes). In the middle layer, the cubes bordering between the front face and each of the side faces, as well as the cubes bordering between the back face and each of the side faces will have 2 faces painted (for a total of 4 more cubes). The bottom layer will be just like the top layer (for a total of 4 more cubes). That's 12 cubes altogether.

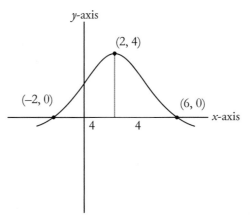

y-axis

(2, 4)

(−2, 0)

(6, 0)

x-axis

4　　4

51.　A　Bear in mind that parabolas (or parabolae, in the Latin) are symmetrical, so the picture must be as shown above. Since the root (6, 0) is located 4 to the right of the vertex, the other root must be 4 to the left of it, which is at (−2, 0).

Trigonometry

52.   **B**   Since this triangle is a 5-12-13 right triangle, the missing side length is 12. (You could calculate this from the Pythagorean Theorem if necessary.) Since cosine is adjacent divided by hypotenuse, we want the angle for which 12 is the adjacent side and 13 is the hypotenuse. This angle is 23°. That is, $\cos(23°) = \dfrac{12}{13}$ from the definition of cosine and the picture, so $23° = \arccos\left(\dfrac{12}{13}\right)$.

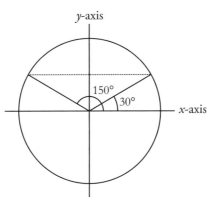

53.   **A**   If $\csc\theta = 2$, then $\dfrac{1}{\sin\theta} = 2$, which means that $\sin\theta = \dfrac{1}{2}$. The usual angle for which this is true is 30°, or $\dfrac{\pi}{6}$. However, this question wants the angle to be greater. From the unit circle shown above, the angle with the same y-value or height (and hence the same value of sine) in the requested range is 150°, or $\dfrac{5\pi}{6}$. Cosine of this angle should be negative, since the x-value is negative, but it should have the same magnitude as $\cos(30°)$. Hence, the answer is (A), the same magnitude as $\cos(30°)$, but negative.

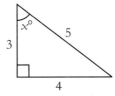

54.   **D**   First, notice that $0 < x < 90°$, which means that x is in the first quadrant. This means that $\tan(x)$ must be positive (eliminate answer choices (A) and (B)). Since cosine is adjacent over hypotenuse, the 3 over 5 can be interpreted as specifying a right triangle with an adjacent side of 3 and a hypotenuse of 5, as shown above. The third side, from the Pythagorean

Theorem, is 4. Since tangent is opposite over adjacent, and since the opposite is 4 and the adjacent is 3, the answer is (D).

55.   **A**   Remember that the area of any triangle can be found from two sides and the angle between them via $A = \dfrac{1}{2}ab\sin\theta$. Hence, in this case, the area of the triangle is given by $A = \dfrac{1}{2}(160)(400)\sin 30°$. Since $\sin 30° = \dfrac{1}{2}$, this becomes $A = \dfrac{1}{2}(160)(400)\dfrac{1}{2}$. Do the arithmetic, and you get 16000, as in (A).

56.   **E**   Looks like a question testing a strange identity, but don't worry. Just Plug In! Let's say that $\theta = 30°$. In that case, $\cos\theta = \dfrac{\sqrt{3}}{2}$. (A) is $\cos(150°) = -\dfrac{\sqrt{3}}{2}$, (B) is $\cos(120°) = -\dfrac{1}{2}$, (C) is $\cos(75°)$ and obscure anyway but clearly not right (as it happens, it's approximately 0.259, but we want approximately 0.866), (D) is $\sin(210°) = -\dfrac{1}{2}$, and (E) is $\sin(60°) = \dfrac{\sqrt{3}}{2}$. Thus, (E) is the only one that works anyway, so (E) is the answer. (By the way, this identity is part of the reason that the exact values of sine and cosine count in opposite directions. That is, $\sin(0°) = \cos(90°)$, $\sin(30°) = \cos(60°)$, etc.)

57.   **E**   Convert this back to degrees, and you get that it's asking about $\sin(135°)$. From the unit circle, this should be at the same height (as in y-value or value of sine) as 45°. Thus, $\sin(135°) = \sin(45°)$, and we know that $\sin(45°) = \dfrac{\sqrt{2}}{2}$. The answer is (E).

NOTES

NOTES

NOTES

NOTES

NOTES

NOTES

NOTES

	Structure	Function
Proteins	Polymers of amino acids (20) 4 levels of structure	Enzymes, hormones, receptors, transporters, antibodies, etc.
Carbohydrates	Polymers of mono-saccharides such as glucose, fructose, galactose	Energy Oxidized in cell respiration Stored in glycogen or starch
Lipids	Hydrophobic Glycerol + fatty acids Steroid/cholesterol derivatives	Phospholipids in membranes Triglycerides store energy Steroid hormones
Nucleic Acids (DNA and RNA)	Polymers of nucleotides $A = T$ and $C \equiv G$	Hereditary/genetic material

GLUCOSE CATABOLISM

Cellular Process	Location	O_2 condition	Major substrates	Net products
Glycolysis	Cytosol	Both	Glucose	2 Pyruvate, 2 ATP, 2 NADH
Fermentation	Cytosol	Anaerobic	Pyruvate, NADH	Lactic acid or Ethanol, NAD^+
Pyruvate decarboxylation	Mitochon-drial matrix	Aerobic	Pyruvate	2 Acetyl-CoA, 2 NADH
Citric acid (Krebs) cycle	Mitochon-drial matrix	Aerobic	Acetyl-CoA	6 NADH, 2 $FADH_2$, 2 GTP
Electron transport chain	Inner mitochondrial membrane	Aerobic	NADH, $FADH_2$, O_2	NAD^+, FAD, H_2O
Oxidative phosphorylation	Inner mitochondrial membrane	Aerobic	ADP, P_i (H^+ gradient)	Euk: 30 ATP Prok: 32 ATP

THE CELL

The plasma membrane: selective permeability barrier consisting of phospholipid bilayer, proteins, and cholesterol.

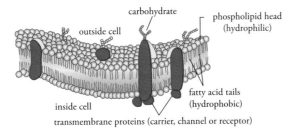

outside cell — carbohydrate — phospholipid head (hydrophilic) — inside cell — fatty acid tails (hydrophobic) — transmembrane proteins (carrier, channel or receptor)

ORGANELLES

- **Ribosome:** protein synthesis via translation
- **Nucleus:** houses the genome
- **Mitochondria:** cell respiration and energy production
- **Rough ER and Golgi:** protein trafficking and modification
- **Lysosome:** autophagy and degradation
- **Peroxisome:** degradation and detoxification
- **Smooth ER:** lipid synthesis

TRANSMEMBRANE TRANSPORT

- **Simple diffusion:** hydrophobic molecules diffuse across the membrane, down their gradient
- **Facilitated diffusion:** hydrophilic molecules through a channel across the membrane, down their gradient
- **Active transport:** energy is used to move molecules across the membrane, against their gradient

PHOTOSYNTHESIS

- Light energy is converted into chemical energy (ATP/ NADPH), which is then used to produce sugars.
- Occurs in chloroplasts.

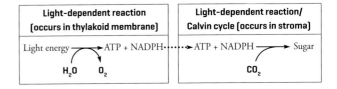

Light-dependent reaction (occurs in thylakoid membrane)	Light-dependent reaction/ Calvin cycle (occurs in stroma)
Light energy → ATP + NADPH H_2O O_2	ATP + NADPH → Sugar CO_2

MOLECULAR GENETICS

NUCLEIC ACID

- **Basic unit:** nucleotide (five-carbon sugar, nitrogenous base, phosphate group(s)).
- Sugar in DNA is deoxyribose; sugar in RNA is ribose.
- 2 types of bases: double-ringed purines (adenine, guanine) and single-ringed pyrimidines (cytosine, thymine, uracil).
- DNA double helix; antiparallel strands joined by hydrogen bonding between base pairs ($A = T$, $G \equiv C$).
- RNA is usually single-stranded: A pairs with U, not T.

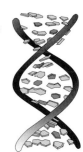

MUTATIONS

Point: One nucleotide is substituted for another. Includes missense, nonsense, and silent mutations.

Missense: One amino acid substituted for another.

Nonsense: Introduces a premature stop codon in the sequence (truncated protein).

Silent: No change in amino acid sequence.

Frameshift: Insertions or deletions of nucleotides not in multiples of three shift the reading frame; the protein can be nonfunctional, of a different length, or not produced.

DNA Replication

- **Semiconserva-tive replication:** parent strand + newly synthesized strand.

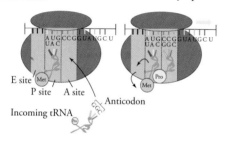

- Key enzymes are helicase (unwinds the DNA), primase (lays down RNA primer), and DNA polymerases (sythesize DNA).

EUKARYOTIC PROTEIN SYNTHESIS

- **Transcription:** RNA polymerase synthesizes hnRNA using DNA, "antisense strand" as a template.
- **Post-transcriptional processing:** Splicing of introns and addition of 5' cap and 3' polyA tail (hnRNA → mRNA); mRNA is then exported out of the nucleus.
- **Translation** occurs on ribosomes in the cytoplasm.

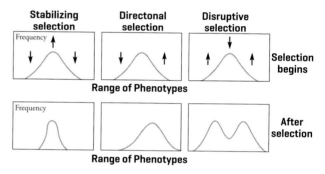

Post-translational modifications: (i.e., disulfide bonds) made before the polypeptide becomes a functional protein.

PROKARYOTIC PROTEIN SYTHESIS

- Occurs simultaneously with transcription because no mRNA processing is required.
- Ribosome is slightly smaller than eukaryotic ribosome.
- mRNA can be polycistronic (code for several different proteins).

CLASSICAL GENETICS

- **Genotype:** the combination of alleles an individual possesses
- **Phenotype:** the physical characteristics of an individual, resulting from their genotype

Law of independent assortment: Alleles of unlinked genes assort independently during meiosis.
- For $Rr \times Rr$: genotypic ratio is 1:2:1, phenotypic ratio is 3:1.
- For $AaBb \times AaBb$: gametes produced are AB, Ab, aB, and ab, and phenotypic ratio is 9:3:3:1

Statistical calculations
- probability of A **and** B = prob (A) × prob (B)
- probability of A **or** B = prob (A) + prob (B) – prob (A and B)

INHERITED DISORDERS IN PEDIGREES
- **Autosomal recessive:** skips generations
- **Autosomal dominant:** appears every generation
- **X-linked (sex-linked):** no male-to-male transmission, and more males affected; can be recessive (red/green colorblindness or hemophilia) or dominant.

POPULATION GENETICS
- **Equation for allele frequency:** $p + q = 1$
- **Equation for genotype frequency:** $p^2 + 2pq + q^2 = 1$

For a population to be in Hardy-Weinberg equilibrium it must be large, be randomly mating, and have no mutation, no natural selection, and no migration.

EVOLUTION

- **Evolution** is driven by natural selection: organisms with advantageous traits survive and reproduce while organisms with disadvantageous traits die out.
- **Fitness** refers to the ability of an organism to successfully pass on its alleles to future generations.

- **Speciation:** creation of new species.
- **Reproductive isolation** is caused by prezygotic barriers that prevent formation of a viable zygote or postzygotic barriers that prevent development, survival, or fertility of the hybrid organism.
- **Homologous structures** in two different organisms have similar functions as a result of common ancestry.
- **Analogous structures** in two different organisms have similar functions but do not share a common ancestry.

DIVERSITY OF LIFE

- **Domain Bacteria:** "true," mostly mesophilic bacteria
- **Domain Archaea:** extremophilic bacteria
- **Domain Eukarya:**
  - **Kingdom Protista:** includes organisms that are plant-like (algae), animal-like (protozoa), and fungus-like (absorptive protists).
  - **Kingdom Fungi:** saprophytes; e.g. yeast, truffles, and mushrooms
  - **Kingdom Animalia:** most diverse kingdom, includes many different phyla.
    - **Vertebrates** include fish, amphibians, reptiles, birds, and mammals.

Kindom Animalis most diverse kingdom, includes many phyla such as poriferans, cnidarians, worms, mollusks, arthropods, echinoderms and chordates

Vertebrates include fish, amphibians, reptiles, birds, and mammals.

Animal Behavior and Interaction:

- **Commensalism:** One organism benefits, the other is unaffected
- **Mutualism:** Both organisms benefit
- **Parasitism:** One organism benefits, the other is harmed
- **Innate behavior:** Preprogrammed, known from birth
- **Learned behavior:** Acquired through interaction with the environment

Viruses

- Acellular structures of double or single-stranded DNA or RNA in a protein coat
- Lytic cycle: virus kills the host
- Lysogenic cycle: virus enters host genome

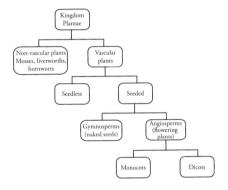

BODY CONTROL AND COMMUNICATION

NERVOUS SYSTEM

- Neurons are the basic cellular unit; they relay signals via an action potential.
- Synapse: junction between a neuron and another neuron/effector organ. Two types: electrical (uses gap junction) and chemical (uses neurotransmitters).
- **Central nervous system:** Brain and spinal cord.
- **Peripheral nervous system:** Somatic nervous system (voluntary, controls skeletal muscle) and autonomic nervous system (involuntary, controls cardiac and smooth muscle).
- **Two branches of autonomic system:** Sympathetic (fight or flight) and parasympathetic (rest and digest).

ENDOCRINE SYSTEM

- **Direct hormones** directly stimulate their effector organs.
- **Tropic hormones** stimulate release of hormones from other endocrine glands.
- Hormones released from the adrenal cortex and the gonads are steroid hormones. All other hormones are peptide hormones.
- Mechanisms of hormone action:
  - **Peptide hormones** bind to their receptor on the PM and activate second messengers like cAMP and IP_3.
  - **Steroid hormones** diffuse across the PM and bind to their receptor in the cytoplasm; the hormone/receptor complex then translocates to the nucleus and regulates transcription of genes.

CIRCULATORY SYSTEM

- Includes the heart (a muscular pump) and blood vessels
- **Heart:**
  - Made of cardiac muscle fibers
  - Has 2 atria (top) and 2 ventricles (bottom)
  - Has its own pacemaker cells (SA node), which spontaneously depolarize and trigger contraction of the heart.
- **Blood vessels:**
  - Arteries: carry blood away from the heart; have thick smooth muscle wall; high pressure vessels
  - Veins: carry blood toward the heart; contain one-way valves; low pressure vessels
  - Capillaries: site of gas, nutrient, and waste exchange
- Blood is 55% plasma (water, ions, sugars, proteins), 45% red blood cells (carry oxygen), and ~1% white blood cells (immunity) and platelets (blood clotting).
- Oxygen is carried through the blood bound to hemoglobin in RBCs
- Carbon dioxide is converted into bicarbonate and dissolves in plasma

IMMUNE SYSTEM

Acquired	B-cells [Humoral immunity]	**Plasma cells**	Make and secrete antibodies (IgG, IgA, IgM, IgD, IgE), which induce antigen phagocytosis	
		Memory cells	Remember antigens, speed up secondary response	
	T-cells [Cell-mediated immunity]	**Cytotoxic T-cells**	Destroy cells directly	
		Helper T-cells	Activate B- and T-cells, and macrophages	
		Memory cells	Remember antigens, speed up secondary response	
Innate	Includes skin, passages lined with cilia, macrophages, low pH in the stomach and vagina, inflammatory response, and interferons (proteins that help prevent the spread of a virus).			

RESPIRATORY SYSTEM

- Two major functions: gas exchange and pH regulation.
- **Conduction zone:** site of air movement (ventilation) only; consists of the nose, pharynx, larynx, trachea, bronchi, and most bronchioles
- **Respiratory zone:** site of gas exchange (respiration); consists of respiratory bronchioles, alveolar ducts, and alveoli.

DIGESTION

- **Mouth:** functions to grind food (mastication) and digest carbohydrates (via salivary amylase)
- **Esophagus:** moves food from mouth to stomach
- **Stomach:** stores food, breaks down proteins (via pepsin)
  - Gastrin stimulates secretion of acid in the stomach
- **Small intestine:** site where most digestion and absorption occurs
  - CCK stimulates bile release and secretin stimulates HCO_3^- release
  - Enterokinase activates trypsin from trypsinogen
- **Large intestine:** site of reabsorption of water and electrolytes, production of vitamin K by colonic bacteria, stores feces

Accessory digestive organs:

- **Liver:** synthesizes and secretes bile for fat emulsification
- **Gallbladder:** stores and concentrates bile
- **Pancreas:** produces digestive enzymes for breakdown of all macromolecules (amylase, trypsin and other proteases, lipase, nucleases) and secretes HCO_3^-

RENAL SYSTEM

- Functions of the kidneys include:
  - urine formation
  - BP and pH regulation
  - ion and water balance
- Basic functional unit: nephron
- Blood filtration occurs at glomerulus
- Modification of the filtrate (reabsorption and secretion) occurs along the PCT, loop of Henle, DCT, and collecting duct.
- Low BP → Posterior pituitary secretes ADH → more water reabsorption in collecting ducts
- Low BP → Kidneys release renin → activates angiotensinogen → produces angiotensin II → vasoconstriction and release of aldosterone → increased BP

MUSCULOSKELETAL SYSTEM

SARCOMERE

- Contractile unit of the fibers in a skeletal muscle cell
- Contains thin actin and thick myosin filaments

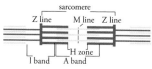

SKELETAL MUSCLE CONTRACTION

- ACh release from a neuron leads to action potential
- Ca^{2+} in the sarcoplasm increases
- Troponin/tropomyosin shift to expose myosin binding sites on actin
- Myosin and actin interact and cause muscle contraction
- Sarcomeres, H zone and I band shorten

BONE FORMATION AND REMODELING

- Regulated by PTH and calcitonin
- Osteoblasts: builds bone
- Osteoclasts: break down bone
- Osteon is the unit of compact bone

REPRODUCTION

Cell division

- G_1: cell growth, organelle and protein synthesis, metabolism
- S: DNA replication
- G_2: similar to G_1
- M: Mitosis via PMAT

SEXUAL REPRODUCTION

Meiosis I

- Replicated homologous chromosomes (each has two chromatids) pair up to form a tetrad in prophase I.
- Crossing over leads to genetic recombination in prophase I.
- Recombined homologous chromosomes are separated into haploid daughter cells.

Meiosis II

- Similar to mitosis.
- Recombined sister chromatids are separated into haploid daughter cells that have a single copy of one set of chromosomes, 23 in humans.

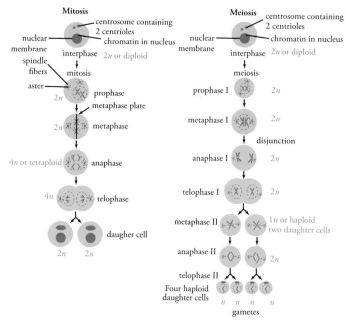

In humans

- Spermatogenesis in males (making sperm in the seminiferous tubules of the testes) and oogenesis (making ova in the ovaries) in females are examples of meiosis.

FOUR STAGES OF EARLY DEVELOPMENT

Cleavage: mitotic divisions of the zygote to form the morula

Implantation: blastocyst (trophoblast and inner cell mass) implant into the endometrial layer of uterine wall

Gastrulation: formation of primary germ layers

Neurulation: formation of the nervous system from germ cell layers.

Organogenesis: formation of all other major organs.

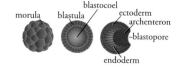

SKIN

Functions in thermoregulation by piloerection and vasoconstriction when cold, and sweating and vasodilation when warm.

GENERAL CHEMISTRY

ATOMIC STRUCTURE

Atomic weight: The weight in grams of one mole (mol) of a given element and is expressed in terms of g/mol.

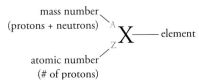

mass number
(protons + neutrons) — A
$_Z^A X$ — element
atomic number — Z
(# of protons)

A **mole** is a unit used to count particles and is represented by **Avogadro's number:** 6.022×10^{23} particles

$$\text{Moles} = \frac{\text{grams}}{\text{atomic or molecular weight}}$$

Isotopes: For a given element, multiple species of atoms with the same number of protons (same atomic number) but different numbers of neutrons (different mass numbers).

Planck's quantum theory: Energy emitted as electromagnetic radiation from matter exists in discrete bundles called quanta.

The Bohr atom: Electrons reside in discreet energy levels around the nucleus. Electrons can absorb energy and move to higher levels of energy or shed energy as photons and settle to lower energy states.

Quantum numbers:

#	Character	Symbol	Value
1st	Shell	n	n
2nd	Subshell	l	From zero to $n - 1$
3rd	Orbital	m_ℓ	Between l and $-l$
4th	Spin	m_s	$\frac{1}{2}$ or $-\frac{1}{2}$

The four subshells corresponding to $l = 0, 1, 2,$ and 3 are known as s, p, d and f, respectively.

ELECTRONIC CONFIGURATION

Electrons are filled in order, from left to right, along the periodic table. The shell in which electrons fall is dictated by their block, and their row. For s and p electrons, n = # of row, for d electrons, n = row # - 1, and for f electrons n = row # - 2.

Hund's rule: Every orbital in a subshell gets one electron (with the same spin) before any orbital gets a second electron.

Valence electrons: Electrons of an atom that are in its outer energy shell or that are available for bonding.

NUCLEAR CHEMISTRY

Unstable nuclei decay, becoming new stable nuclei through the emission of a number of different particles (α, β, γ, etc). In any nuclear chemistry reaction the total mass and total atomic number in the reactants must equal the total mass and atomic number of the products.

Summary of Radioactive Decay		
$N\downarrow Z\downarrow$	Alpha Decay	$_Z^A X \xrightarrow{\alpha} {}_{Z-2}^{A-4}Y + {}_2^4\alpha$
$N\downarrow Z\uparrow$	Beta Minus Decay	$_Z^A X \xrightarrow{\beta^-} {}_{Z+1}^{A}Y + {}_{-1}^{0}e^-$
$N\uparrow Z\downarrow$	Beta Plus Decay	$_Z^A X \xrightarrow{\beta^+} {}_{Z-1}^{A}Y + {}_{+1}^{0}e^+$
$N\uparrow Z\downarrow$	Electron Capture	$_Z^A X + {}_{+1}^{0}e^- \xrightarrow{EC} {}_{Z-1}^{A}Y$
	Gamma Decay	$_Z^A X^* \xrightarrow{\gamma} {}_Z^A X + \gamma$

N = # of neutrons; Z = atomic number/ # of protons; A = N + Z

Half life $t_{1/2}$: the amount of time it takes for a sample to decay to half its original mass.

MOLECULAR GEOMETRY AND SHAPE

Geometric Family	# Electron Pairs on Central Atom	Shape		Bond Angles
Linear	0	Linear	O—●—O	180°
Trigonal Planar	0	Trigonal Planar		120°
Trigonal Planar	1	Bent		116°
Tetrahedral	0	Tetrahedral		109.5°
Tetrahedral	1	Trigonal Pyramidal		107°
Tetrahedral	2	Bent		104.5°
Trigonal Bipyramidal	0	Trigonal Bipyramidal		90° 120° 180°
Octahedral	0	Octahedral		90° 180°

BONDING AND CHEMICAL INTERACTIONS

Formal charges

$$\text{Formal Charge} = \text{Valence electrons} - \frac{1}{2}N_{\text{bonding}} - N_{\text{nonbonding}}$$

INTERMOLECULAR FORCES

1. **Hydrogen bonding:** Between H and lone pair of electrons in N, O, F
2. **Dipole-dipole interactions:** Between δ^+ and δ^- in a polar molecule
3. **Dispersion forces:** present in all molecules; due to transient unequal sharing of electrons in a bond.

GASES

1 atm = 760 mm Hg = 760 torr
STP: 273K, 0°C, 1 atm, 1 mole of gas = 22.4L, used for gases

Standard state: 298K or 25°C, 1 atm, 1M, used in thermodynamics, equilibrium, electrochemistry

Boyle's law

$$PV = k \text{ or } P_1 V_1 = P_2 V_2$$

Law of Charles and Gay-Lussac

$$\frac{V}{T} = k \text{ or } \frac{V_1}{T_1} = \frac{V_2}{T_2}$$

Avogadro's principle

$$\frac{n}{V} = k \text{ or } \frac{n_1}{V_1} = \frac{n_2}{V_2}$$

Ideal gas law

$$PV = nRT$$

GRAHAM'S LAW OF DIFFUSION AND EFFUSION

Diffusion occurs when gas molecules diffuse through a mixture.

Effusion is the flow of gas particles under pressure from one compartment to another through a small opening. Both diffusion and effusion have the same formula.

$$\frac{r_1}{r_2} = \left(\frac{M^2}{M^1}\right)^{\frac{1}{2}}$$

SOLUTIONS

UNITS OF CONCENTRATION

Percent composition by mass: $= \dfrac{\text{Mass of solute}}{\text{Mass of solution}} \times 100 \, (\%)$

Mole fraction: $\dfrac{\text{\# of mol of compound}}{\text{total \# of moles in system}}$

Molarity: $\dfrac{\text{\# of mol of solute}}{\text{liter of solution}}$

Molality: $\dfrac{\text{\# of mol of solute}}{\text{kg of solvent}}$

PHASES AND PHASE CHANGES

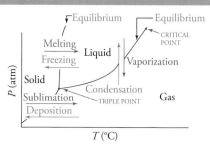

Colligative properties: These are physical properties derived solely from the number of particles present, not the nature of those particles. These properties are usually associated with dilute solutions.

Freezing point depression $\Delta T_f = K_f im$

Boiling point elevation $\Delta T_b = K_b im$

Osmotic pressure $\Pi = iMRT$

Van't Hoff factor (i): the number of particles a given substance will form in solution. For binary salts (e.g., NaCl) $i = 2$.

Vapor-pressure lowering (Raoult's law) $P_A = X_A P^o_A$; $P_B = X_B P^o_B$

Solutions that obey Raoult's law are called ideal solutions.

KINETICS

For $xA + yB \rightarrow C$, Rate $= k\,[A]^x[B]^y$

- Rate = determined experimentally; units = M/sec
- k = rate constant; unit varies
- $x + y$ = reaction order

Factors that affect reaction rates: [R] in rate limiting step, T, catalysts

Catalysts: ↑ reaction rate, ↓ E_a, not consumed

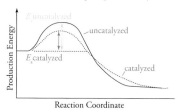

Law of mass action

$$a\,A + b\,B \rightleftharpoons c\,C + d\,D$$

$$K_c = \frac{[C]^c[D]^d}{[A]^a[B]^b}$$

K_c is the equilibrium constant. (c stands for concentration.)

Properties of the Equilibrium Constant

- K: don't include pure (s) and (l)
- K_{eq} for a specific system at a given T
- If $K_{eq} \gg 1$, then [P] $\gg$ [R]
- If $K_{eq} \ll 1$, then [P] $\ll$ [R]
- If $K_{eq} = 1$, reaction is at equilibrium, [P] = [R]

Reaction quotient (Q): Once a reaction commences, the standard state conditions no longer hold. For the reaction,

$$a\,A + b\,B \rightleftharpoons c\,C + d\,D \qquad\qquad Q = \frac{[C]^c[D]^d}{[A]^a[B]^b}$$

A + B $\rightleftharpoons$ C + heat	
Will Shift to the Right	**Will Shift to the Left**
1. if more A or B added	1. if more C added
2. if C taken away	2. if A or B taken away
3. if pressure applied or volume reduced (assuming A, B, and C are gases)	3. if pressure reduced or volume increased (assuming A, B, and C are gases)
4. if temperature reduced	4. if temperature increased

ACIDS AND BASES

	Acid	**Base**
Arrhenius	Produces H^+ in (*aq*) solution	Produces OH^- in (*aq*) solution
Bronsted-Lowry	Donates H^+	Accepts H^+
Lewis	Accepts e^-	Donates e^-

Properties of Acids and Bases

$$pH = -\log[H^+]$$
$$pH = -\log[OH^-]$$
$$H_2O(l) \rightleftharpoons H^+(aq) + OH^-(aq)$$
$$K_w = [H^+][OH^-] = 10^{-14}$$
$$pH + pOH = 14$$

Weak Acids and Bases

$$HA(aq) + H_2O(l) \rightleftharpoons H_3O^+(aq) + A^-(aq)$$
$$K_a = \frac{[H_3O^+][A^-]}{[HA]}$$
$$K_b = \frac{[B^+][OH^-]}{[BOH]}$$
$$pH = pK_a + \log\frac{[\text{conjugate base}]}{[\text{weak acid}]}$$
$$pOH = pK_b + \log\frac{[\text{conjugate acid}]}{[\text{weak base}]}$$

Neutralization:

$$\underset{\text{(acid)}}{HA} + \underset{\text{(base)}}{BOH} \longrightarrow \underset{\text{(salt)}}{BA} + \underset{\text{(water)}}{H_2O}$$

Titration and Buffers

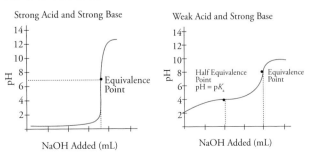

Titration is a technique used to determine concentration of an acid or a base using a solution of known concentration to neutralize it.

THERMOCHEMISTRY

Specific heat

$$Q = mc\Delta T$$

- Q is heat absorbed or released; units: joules or calories
- m = mass, c = specific heat, ΔT = change in temperature
- Can only be used when phase is not changing
- $Q > 0$ = heat is absorbed
- $Q < 0$ = heat is released

Heat of transformation: the quantity of heat required to change the **phase** of 1 kg of a substance.

$$q = n \times \Delta H_{\text{phase change}}$$
$$q = m \times \Delta H_{\text{phase change}}$$

Phase changes are isothermal processes

First law of thermodynamics: $\Delta E = q + w$

- **Enthalpy** (H): change in heat energy at constant pressure.
- **Standard heat of formation** (ΔH°_f): the change in enthalpy when one mole of a compound is formed from its elements in their standard states.
- **Standard heat of reaction** ($\Delta H^\circ_{\text{rxn}}$) = (sum of $\Delta H^\circ_{\text{rxn}}$ of products) – (sum of $\Delta H^\circ_{\text{rxn}}$ of reactants)
- **Hess's law:** enthalpies of reactions are additive.
- **Bond dissociation energy:** energy required to break a particular type of bond in one mole of gaseous molecules.
- **Entropy** (S): the measure of the disorder, or randomness, of a system. ΔS universe = ΔS system + ΔS surroundings
- **Gibbs free energy** (ΔG) = $\Delta H - T\Delta S$
- $\Delta G < 0$ = spontaneous reaction
- $\Delta G > 0$ = nonspontaneous reaction
- $\Delta G = 0$ = reaction is in equilibrium

REDOX REACTIONS AND ELECTROCHEMISTRY

Oxidation: loss of electrons

Reduction: gain of electrons

Oxidizing agent: causes another atom to undergo oxidation, and is itself reduced.

Reducing agent: causes another atom to be reduced, and is itself oxidized.

Galvanic cell: electrons flow **spontaneously** from anode (–) to cathode (+). E = **positive**

Electrolytic cell: electrons are forced to flow from anode (+) to cathode (–) using external power source (**non-spontaneous**). E = **negative**.

NOMENCLATURE

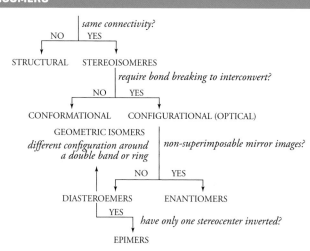

t-butyl   neopentyl   isopropyl   *sec*-butyl   isobutyl

Functional Group	Suffix	Functional Group	Suffix
Carboxylic Acid	-oic acid	Ketone	-one
Ester	-oate	Thiol	-thiol
Acyl halide	-oyl halide	Alcohol	-ol
Amide	-amide	Amine	-amine
Nitrile/ Cyanide	-nitrile	Imine	-imine
Aldehyde	-al	Ether	-ether
Alkene	-ene	Alkyne	-yne

ISOMERS

```
                    same connectivity?
          NO              YES
           ↓               ↓
     STRUCTURAL      STEREOISOMERES
                  require bond breaking to interconvert?
                   NO            YES
                    ↓             ↓
           CONFORMATIONAL   CONFIGURATIONAL (OPTICAL)
        GEOMETRIC ISOMERS
     different configuration around    non-superimposable mirror images?
        a double band or ring
                              NO        YES
                               ↓         ↓
                  DIASTEROEMERS      ENANTIOMERS
                         YES    have only one stereocenter inverted?
                          ↓
                       EPIMERS
```

Newman Projections:

staggered and anti   gauche and staggered   eclipsed   totally eclipsed

Conformations of Cyclohexane:

chair   boat   twist boat

BONDING

Bond order	Single	Double	Triple
Bond type	Sigma	Sigma / pi	Sigma / 2 pi
Hybridization	sp^3	sp^2	sp
Angles	109.5°	120°	180°
Example	C-C	C=C	C≡C

STABILIZATION

Induction: electron deficient group (radicals and C⁺) are more stable when substituted with EDG

Electron rich groups (C⁻) are more stable when less substituted, or by EWG.

Resonance: delocalization of π electrons and charge leads to stabilization.

Charge must be adjacent to π bond for resonance to occur.

ALKANES

REACTIONS

Free radical halogenation

- initiation (↑ # radicals)
- propagation (no change # radicals)
- termination (↓ # radicals)

Combustion

$$C_3H_8 + 5O_2 \rightarrow 3CO_2 + 4H_2O + heat$$

Types of Carbons: 1° → CH_3, 2°, 3°

ALKYL HALIDES SYNTHESIS

$$+OH + HBr \rightarrow +OH_2^+ + Br^-$$

$$Br^- + +OH_2^+ \rightarrow +Br + H_2O$$

tosyl chloride

SUBSTITUTIONS REACTIONS

$$X + Nuc^- \rightarrow Nuc + X^-$$

S_N1	S_N2
2 steps, rearrangements possible	1 step, backside attack
3° > 2° >1° >methyl	Methyl > 1° > 2° > 3°
Racemic products	Optically active and inverted products
Rate = $k[RX]$	Rate = $k[Nu^-][RX]$
Strong nucleophile not required	Favored with strong nucleophile
Favored in polar protic solvents	Favored in polar aprotic solvents

ELIMINATION REACTIONS

$$X + Base \xrightarrow{\Delta} + BH^+ + X^-$$

E1	E2
2 steps, rearrangements possible	1 step, antiperiplanar H and LG
3° > 2° > 1°	3° > 2° >1°
Zaitser (most substituted) product forms; trans > cis	Stereochemistry of double bond determined by starting conformation
Rate = k [substrate]	Rate = k [substrate][base]
Favored with heat and weak base	Favored with heat and strong base; small base gives most substituted DB; bulky base gives least substituted DB

ALKENES

Electrophilic addition of HX (Markovnikov)

Free radical addition (anti-Markovnikov)

most stable radical

Electrophilic addition of X_2

Anti-addition

Electrophilic addition of H_2O (Markovnikov)

Hydroboration (anti-Markovnikov, *syn* orientation)

1. BH_3
2. H_2O_2, OH^-

Catalytic reduction

syn

$\dfrac{H_2}{Pd/Pt}$

Oxidation with $KMnO_4$

cold dilute $KMnO_4$

Oxidation with O_3

1) O_3, CH_2Cl_2
2) Zn/H_2O

ALKYNES

Reduction with Lindlar's catalyst or Na in liquid ammonia

$CH_3C \equiv CCH_3$
2-butyne

$\dfrac{H_2, Pd/BaSO_4}{\text{Quinoline (Lindlar's Catalyst)}}$

cis-2-butene

$CH_3C \equiv CCH_3$
2-butyne

$\xrightarrow{Na, NH_3(liq)}$

trans-2-butene

ALCOHOLS

- Higher boiling points than alkanes
- Weakly acidic hydroxyl hydrogen

Synthesis
- Addition of water to double bonds
- S_N1 and S_N2 reactions
- Reduction of carboxylic acids, aldehydes, ketones and esters
  - Aldehydes and ketones with $NaBH_4$
  - Esters and carboxylic acids with $LiAlH_4$

REACTIONS

E1 dehydration reactions in strongly acidic solutions

$\dfrac{H_2SO_4}{\Delta}$

Hydride Shift

Major, Zaitsev   Minor, Hoffman

Minor, Hoffman

Oxidation
- PCC takes a primary alcohol to an aldehyde.

$\xrightarrow{PCC}$

- CrO_3, $KMnO_4$ and dichromate salts will convert secondary alcohols to ketones, and primary alcohols to carboxylic acids.

$\dfrac{Na_2Cr_2O_7}{H_2SO_4}$

- Tertiary alcohols cannot be oxidized without breaking a carbon to carbon bond.

ALDEHYDES AND KETONES

The dipole moment of carbonyl compounds causes an elevation of boiling point, but not as high as alcohols since there is no hydrogen bonding.

Synthesis
- Oxidation of primary or secondary alcohols
- Ozonolysis of alkenes

Nucleophilic addition

Commonly used
$Nu^- = RMgBr$, ROH, RNH_2

When $Nu^- = H^-$, this reaction is a reduction.

Aldol condensation

An **aldehyde** acts both as nucleophile (enolate) and electrophile (keto form).

Reactions of enolates (Michael additions)

Base

$+ H$ Base$^+$

$+$ Base

Oxidation and reduction

O → (LiAlH₄ / NaBH₄) → OH

CH₃CH (O) → (KMnO₄, CrO₃) → CH₃COH (O)

CARBOXYLIC ACIDS

Carboxylic acids have pK_a's of around 5 due to resonance stabilization of the conjugate base. Electronegative atoms increase acidity with inductive effects. Boiling point is higher than alcohols because of the ability to form two hydrogen bonds.

Synthesis
Oxidation of primary alcohols with KMnO₄

$$\text{—OH} \xrightarrow{\text{KMnO}_4} \text{—COOH}$$

Organometallic reagents with CO_2 (Grignard)

Br → (Mg, ether) → MgBr → (1) CO_2 gas, 2) H⁺, H_2O) → COOH

Reactions
Formation of soap by reacting carboxylic acids with NaOH; arrange in micelles

nonpolar tail — O⁻Na⁺ polar head

Reduction to alcohols

carboxylic acid → aldehyde → alcohol

CARBOXYLIC ACID DERIVATIVES

All derivatives go through additional-elimination mechanisms when they are interconverted.

Nu⁻ + (C=O, LG) —Addition→ (tetrahedral) —Elimination→ Nu + LG⁻

All derivatives can be synthesized from an appropriate nucleophile and a more reactive derivative.

Relative reactivity of derivatives

$$\text{R—C(O)—Cl} > \text{R—C(O)—O—C(O)—R} > \text{R—C(O)—OR} > \text{R—C(O)—NR}_2$$

Amides Amine + acid chloride, anhydride, or ester

:NH₃ + (C=O, Cl) → (ÖH, NH₂, Cl) → (C=O, NH₂) + Cl⁻

Esters
Alcohol + acid chloride or anhydride

Acid Anhydride

Carboxylate + acid halide

(mechanism) → R—C(O)—O—C(O)—R + Cl⁻

Acid halide can only be synthesized from acid directly.

RCOOH + SOCl₂ → R—C(O)—Cl

LAB TECHNIQUES

Extractions: separates based on solubility.
- RNH₂ extracted with HCl
- RCOOH extracted with NaHCO₃
- PhOH extracted with NaOH

Chromatography separates based on polarity.

High polarity = low R_f values
Low polarity = high R_f values

Gas chromatography separates based on boiling point.

High boiling point comes off column late
Low boiling point comes off column early

Distillation separates based on boiling point.

Simple-solvents with very different BPs
Fractional-solvents with similar BPs

Spectroscopy: IR

Functional group	Wave number
C = O	1720 cm⁻¹
C = C	1650 cm⁻¹
O-H	3200-3600 cm⁻¹
C≡C, C≡N	2100-2260 cm⁻¹

'H NMR–spectrum tells four things about structure.

1. # of nonequivalent Hs = # signals
2. # of Hs in each signal = integration
3. # of nonequivalent neighboring Hs = splitting pattern (follows $n + 1$ rule where n = # neighboring Hs)
4. chemical environment of Hs = chemical shift

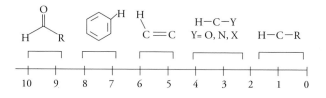

READING COMPREHENSION TEST (RCT)

- **Rank the passages:** look at topic and readability so you work on the easiest passage first and save the hardest one for last

- Skim read the passage in 1-4 minutes

- Generate a passage map by writing down the topic of each paragraph

- Highlight or circle key words in the passage

- Answer straight forward questions first

- Leave harder or open-ended questions for later

- Make sure you understand what the question is asking

- Go back to the passage and answer questions based on information in the passage

- **Do process of elimination (POE):** eliminate incorrect answer choices by striking them out

- **Retrieval questions:** the correct answer will be exact words from the passage or a close paraphrase

- **Inference questions:** the correct answer will be something implied by the passage (but maybe not directly stated)

- Stick to the content, tone and scope of the passage when answering questions

- **Know when to move on:** if you're spinning your wheels, cut your losses, answer the question with your letter of the day, and move on

- Make sure you have an answer selected for all 50 questions before time is up!

PHYSICS

LINEAR KINEMATICS

- **THE BIG FIVE**

    - $d = \frac{1}{2}(v_0 + v)t$

    - $v = v_0 + at$

    - $d = v_0 t + \frac{1}{2}at^2$

    - $d = vt - \frac{1}{2}at^2$

    - $v^2 = v_0^2 + 2ad$

- **PROJECTILE MOTION**

	Horizontal	Vertical
Displacement	$x = v_{0x}t$	$y = v_{0y}t - \frac{1}{2}gt^2$
Velocity	$v_x = v_{0x}$	$v_y = v_{0y} - gt$ $v_y^2 = v_{0y}^2 - 2gy$
Acceleration	$a_x = 0$	$a_y = -g$

STATICS DYNAMICS

- **NEWTON'S LAWS**

    - $\vec{F}_{net} = 0 \Leftrightarrow \vec{v} \; constant$

    - $\vec{F}_{net} = m\vec{a}$

    - $\vec{F}_{1 \, on \, 2} = -\vec{F}_{2 \, on \, 1}$

- **GRAVITY**

    - Local Gravity: $F_g = mg$

    - Universal Gravity: $F_G = \frac{GMm}{r^2}$

    - $g = \frac{GM}{r^2}$

- **FRICTION**

    - Static Friction: $F_{fs} \leq \mu_s F_N$

    - Kinetic Friction: $F_{fk} = \mu_k F_N$

- **ROTATION**

    - Centripetal Acceleration: $a_c = \frac{v^2}{r}$

    - Centripetal Force: $F_c = \frac{mv^2}{r}$

    - $v = \omega r$

    - $a_t = \alpha r$

    - Torque: $\tau = rF\sin\theta = lF$

EQUILIBRIUM

- **EQUILIBRIUM**

    - $F_{net} = 0$

    - $\tau_{net} = 0$

- **Center of Mass:**

    - $x_{CM} = \frac{m_1 x_1 + m_2 x_2 + m_3 x_3 + \dots}{m_1 + m_2 + m_3 + \dots}$

    - $x_{CM} = x_{CG}$

ENERGY & MOMENTUM

- **Work:** $W = Fd\cos\theta$
- **Power:** $P = \frac{W}{t}$
- **Work-Energy Theorem:** $W_{net} = \Delta KE$
- **Kinetic Energy:** $KE = \frac{1}{2}mv^2$
- **Gravitational Potential Energy:**

    - $W_{by \; g} = -\Delta PE_g$

    - $PE_g = mgh$

- **CONSERVATION OF ENERGY**

    - Total Energy: $E_{net} = KE + PE$

    - $E_i = E_f$

    - $KE_i + PE_i = KE_f + PE_f$

    - $\Delta KE = -\Delta PE$

- **CONSERVATION OF MOMENTUM**

    - Momentum: $\vec{p} = m\vec{v}$

    - $\vec{p}_i = \vec{p}_f$

- **COLLISIONS**

	Momentum	Kinetic Energy
Perfectly Inelastic	Conserved	NOT Conserved
Inelastic	Conserved	NOT Conserved
Elastic	Conserved	Conserved

FLUID STATICS

- Density: $\rho = \dfrac{m}{V}$

- Specific Gravity: $sp.\ gr. = \dfrac{\rho}{\rho_{water}}$

- $\rho_{water} = 1000\dfrac{kg}{m^3} = 1\dfrac{g}{cm^3}$

- **PRESSURE**
  - $P = \dfrac{F_\perp}{A}$
  - Gauge: $P_{gauge} = \rho_f gD$
  - Total: $P_{net} = P_{surface} + P_{gauge}$
  - $P_{atm} \approx 100\ kPa$

- Buoyant Force: $F_b = \rho_f V_{sub} g$

- Pascal's Law: $\dfrac{F_1}{A_1} = \dfrac{F_2}{A_2}$

ELECTROSTATICS

- **Elementary Charge:** $e = 1.6 \times 10^{-19}\ C$

- **ELECTROSTATIC FORCE**
  - Coulomb's Law: $F_E = \dfrac{k|Q\|q|}{r^2}$
  - Opposite charges attract; like charges repel
  - $k = 9 \times 10^9\ \dfrac{Nm^2}{C^2}$
  - $\vec{F}_E = q\vec{E}$
  - Electric field: $E = \dfrac{k|Q|}{r^2}$
  - Positive charges accelerate with $\vec{E}$; negative charges accelerate against $\vec{E}$

- **Electrostatic Potential Energy:**
  - $W_{by\ E} = -\Delta PE_E$
  - $\Delta PE_E = q\,\Delta\varphi = qV$
  - Electric Potential: $\varphi = \dfrac{kQ}{r}$

- **CONDUCTORS**
  - Inside: $\vec{E} = 0$
  - Charge rests on the outer surface

D.C. CIRCUITS

- **Current:** $I = \dfrac{Q}{t}$

- **RESISTANCE**
  - Resistance: $R = \rho\dfrac{L}{A}$
  - Ohm's Law: $V = IR$
  - Power: $P = IV = I^2 R = \dfrac{V^2}{R}$

- **EQUIVALENT RESISTANCE**
  - Series: $R_{eq} = R_1 + R_2 + \ldots$
  - Parallel: $\dfrac{1}{R_{eq}} = \dfrac{1}{R_1} + \dfrac{1}{R_2} + \ldots$

- **CAPACITORS**
  - Capacitance: $C = \kappa\dfrac{\varepsilon_0 A}{d}$
  - $\kappa_{vacuum} = \kappa_{air} = 1$
  - $Q = CV$
  - $PE = \dfrac{1}{2}QV = \dfrac{1}{2}CV^2 = \dfrac{Q^2}{2C}$
  - $V = Ed$

- **EQUIVALENT CAPACITANCE**
  - Series: $\dfrac{1}{C_{eq}} = \dfrac{1}{C_1} + \dfrac{1}{C_2} + \ldots$
  - Parallel: $C_{eq} = C_1 + C_2 + \ldots$

SHM & WAVES

- **Period and frequency are independent of amplitude**
  - $T = \dfrac{1}{f}$

- **SPRING-MASS SYSTEM**
  - Hooke's Law: $\vec{F} = -k\vec{x}$
  - $PE_{elastic} = \dfrac{1}{2}kx^2$
  - $v_{max} = A\sqrt{\dfrac{k}{m}}$
  - $T = 2\pi\sqrt{\dfrac{m}{k}}$ & $f = \dfrac{1}{2\pi}\sqrt{\dfrac{k}{m}}$

- **SIMPLE PENDULUM**
  - $v_{max} = \sqrt{2gh}$
  - $T = 2\pi\sqrt{\dfrac{L}{g}}$ & $f = \dfrac{1}{2\pi}\sqrt{\dfrac{g}{L}}$

- **Wave speed:** $v = \lambda f$

- **TWO BIG RULES FOR WAVES**
  - Wave speed depends on the type of wave and the medium
  - Frequency stays the same as a wave passes between media

- Photon energy: $E = hf = \dfrac{hc}{\lambda}$
  - $c = 3 \times 10^8 \dfrac{m}{s}$
- Law of Reflection:
  - The angle of incidence is equal to the angle of reflection
  - $\theta_{incidence} = \theta_{reflection}$
- **REFRACTION**
  - Snell's Law:

    $n_1 \sin \theta_1 = n_2 \sin \theta_2$
  - $n = \dfrac{c}{v}$
  - $n_{vaccum} = n_{air} = 1$
  - Total Internal Reflection: $\sin \theta_{crit} = \dfrac{n_2}{n_1}$
- Mirror/Lens Equation: $\dfrac{1}{f} = \dfrac{1}{i} + \dfrac{1}{o}$
- Magnification: $m = -\dfrac{i}{o}$
- Focal Length: $f = \pm\dfrac{R}{2}$
- Lens Power: $P = \dfrac{1}{f}$
- Focal length is positive for converging optics and negative for diverging optics
- Object distance is always positive
- Image distance is positive where light actually goes
- Positive i: Real and Inverted
- Negative i: Virtual and Upright

- **HEAT TRANSFER**
  - Positive Q means heat is transferred into the system; negative Q means heat is transferred out of the system
  - Constant Phase: $Q = mc\Delta T$
  - Phase Change: $Q = mL$
  - Mechanisms of heat transfer include conduction, convection, and radiation
- **THERMAL EXPANSION**
  - Linear: $\Delta L = \alpha L_i \Delta T$
  - Volume: $\Delta V = \beta V_i \Delta T$
- Ideal Gas Law: $PV = nRT$
- Kinetic Theory of Gases: $KE_{avg} = \dfrac{3}{2} k_B T$
- **FIRST LAW OF THERMODYNAMICS**
  - $\Delta E_{internal} = Q - W$
  - Positive W is work done BY the system; negative W is work done ON the system
  - Work can be found from the area under a P-V diagram
- **THERMODYNAMIC PROCESSES**
  - Isobaric: $\Delta P = 0$ & $\Delta E_{internal} = Q - P\Delta V$
  - Isochoric: $\Delta V = 0$ & $\Delta E_{internal} = Q$
  - Isothermal: $\Delta T = 0$ & $\Delta E_{internal} = 0 \Rightarrow Q = W$
  - Adiabatic: $Q = 0$ & $\Delta E_{internal} = -W$
- Thermal Efficiency: $e = 1 - \dfrac{|Q_C|}{Q_H}$

GLOBAL TECHNIQUES

- Two-pass system
- P.I. or P.I.T.A.
- Rounding/Estimation

ALGEBRA

- To solve simultaneous equations, usually you must add or subtract one equation from the other.
- **Common Quadratics**
  - $(x + y)(x + y) = x^2 + 2xy + y^2$
  - $(x - y)(x - y) = x^2 - 2xy + y^2$
  - $(x + y)(x - y) = x^2 - y^2$
- To solve inequalities, solve just like equations, except that if you multiply or divide by a negative number, you must reverse the direction of the inequality.
- **Exponent Rules**
  - MADSPM
  - $x^0 = 1, x \neq 0$
  - $x^{a/b} = \sqrt[b]{x^a}$
  - $x^{-a} = \dfrac{1}{x^a}$
- **Logarithm Rules**
  - $a^b = c \Leftrightarrow b = \log_a c$
  - $\log a + \log b = \log(ab)$
  - $\log a - \log b = \log(a/b)$
  - $\log a^b = b \log a$
- **Absolute Value:** the magnitude of a number (its value without a negative sign).
- To solve ratio problems, use the Ratio Box.
- To solve mixture and weight average problems, use the weighted average formula.
- **Direct variation:** $y = kx$, k is constant
- **Indirect variation:** $y = \dfrac{k}{x}$, k is constant

NUMERICAL CALCULATIONS

- To add or subtract fractions, find a common denominator and then add or subtract the numerators.
- To multiply fractions, multiply the numerators and multiply the denominators.
- To divide fractions, multiply by the reciprocal of the fraction that was in the denominator.
- To add or subtract decimals, line up the decimal points.
- To multiply decimals, simply multiply as usual. Then count the number of digits after the decimal point in the two numbers being multiplied, and place the decimal point so that there are as many digits after the decimal point in the result.
- percent change $= \dfrac{difference}{original} \times 100$
- When putting a number in scientific notation, each shifting the decimal point once to the left (right) means increasing (decreasing) the exponent on the factor of 10 by 1.

CONVERSIONS

- T (in K) $= T$(in °C) $+ 273.15$
- 1 minute = 60 seconds
- 1 hour = 60 minutes
- 1 day = 24 hours
- 1 pound (lb.) = 16 ounces (oz.)
- 1 ton = 2000 pounds
- 1 foot = 12 inches
- 1 yard = 3 feet
- 1 mile = 5,280 feet

PROBABILITY AND STATISTICS

- **Arithmetic mean:** the normal average. To solve average problems, use the Average Pie.
- **Median:** the middle number or the average of the two middle numbers (when numbers are arranged in order).
- **Mode:** the number that occurs most frequently.
- **Variance and standard deviation:** describe the spread of the data. A larger variance or standard deviation means that the values are farther apart from each other than a smaller variance or standard deviation indicates.

- **Factorial:** written with a !, means multiply by the integers decreasing to 1.

- **Permutations, combinations, and other arrangements:** to determine how many ways something can be done, write out blanks for each thing to be done and the number of ways each can be done. (If the things are not in any particular order, divide by integers starting with the number of blanks and counting down.) Then multiply.

- Probability $= \dfrac{\#\ of\ outcomes\ you\ want}{\#\ of\ outcomes\ possible}$

GEOMETRY

- When two non-perpendicular lines cross, they form two types of angles: big angles and small angles. The big angles are equal, and the small angles are equal. Big + Small = 180°. Adding another line in parallel to the first two creates more equal angles.

- $m = \dfrac{y_2 - y_1}{x_2 - x_1}$

- $y = mx + b$, b is the y-intercept

- $d = \sqrt{\left(x_2 - x_1\right)^2 - \left(y_2 - y_1\right)^2}$

- Area of a triangle $= \dfrac{1}{2} bh$

- Area of a triangle $= \dfrac{1}{2} ab \sin \theta$

- Area of a rectangle $= bh$

- Area of a trapezoid $= \dfrac{1}{2}(b_1 + b_2)h$

- **Pythagorean Theorem:** $a^2 + b^2 = c^2$
  - $3^2 + 4^2 = 5^2$
  - $5^2 + 12^2 = 13^2$
  - $7^2 + 24^2 = 25^2$

- **Special Triangles** (angles and sides)
  - 30°:60°:90° and $1{:}\sqrt{3}{:}2$
  - 45°:45°:90° and $1{:}1{:}\sqrt{2}$

- $\dfrac{central\ angle}{360°} = \dfrac{arc\ length}{2\pi r} = \dfrac{sector\ area}{\pi r^2}$

- The sum of the angles inside a polygon with n sides is given by $(n-2)180°$.

- S.A. of a box $= 2lw + 2lh + 2wh$

- S.A. of a cylinder $= 2\pi r^2 + 2\pi rh$

- Volume of a box $= lwh$

- Volume of a cylinder $= \pi r^2 h$

- Volume of a cone $= \dfrac{1}{3}\pi r^2 h$

TRIGONOMETRY

- SOHCAHTOA

- $\tan \theta = \dfrac{\sin \theta}{\cos \theta}$

θ	0°	30°	45°	60°	90°
sin θ	$\dfrac{\sqrt{0}}{2}$	$\dfrac{\sqrt{1}}{2}$	$\dfrac{\sqrt{2}}{2}$	$\dfrac{\sqrt{3}}{2}$	$\dfrac{\sqrt{4}}{2}$
cos θ	$\dfrac{\sqrt{4}}{2}$	$\dfrac{\sqrt{3}}{2}$	$\dfrac{\sqrt{2}}{2}$	$\dfrac{\sqrt{1}}{2}$	$\dfrac{\sqrt{0}}{2}$
tan θ	$\dfrac{\sqrt{0}}{\sqrt{4}}$	$\dfrac{\sqrt{1}}{\sqrt{3}}$	$\dfrac{\sqrt{2}}{\sqrt{2}}$	$\dfrac{\sqrt{3}}{\sqrt{1}}$	$\dfrac{\sqrt{4}}{\sqrt{0}}$

- $\csc \theta = \dfrac{1}{\sin \theta}$

- $\sec \theta = \dfrac{1}{\cos \theta}$

- $\cot \theta = \dfrac{1}{\tan \theta}$

- π radians = 180°

- $\sin^2 \theta + \cos^2 \theta = 1$